The Voice and Its Disorders

5th Edition

The Voice and its Disorders

5th Edition

Margaret C. L. Greene

formerly Head of the Department of Speech Therapy
St. Bartholomew's Hospital
London

Lesley Mathieson

Visiting Lecturer
Voice Pathology
Department of Linguistic Science
University of Reading

W

Whurr Publishers
London and New Jersey

Whurr Publishers Ltd
19b Compton Terrace
London N1 2UN
England

First published 1989
Reprinted 1991

British Library Cataloguing in Publication Data

Greene, Margaret C.L. (Margaret Cicely Langton)
The voice and its disorders.—5th ed.
1. Man. Voice disorders
I. Title II. Mathieson, Lesley
616.2'2

ISBN 1-870332-25-3
ISBN 1-870332-30-X (soft cover)

For information about our audio products, write to us at:
Newbridge Book Clubs, 3000 Cindel Drive, Delran, NJ 08370

Typeset by Maggie Spooner Typesetting, London
Printed in Great Britain by Athenaeum Press,
Newcastle upon Tyne

Preface to 5th edition

After the publication of the fourth edition in 1980 the last thing that was envisaged was another edition of *The Voice and Its Disorders*. However, as a decade progressed, far from falling into oblivion, requests for the book increased. These requests came mainly from qualified speech therapists confronted with the problems of planning and executing treatment for dysphonia.

Undergraduate speech therapists are given theoretical understanding of voice production and voice pathology in addition to important clinical experience. This alone is not sufficient preparation for their therapeutic role. They have little practical instruction in the production of their own voices which is an essential requirement for real insight into the perception and clinical treatment of dysphonic patients. Whilst we have explored theories and the latest research and instruments which can be used in objective assessment, we have been at pains to emphasise the practical approach to the rehabilitation of the dysphonic patient. We have asked ourselves, 'What do we do with this patient?'. The answers can often be found in the case histories we have quoted which endeavour to explain the problem and the measures which helped.

In the first edition (1957) the preface began thus: 'The chief motive in writing this book was the desire to provide a guide to treatment of voice disorders, simple yet comprehensive enough to serve not only speech therapists but doctors and laryngologists, and, more especially, those in many countries of the world where speech therapy is unknown and unpractised.' We have included therefore some pathologies not encountered in the Western World but still endemic in the less developed countries where such conditions as diphtheria and syphilis of the larynx still occur.

At risk of being over-repetitive we would like to comment here on a point frequently made in the text. No machine can replace the expertise and empathy of the experienced speech therapist. Increasingly sophisticated instrumentation for the analysis of vocal function and for monitoring response to treatment gives us interesting new insights but it is only one aspect of intervention. Effective therapy is soundly based upon clinical experience and is comprised of an amalgam of watching and of listening to the voice and the complaints of the dysphonic patient. It is linked into a network of anatomical, physiological, neurological, cultural and pathological cues, and presents a holistic picture against which particular acoustic measurement falls into proper perspective. To speech therapists without the instrumentation we describe we wish to extend the consolation that we have also worked extensively in situations where it has been unavailable. This lack has not prevented us from providing successful voice therapy to a large number of patients.

We must acknowledge our appreciation of all those who have helped us over some of our worries with advice and discussion. Not least we must thank all those writers of excellent books and papers encapsulating their research and the wisdom of their experience which we acknowledge in our references throughout the text. Particular thanks must be made to Eva Carlson who has been most generous in providing laryngograph waveforms and analyses.

We are greatly indebted to Mr D. Garfield Davies, FRCS, Director of the Ferens Institute of Otolarynology, The University College and Middlesex School of Medicine, London who provided many photographs and diagrams of the larynx to illustrate pathological conditions of the vocal folds. He helped in their selection and gave invaluable advice and encouragement.

We also wish to thank Dr Frances MacCurtain for giving permission to reproduce the xeroradiographs of our patients.

We are indebted to Brüel and Kjaer Ltd in Denmark and the UK and to Kay Elemetrics Corporation in the USA for providing an excellent selection of slides and photographs from which we were able to choose suitable illustrations.

Finally, we must thank Mark Mathieson who organised our disk filing system and wrote appropriate computer programs for producing flow charts, waveforms and index lists, while convincing us that sanity could prevail.

Margaret Greene, Wingrave
Lesley Mathieson, Chalfont St Giles
June 1989

Preface to 4th edition

This, the fourth edition of *The Voice and its Disorders*, appears 7 years after the third and 22 years after the first. Dr Anne Mcallister, one of the early pioneers of speech therapy whose opinion I greatly value, said that the first edition excelled as a manual for students but that successive editions lost much of value regarding guidance in treatment. Bearing this remark always in mind, I have endeavoured valiantly to emphasise treatment or therapy while incorporating information concerning advances in knowledge of function, in technology and scientific assessment and diagnosis which lay the foundations on which suitable and successful therapy must be based.

In this edition, apart from the rearrangement of certain sections and some omission of historical data in the interests of brevity, the two chief areas requiring revision were those of surgery and electronic 'hardware'.

Advances in surgery include the operation by Dedo of section of the recurrent laryngeal nerve for alleviation of spastic dysphonia. There are also new procedures in use for laryngeal palsy. The fibreoptic nasendoscope used in assessment of palatopharyngeal incompetence and promoted by Pigott is widening selection of suitable secondary operations in cleft palate. A swing back to conservation or conservative surgery, as opposed to radical surgery, in management of carcinoma of the larynx and the search for viable fistula speech reaches into the future.

Developments in surgery and electronic microprocessors linked to the relatively new concept of biofeedback and self-teaching pose a real threat to traditional speech therapy. One can envisage that speech clinics of the future will be akin to laboratories furnished with robot-like machines and staffed by technologists whose clients monitor visual displays programmed from computerised data from yet other machines. In this depressing outlook the speech therapist can seek consolation in certain facts. Science and statistics are often found wanting particularly in the realms of unpredictable and idiosyncratic human behaviour. Machines may accurately focus upon isolated features in dysphonia and may also be useful in teaching but they cannot heal. Speech therapy is more art than science and must remain so. The art is based upon experience and sound clinical observation tied to all the facts at the therapist's disposal from other allied disciplines; it transcends scientific explanation and embraces the personality of the therapist in relation to that of the patient. Communication is established between the two which inspires confidence, hope and faith in recovery which ultimately is the greatest healer of all . . . a simple truth from which modern man has been led astray in the pursuit of the fruits of his intelligence and so lost himself.

For the rest I have endeavoured to keep my narrative clear and simple and as interesting as possible hoping that the new ideas which have excited me will infect the reader with the same enthusiasm for this fascinating facet of behaviour which is dysphonia. I have also indulged myself here and there in a touch of humour to liven the text and to relieve the sadness of compassion. I have resolutely steered away from current fashions in linguistic contortion which it is only too easy to emulate. When finding myself slipping, I have asked myself severely, What does it mean? What does 'interjudge and intrajudge reliability ratings' really mean? Or this gem? 'Final transfer of postural quality learning to spoken style should be simple if generalisation has been achieved in these simple procedures.' On the other hand I have derived much pleasure from the utter clarity and economy in words of surgical English which I can understand despite the fact that I am a layman. Surgeons enjoy the security of professional status reaching back to the Hippocratic oath while technocrats, among whom we can include clinical psychologists and speech pathologists, suffer from the insecurity of an adolescent profession aspiring to impress with a neolinguistic hyperbole all its own.

My editor does not favour the printing of the previous three prefaces, but I am loathe to omit the contributions of previous kind and helpful colleagues whose teaching is still present in the text. I acknowledge with abiding gratitude the advice of the laryngologists, Sir Victor Negus and Professor F.C. Ormerod, Professor T. Pomfret Kilner, plastic surgeon Professor Linford Rees and Professor Frits Grewel of Amsterdam, neurologist, psychiatrist and orthopedagogue.

For the present edition, I thank Professor Bernard Watson, Department of Applied Medical Electronics, St Bartholomew's Hospital, and Mr Robin McNab Jones and Juliet Glover. I also wish to remember the opportunities provided in continued study and treatment of voice cases by Margaret Thorndike in Hertfordshire after my retirement from St Bartholomew's, and to record my gratitude for all her help.

I am also most grateful to all those who have generously given permission for the reproduction of diagrams and illustrations: Mr Lavell, Mr Gareth Piggott, Mr Nigel Edwards, Mr Shah, Yvonne Edels and Professor Adrian Fourcin.

My acknowledgements would not be complete without mention of the honour accorded me by the New Zealand Speech Therapists Association and the Department of Education in 1978 in inviting me to take part in their biennial conference and refresher course and a lecture tour with clinical workshops, the fruits of which I hope are apparent in my text, especially in connection with childhood dysphonia. At the same time I was invited speaker to the Australian Association of Speech and Hearing Conference in Tasmania which also led to exposure to new attitudes to treatment and widened my horizon beneficially. The hospitality and generosity of my colleagues in the Antipodes went far beyond the requirements of professional duty and provided a heart-warming recognition and climax to my career.

M.C.L. Greene
Wingrave, March 1979

Contents

Phonetic symbols used in the text

Vowels

/ɪ/	as in it
/i:/	as in eat
/e/	as in bed
/æ/	as in at
/ɑ:/	as in arm
/ɜ:/	as in her
/ə/	as in supper
/ʌ/	as in cut
/ɒ/	as in not
/u:/	as in pool

Consonants

/m/	as in me
/n/	as in no
/ŋ/	as in sing
/p/	as in pea
/b/	as in bat
/t/	as in to
/d/	as in day
/k/	as in cat
/g/	as in go
/f/	as in fit
/v/	as in vim
/θ/	as in think
/ð/	as in that
/r/	as in red
/j/	as in yet
/s/	as in so
/z/	as in zoo
/ʃ/	as in shoe
/tʃ/	as in chat
/ʤ/	as in jam
/ʒ/	as in leisure
/h/	as in he

Diphthongs

/ɑʊ/	as in house
/ei/	as in day
/aɪ/	as in lie

Part I

Normal Voice

Chapter 1 Communicative Functions of the Voice – An Introduction

The importance of the voice in rendering verbal communication audible is generally recognised since most people have lost their voices at some time and remember the misery this caused. It is also generally recognised that voices are identifiable as belonging to particular people; they are uniquely personal like faces. The voice, however, conveys a wealth of further information about a speaker and what the listener hears depends upon experience and sensitivity. A speech therapist or linguist will be aware of nuances which may evade the non-professional. The voice of an infant can be recognised by the mother, also degrees of distress and well-being. Throughout life emotions colour the voice and infuse the personality. As infant vocalisation progresses and babbling develops as a preliminary to speech, the intonation patterns of the home language are absorbed and form musical patterns into which words and phrases gradually fit.

As the social and emotional boundaries of a child's life expand, the voice picks up characteristics of the socioeconomic groups encountered, the peculiarities of regional dialect and class. The voice thus embraces an extraordinary amalgam of personal information, presenting a cameo of life history carved into paralinguistic and linguistic channels.

Our overview of the communicative functions of the human voice will be explained and expanded in this introduction. But to understand the wonders of the voice it is necessary to know how it is produced, how the anatomy and physiology of lungs, larynx and the resonators relate to the laws of acoustics and coordinate under control of the nervous system, the brain and its language centres. Subsequent chapters deal with these matters and the normal voice in detail. This study of the normal voice must precede study of voice disorders and their remediation, and this forms the second part of the book.

Facets of Vocalisation

The voice transmits a wealth of information concerning the speaker through changes of vocal tone registered in the diverse attitudes evoked by different social contexts. Vocal behaviour is one aspect of the total image presented by an individual which is a composite of dress, grooming, posture, gesture and facial expression. Listeners draw inferences from the voice regarding sex, age, intelligence, regional and socioeconomic origins, education and occupation (Ryan, Giles and Sebastian, 1982). A cross-disciplinary approach and the study of various attitudes in social settings is recognised as necessary in any comprehensive evaluation of communicative behaviour (Edwards, 1982). This is the core construct of the rapidly developing discipline of socio-linguistics which provides an integrative approach to social psychology. These aspects of voice from which inferences are drawn are known as paralinguistic features; they run parallel to the linguistic message and are important in placing it in context.

This introduction to vocal function will be directed broadly into these two areas: paralinguistic and linguistic - although in practice the two aspects are not always clearly defined and frequently overlap and fuse.

Voice Permanence

Every voice is unique to the speaker. The distinctive voice quality by which each person is identifiable is dependent upon anatomical features and the vocal setting giving it permanence.

Anatomical features

The dimensions of the vocal tract and resonating system of each individual are unique. They impart the particular vocal quality which distinguishes one individual from all others and by which the speaker is recognised. It is these anatomical features which result in the permanent voice quality over which there is little control and which cannot be completely suppressed or disguised. Actors and actresses play different dramatic characters but well-known voices, such as that of Laurence Olivier or Vanessa Redgrave, remain recognisable whatever role they assume.

Vocal settings

Superimposed upon the permanent anatomical voice features is the highly variable range of possible 'voice settings'. These are the muscular tension adjustments of the vocal tract which are learned unconsciously in the family and, later on, in the school, social, professional or occupational group. The voice settings, besides the adjustments in the vocal tract affecting tone, also include characteristic levels of volume and pitch. They become habitual, and there is no awareness of them in the majority of speakers but they may be controlled by the individual. These settings can be assumed and imitated and are peculiar to different groups within regional and local populations. An interesting illustration of this is the evidence which suggests that many American males have learned to use a lower part of the pitch range than British males (Giles and Powesland, 1975) (see 'Contact ulcers', p. 125).

The sociolinguistic implications of an individual's speech patterns are acknowledged in the literature. The class-conscious British detect the background of a speaker very readily (Scherer and Giles, 1979). It is agreed that 'received pronunciation' (RP) is the most prestigious standard accent in the United Kingdom (Kramarac, 1982), with high status and competence connotations, placing speakers in a socially superior position to those with apparently less advantageous antecedents. However, studies of voice quality and social grouping are less common and appear to be less frequently considered. A study in Edinburgh (Scherer and Giles, 1979) produced results showing a correlation between social status and voice settings. Higher social status was associated with more 'creaky' phonation while lower social status revealed voices with more whispering and harshness.

The English are reputed to be the most class-conscious race in Europe, unlike the Americans who recognise regional differences but not as markers of social class. In Italy, Tuscan accent is quite different from that of the north or south. It is appreciated for its beauty of tone but does not place these Italians on a higher social plane although it has great cultural status.

It is suggested by some writers that future academic success can be predicted by voice pitch and range. Scherer and Giles (1979) cite a study by Freuder, Brown and Lambert in which teachers evaluating young school children judged slow speech at a low pitch to be indicative of school failure. This study was confirmed by Edwards (1982). It was found that the academically successful pupils of low socioeconomic status did actually use higher pitch, less volume and more appropriate intonation than their unsuccessful peers.

The judgement of an individual's abilities and intelligence from the voice is obviously highly dubious. Some teachers and many other members of society hold stereotyped and often negative views of certain ethnic and social groups unconsciously. Inappropriate predictions should not become prophecies. Much help can and should be given to raise the performance levels of underprivileged groups. The adverse effect on highly intelligent children of adverse environmental factors is well known.

Paralinguistic Features

In contrast to the long-term nature of the anatomy and voice settings which combine to make voice permanence, there are paralinguistic features of voice which change with emotion. Shades of feeling are reflected in the voice and are inextricably linked with the verbal message and may over-ride it. These features are recognised as timbre, tone of voice or vocal quality. Crystal (1980) refers to them as voice qualifiers. Such changing vocal settings are difficult to measure but that the voice changes colour with changing emotion is universally recognised. This is reflected in the way a remark is delivered, not how it is worded: 'It wasn't what she said but the way that she said it that made me mad' or 'I know perfectly well what she meant although she didn't say it in so many words' etc. An impartial judge may be totally bewildered by the feelings of bitterness and agression which arise between contestants and how innocent words can be apparently so misinterpreted.

In more subtle emotional contexts, such feelings as sadness, disappointment, happiness, love and joy are reflected. The sincerity and empathy of a speaker are conveyed to the listener, and words not sincerely felt may be recognised as false. The paralinguistic features of voice allow us to communicate feeling without being explicit. Siegman (1987) suggests that in this way we can express feelings without taking full responsibility for them.

Social group differences

Paralinguistic features of voice are not necessarily interpreted correctly between individuals of different ethnic groups. Scherer and Giles (1979) observed that West Indians in normal calm conversation will suddenly alter pitch and increase loudness of the voice for emphasis. This may be interpreted as an angry outburst by those of other groups, and emphatic speech may be incorrectly regarded as angry or aggressive. The potential dangers to relationships between different ethnic and social groups is only too obvious (Bourhis, 1985).

Personality indicators

Inferences can be drawn about a speaker's personality from voice quality although the same inference is not necessarily made by each listener. For example, relatively high vocal pitch may indicate positive aspects of personality such as competence, dominance and assertiveness to one listener, but another may conclude that the speaker is nervous and deceitful (Ryan, Giles and Sebastian, 1982). There seems to be a general assumption that a speaker is dynamic and extravert if the pitch shows marked variability. A loud voice can indicate extraversion but if the voice is inappropriately loud it may signal insensitivity to the situation and embarrass the listener. Addington (1968) says that nasality is strongly linked with negative attributes such as unattractiveness and neuroticism.

Psychiatrists recognise the voices of anxiety, depression and despair. Moses (1954) emphasised the vocal symptoms emitted by distressed individuals. Ostwald (1963) emphasised the need to listen to the different vocal qualities such as hollow tone and flat intonation compared to the 'robust' voice. Low vocal pitch in association with slow speech is recognised as indicating depression, while the breathy, irregular voice accompanying rapid speech is indicative of anxiety (Gudykunst, 1986).

Voice loudness

Loudness is a parameter of voice which varies from one individual to another and will vary at different times within the same individual according to the emotional or linguistic content of the communication. There appear to be differences of voice volume between the sexes with men generally talking more loudly, although women are more likely to compensate for external noise by increasing vocal intensity (Scherer and Giles, 1979). It is suggested that both sexes tend to talk more loudly to members of the opposite sex.

The ability to vary vocal volume allows the speaker considerable control over the behaviour of others. Increasing loudness is an effective way of establishing the speaker's turn in a conversation and will also deter the intervention of other speakers. Margaret Thatcher's dominant role in the House of Commons demonstrates this publicly, but increased vocal volume has a similar effect in other contexts. The loud voice used for commanding, calling, warning and attracting attention cannot be ignored by the listener very easily, while the whisper or very quiet voice signals the appropriate behaviour for the listener. In anger the amplitude of the voice may be the dominant feature in communicating the heart-felt message.

Non-verbal communication

A description of paralinguistic aspects of voice is not complete without acknowledging the part played by non-verbal communication, or body language, which is another paralinguistic feature of great importance. From the purely physiological viewpoint, body postures change the tensions and dimensions of the resonators and therefore reflect what is meant beneath the verbal signals. Facial, hand and arm gestures and body postures are an integral part of communication which vary between individuals and between social and ethnic groups. There are also differences in the same individual according to mood and the relative degree of formality of a situation. In general, movements are less animated when an individual is depressed or very relaxed or when the occasion is particularly formal. Even complete lack of both facial expression and active body gesture is an aspect of this communication.

MacDonald Critchley (1939b) in his study *The Language of Gesture* examined this aspect of communication very thoroughly. Psychologists and sociolinguists now examine the sequence of events and patterns of behaviour in various social situations. The posture of participants in a job interview, for instance, marks the dominant role of the employer and the submissive role of the applicant. The former may lean back in his chair and the latter sit stiffly erect or lean forward, ingratiatingly. The questions and answers, of course, guide the conversation (Cappella and Street, 1985) and allied to this are the vocal undertones. Following the tenor of the interview, hesitancy or fluency occurs as confidence swells and recedes. The posture, eye contact or avoidance, head movement, shifting or fidgeting all play a part. However, during conversation some individuals model their own behaviour on that of the person to whom they are talking, particularly if they are in agreement. This behaviour is referred to by Argyle (1970) as 'response matching'.

Set patterns of social conduct greatly influence communication and enable individuals to influence attitudes and change them radically. Kalin (1982) has reviewed the social significance of speech in medical, legal and social settings and the 'set' registers which maintain dominant and subservient roles and which differ greatly in colloquial contexts. Manipulation of attitude can reassure and antagonise; empathy can be established or confidence and trust destroyed. This aspect of communication is of enormous importance for the speech therapist in establishing rapport with the patient and is crucial in successful rehabilitation (Morris, 1985), assisting integration in the professional or educational team.

In the widely acclaimed book by Skynner and Cleese (1983) entitled *Families and How to Survive Them*, a discussion arises concerning why strangers selected for group therapy paired off as they did when left to chat to each other. It emerged that this unconscious attraction was due to shared common backgrounds and experiences. This recognition was achieved initially without verbal exchanges of personal information. Skynner explains, 'We're giving off information the whole time about what sort of people we are. It's conveyed by our facial expression and the way we use our bodies - all that body language stuff we've heard about recently'. Skynner goes on to point out that it is not only movements we make, but how we make them and how often. Facial expression etches lines on the face which match posture and the way we walk. The depressed person presents a different picture from one who is happy. People are unconsciously attracted by similarities to themselves in others. They recognise immediately, on the other hand, lack of sympathy and hostility in others without any other communication than the visual clues.

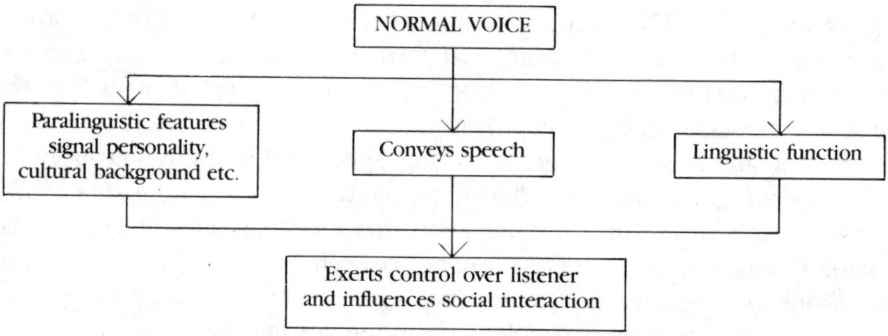

Figure 1.1. Normal voice in social interaction.

Linguistic Vocal Features

Segmental phonology

The voice is an integral part of individual phonemes and in this context is part of the structure of pronunciation as opposed to the system of language (Abercrombie, 1967; Grunwell, 1982). It can be analysed and described in relation to each phonological segment. Coordination of phonation with articulation is essential; if phonemes which should be voiced are produced without voice, and vice versa, word-meaning is changed.

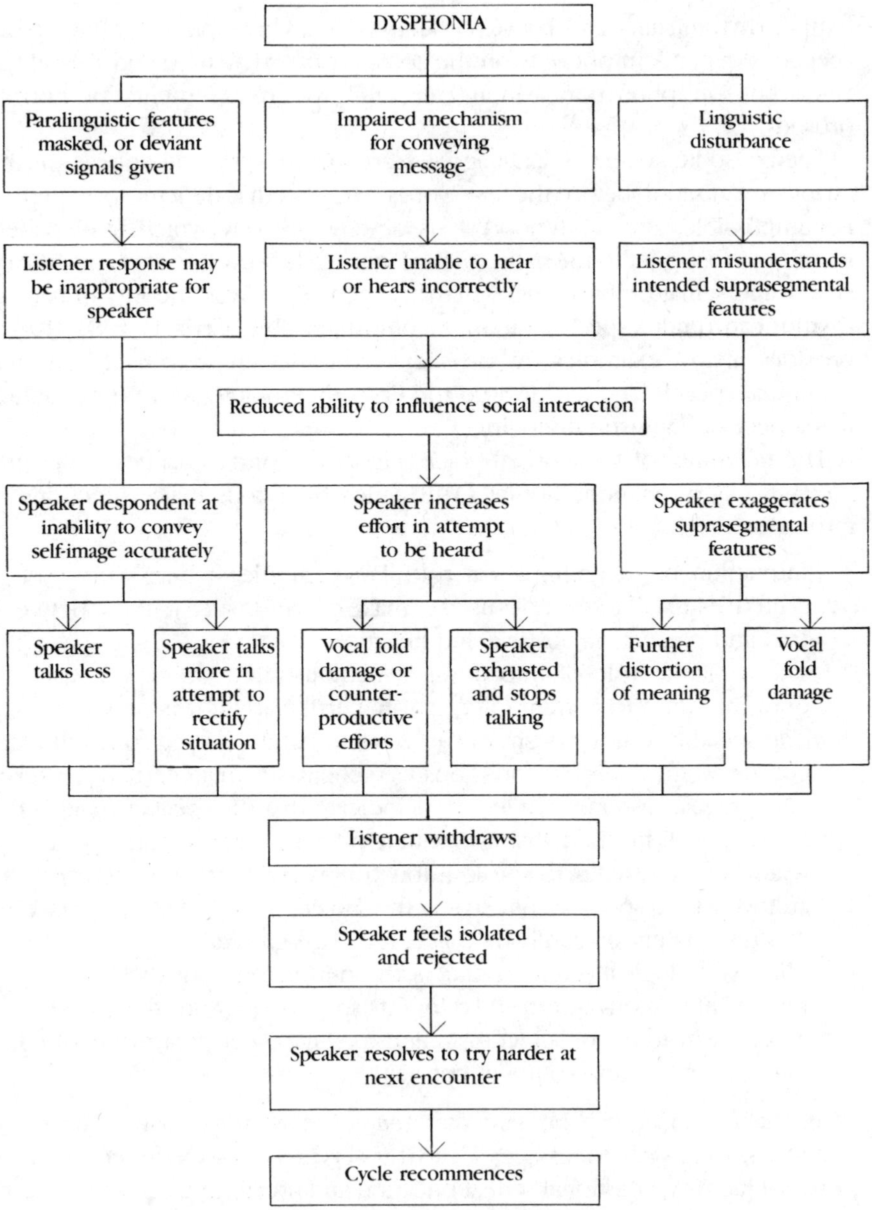

Figure 1.2. Dysphonia in social interaction.

Non-segmental phonology (suprasegmental phonology)

The voice plays a crucial role in the linguistic conveyance of meaning in non-segmental phonology. This can be considered separately from the para-linguistic aspects previously described which convey the emotional context of the message. In non-segmental phonology voice contributes to 'linguistic contrastivity' (Crystal, 1981) which is based on the variables of pitch, stress, tempo, rhythmicality and pause, collectively known as prosody. Intelligible speech is dependent not only on the accuracy of articulation and an audible voice but on phonation which can fulfil the requirements of normal prosody.

The prosodic system of language is learned very early and appears in the infant's vocalisation before the first words. The system is difficult to acquire, if not impossible, after childhood. It is deviant prosody which immediately identifies a foreigner to the native of the language however perfect vocabulary, syntax and semantic proficiency may be. Incorrect stress and loss of natural rhythm can render speech almost incomprehensible. Crystal (1981, 1982) provides many examples of prosodic contrasts in conversational and colloquial speech, and has devised the Prosody Profile (PROP) for profiling this aspect of linguistic disability.

The flexibility of the normal voice allows the pitch changes which we recognise as intonation. Crystal (1981) describes four major functions of intonation:

1. Intonation has a grammatical role. For example, it marks the end of sentences and clauses and is used to make contrasts such as those between past and present or positive and negative.
2. The semantic role of intonation is demonstrated when it is used to draw attention to certain information, particularly if it is new.
3. The social role is apparent in the way intonation is used to manipulate conversation. It is unconsciously recognised that certain patterns encourage a response while others indicate that the speaker regards the interaction as finished. Rising or falling pitch indicates that the speaker is ready for the listener to speak. Intonation will also frequently reveal the attitude of the speaker concerning the subject matter of the utterance so that uncertainty or confidence is readily recognised.
4. The psychological function affects the performance of the listener. By varying intonation pattern and relevant aspects of prosody the speaker can influence attitude, recall, comprehension and other parameters of communication in conversational contexts.

In conclusion, it can be said that the voice is more than a means of communicating verbal messages clearly. It serves as a powerful conveyor of personal identity, emotional state, education and social status. It is because of this that impairment of vocal function or complete loss of voice is so distressing to any individual. Voice constitutes the matrix of verbal communication, infusing all parameters of human speech and the unique self we present to the world.

Chapter 2
Anatomy and Physiology of Respiration

The Lungs

The primary function of respiration is to carry air into the lungs via the trachea, bronchi and alveoli where the transfusion of gases takes place. Oxygen enters the venous blood stream and carbon dioxide moves out through the capillaries wrapped around the very thin membrane which encloses the air sacs (alveoli). The lungs are sponge-like and there are roughly 300 million alveoli approximately 0.3 mm in diameter (West, 1979). Breathing is vital to the maintenance of life and the term 'breath of life' is no romantic notion but a reality. Without breathing life rapidly expires - suffocation taking 4-5 minutes.

The lung, besides the function of gas interchange, has other uses such as the filtering out of toxic particles from polluted air. These are swept out in a flow of mucus by the ciliated epithelium lining the bronchial walls. Large particles are filtered out by the nasal passages. Some particles settle in the alveoli and diminish their efficiency. Coal dust and smoke permanently damage the lungs (Cotes, 1979). Healthy lungs are essential for good health. Cilia can be destroyed by toxic gases and nicotine: the alveoli clog up and lose their elasticity with resultant emphysema.

The Thorax

The thoracic skeleton or rib cage houses the lungs and provides a movable scaffold for the attachment of the muscles of respiration. The rib cage consists of 12 pairs of ribs in both male and female. That a female has fewer is pure mythology. The first pair of ribs is immobile, being attached to the spinal vertebra posteriorly and to the manubrium (handle) of the sternum (breast bone) anteriorly. The second to seventh pairs are attached to the vertebrae posteriorly and to the sternum anteriorly by synovial joints which allow smooth rotation. The eighth to tenth pairs are attached to each other anteriorly by flexible cartilage and fibrous bands and only indirectly to the sternum because the eighth pair of ribs is bound to the seventh. These are known as false ribs. The eleventh and twelfth pairs are known as 'floating ribs' because the anterior attachment is not to the sternum but to the abdominal wall by fibrous membranes or fascia.

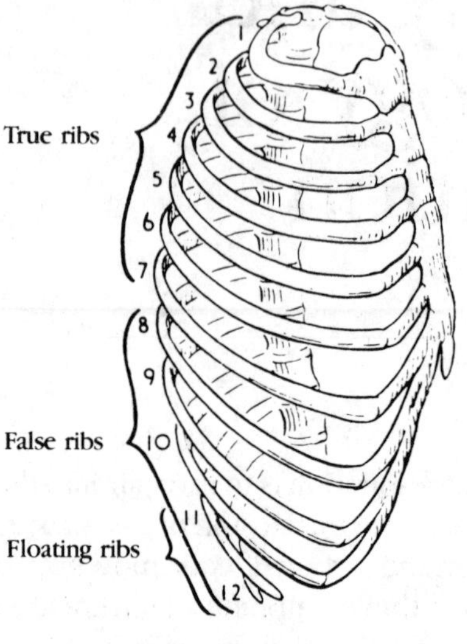

Figure 2.1. Skeleton of the thorax.

Thoracic movement

The movement of the second to sixth pairs of ribs about their axis increases the anteroposterior dimensions of the chest by lifting the sternum. Cotes (1979) likens the movement to that of a farmyard pump handle. The seventh to tenth pairs of ribs act like bucket handles and as they rotate about the anteroposterior axis they widen the chest dimension. The floating ribs follow the movements of the abdomen, mainly backwards and forwards and in this region expansion of the lungs is greatest.

Muscles of Respiration

The thoracic skeleton provides surfaces for insertion of the muscles of respiration. These activate expansion and contraction of the chest and lungs and maintain the rhythmic excursions of inspiration and expiration.

Inspiration

The muscles active in inspiration are the diaphragm and the external intercostal muscles. The diaphragm is a dome-shaped muscle which divides the thoracic from the abdominal cavity. The fibres of the diaphragm originate in the circumference of the thorax, the sternum, the ribs and the vertebral column. The muscle fibres are inserted in a trilobed central tendon which acts like a piston. The diaphragmatic aponeurosis operates much like the diaphragm of a bellows. The rise and fall of the diaphragm fills and empties air from the lungs. Its movement is passive and controlled by the abdominal and intercostal muscles. It is devoid of proprioceptive nerve endings (unlike the rest of the respiratory muscles). The breather is therefore unaware of the rise and fall of the diaphragm taking place within the chest cavity and experiences sensation from the chest wall and abdomen only (Agostini and Sant' Ambrogio, 1970). The external intercostals fill in the interstices between the ribs and elevate them on contraction thus increasing the dimensions of the thorax.

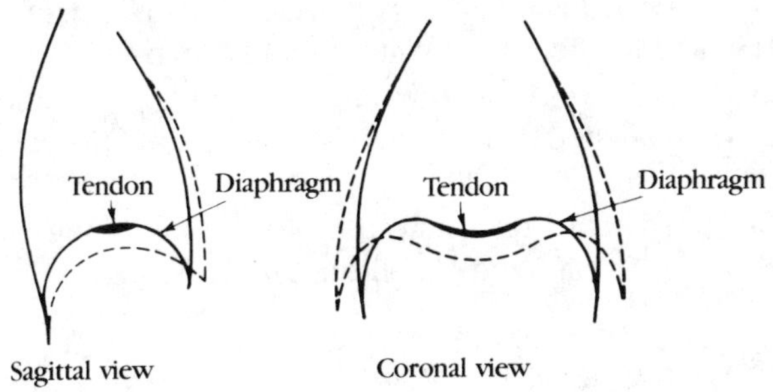

Figure 2.2. Diagrams illustrating enlargement of the thorax during inspiration.

Expiration

The muscles of expiration are the internal intercostal and abdominal muscles. The internal intercostals oppose the external intercostals and pull the ribs down, diminishing the size of the thoracic cavity.

The abdominal muscles are the rectus abdominis, external and internal oblique, and transversus abdominis. When the abdominal wall contracts and exerts pressure on the viscera the diaphragm is pushed upwards, the lungs are compressed and air is expelled. The diaphragm is operated by more forceful action of the abdominal muscles in coughing, defaecation, hiccup and vomiting.

Expiration is largely passive, brought about by the elastic recoil of the inspiratory muscles as they relax. In normal vegetative or tidal breathing the diaphragm's height changes approximately only 1.5 cm, but in forced inspiration and expiration a total excursion of 10 cm may occur (West, 1979). This is accompanied by increased movement of the chest wall and abdomen. Hixon, Mead and Goldman (1976) stress the fact that the diaphragm and abdomen behave as a single unit since, as the diaphragm descends, the abdominal contents (viscera) press the abdominal wall forward. The reverse is the case on expiration.

The accessory muscles of respiration are those of the shoulder girdle - the scaleni and sternomastoid muscles in particular (Campbell, 1974). These muscles assist in elevation of the ribs and are only called into play normally during exercise. This forceful breathing occurs with maximum expansion of the rib cage in all directions to accommodate the ballooning of the lungs.

Lung Ventilation and Volume

The volumes of air ventilating the lungs at rest and in various activities - speaking, singing, athletics of all sorts - are difficult to measure and need sophisticated laboratory equipment and technicians (West, 1979; Hixon, 1987) (see p. 110).

Lung capacity varies considerably among individuals. There are measurable differences between male and female. Age, exercise, size, weight, posture, health and smoking affect lung volumes and function (Cotes, 1979). Hixon (1987) says that 'it is more relevant to obtain information about single individuals when needed than to establish scientific statistical data concerning mean values'.

A number of standard terms are used to describe lung capacity variation (Campbell, 1974; Slonim and Hamilton, 1976).

Tidal capacity (TC)

There appears to be agreement that 500 ml is the average volume of air inspired and expired in normal breathing at rest. This is known as tidal capacity. This volume can be doubled or trebled according to the needs and activity of the individual.

Expiratory reserve volume (ERV)

Maximum volume of gas expired at the end of spontaneous expiration.

Residual volume (RV)

The volume of gas left in the lungs after maximum expiration.

Inspiratory reserve volume (IRV)

The volume that can be inspired at the end of tidal inspiration; it is the reserve which is available for increasing the tidal volume.

Functional residual capacity (FRC)

The volume of gas in the lungs after normal expiration.

Vital capacity (VC)

The exhaled volume after maximal inspiration. This is also described by Cotes (1979) as the extent to which total lung capacity exceeds the residual volume. Vital capacity in healthy males is in the range 2.0–6.6 litres. The range for the healthy female is 1.4–5.6 litres. Height, weight and age affect vital capacity.

Total lung capacity (TLC)

Volume of gas in the lungs at the end of maximal inspiration, i.e. the maximum volume of gas that the lungs can obtain.

Total ventilation (TV) and minute volume (MV)

The volume of air exhaled in a minute. There are on average approximately 15 breaths per minute (15 × tidal volume is equal to 7500 ml/min).

Use of these terms varies somewhat with different authors and it is to be hoped that in reports on all research projects what exactly has been measured is clearly defined.

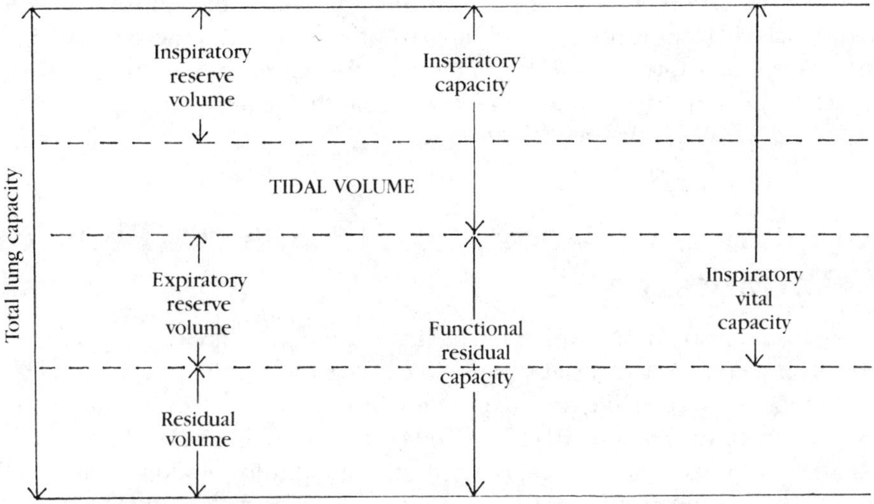

Figure 2.3. Ventilatory lung function: subdivisions of total lung capacity. (After Cotes, 1979.)

Dual Control of Respiration

Reflex control

As already noted, the chief function of respiration is to oxygenate the blood and to remove excess carbon dioxide. This vegetative, automatic process is carried on continuously throughout life whether asleep or awake. It needs no conscious attention. The respiratory muscles work in a finely coordinated rhythmic fashion which is controlled by the 'central controller' (West, 1979) or the respiratory centres, the collection of neurones in the pons and medulla. The level of ventilation is exactly controlled by sensors or chemoreceptors which instantaneously feed back information to central control regarding the oxygen and carbon dioxide balance in the arterial blood. This balance is constantly changing with bodily activity but is adjusted by the central control which programmes ventilation and action of the respiratory muscles. The rate of breathing is correlated with stress factors as well as physical demands (Lenneberg, 1967).

Failure in coordination can occur as when the inspiratory muscles operate as antagonists to the expiratory muscles. This may occur in premature babies when asleep. Respiration in at-risk infants needs careful monitoring as certain respiratory abnormalities are thought to be related to sudden infant death syndrome (SIDS).

Voluntary control

Breathing is also under voluntary control and the cortex can take over control of the respiratory centres to some extent. Breath can be held, for example, or respiration be slowed down or greatly accelerated causing the distressing experience of hyperventilation (hypocapnia). Should an individual lose consciousness, the respiratory centres will take over control and the individual will resume normal breathing. Breathing pattern is altered at will by attention being directed to movements of the chest and abdomen. This awareness is developed to a high level during the acquisition of particular breathing methods for speech and song.

Adaptation of Respiration to Speech (Phonic Respiration)

In vegetative respiration, expiration and inspiration times are equal (approximately 2 seconds) with a slight pause occurring at the end of expiration. In respiration for speech, the rhythm changes. Inspiration is relatively quick and expiration is prolonged to 10–15 seconds (Fry, 1979). Immediately prior to phonation the vocal folds are abducted during rapid inspiration, while the larynx is simultaneously lowered in the vocal tract. This is described by Wyke (1983) as the pre-phonatory inspiratory phase. It is followed by the pre-phonatory expiratory phase as the diaphragm and intercostal muscles relax. Intake of air is matched to phrasing. A monosyllable, it is true, may not require any change in breathing pattern, but a shout or peroration will need more air pressure to achieve adequate intensity and length. As the nasal passages are too narrow for the rapid inspiration necessary for speech, breathing becomes oral. Abdominal muscles are of particular importance in connected speech as they time the ascent of the diaphragm and phonic expiration (Hixon, Mead and Goldman, 1976). The lung volume required for the initiation of speech is 50% of the vital capacity.

Development of phonic respiration

Breathing for speech develops from the first cry of the neonate and the uncoordinated gasps and spluttering of the infant. Control of breath for speech develops on a continuum as the child begins to produce babble sounds and as muscular and neurological control systems mature (Langlois, Baken and Wilder, 1980). Voluntary control emerges gradually and becomes automatic, almost reflex. This is important to note because it explains why individuals suffering from vocal strain commonly do not associate their problems with breathing nor realise that breath provides energy source for voice.

The relationship between volume of air expired and the subglottic pressure controlled by tension in the vocal folds is crucial in determining volume, pitch and tempo. But it is also related to vocal quality since the vibration of the vocal folds, as we shall see, is exceedingly complex. Harmonics are created by the fundamental frequency and contained within the resonated tone.

Prosody and respiration

Another factor in airflow is the part it plays in the prosodic features of speech to mark stress, prominence, intonation and rhythm. These features are monitored by the linguistic system which influences the action of the expiratory muscles. Stressed syllables, for example, require an increase in subglottic pressure obtained by the internal intercostal muscles (Ladefoged, 1974). In connected speech the abdominal muscles contribute to the control of expiration. A baseline pressure in the lungs is established in order to produce sequences of speech segments. It is dependent on the intercostal muscles and the diaphragm interacting with the elastic recoil of the lungs. The muscles make adjustments to keep this pressure constant as the lung volume diminishes (Gould, 1981).

Control of phonic breathing

In ordinary everyday conversation, natural breathing proceeds without thought or training. Minimal adjustments in tidal airflow take place but do happen. Inspiration time quickens and expiration time lengthens with fluctuations in the activity of the respiratory muscles. The variations in the degree of effort required will go largely unnoticed in the normal untrained speaker. These variations depend not only on whether a whisper or a shout is being produced but also on the lung volume. Considerable effort will be needed to produce even quiet voice if the residual volume is low. Voice is produced effortlessly when the vital capacity is high (Gould, 1981).

From time immemorial training in 'correct' breathing method aimed at increasing control of the voice has been deemed essential for public speakers, actors and singers. In the past, singers strengthened their abdominal muscles by lying prone and lifting weights up and down on their stomachs. The abdomen's control of the ascent of the diaphragm was recognised. So also was the need to economise airflow and to this end the practice of singing a vowel before a lighted candle, without exciting a flicker, was advocated.

The complicated aerodynamic studies carried out in phonetic laboratories in the last 30 years using sophisticated electronic instruments (see p. 110) has disproved some briefs and verified others. Big expansions of the chest and the expulsion of great volumes of air are not necessary in order to produce good voice. Slight abdominal contraction is apparently essential as part of the adjustments made by the chest wall prior to phonation, although rib cage movements may vary (Wilder, 1983). Scientists reporting their researches into airflow and pressure levels have never suggested that control of phonic respiration is not important nor that training in correct use of the respiratory muscles is not necessary in rehabilitation.

Luchsinger (1965c), having drawn attention to the changed rhythm in respiration at rest and in speaking or singing, writes with commendable logic:

> The longer the available air lasts, the more can be said or sung on one breath. Here is the essential secret of breath control for speaking and singing: to achieve prolonged phonic expiration through proper muscular co-ordination. Obviously, singing and speaking require much deeper inspirations than does quiet breathing.

It has become fashionable among some speech pathologists to deride 'breathing exercises' in rehabilitation of dysphonic patients and the instruction 'to breath naturally' is considered enough to cure voice disorders. We do not like the term 'breathing exercises'. The process by which breath control and increased capacity are developed consists of increased understanding of the respiratory process and its relevance to phonation. The practice of appropriate respiration for speech establishes new kinaesthetic and proprioceptive patterns which are incorporated into voice production. Individuals suffering from clinically diagnosed voice disorders frequently do not breathe normally and naturally. Their breathing has become constrained by anxiety and tension and the problem is compounded by the compensatory strategies which they subsequently evolve in an attempt to produce useful voice. Training in relaxation, respiration and phonation is the foundation of correct voice production. Not least is the development of sensory awareness of strain and the conscious control of expiration. We agree with Wilder (1983) that modification of respiratory patterns is an important issue in voice therapy.

Posture

The traditional view that posture has a significant effect on breathing is confirmed by recent studies (Hixon, 1987). In the upright position the vital capacity is at its greatest because the abdominal contents are pulled down by gravity, allowing full descent of the diaphragm. Sitting and supine positions reduce the vital capacity. Gould's conclusions (1981) summarise the views of many of the workers in the field of phonic respiration. He states: 'defects in or misuse of the pulmonary apparatus lead to laryngeal dysfunction. A clear understanding of the pulmonary laryngeal system is needed so that preventive or corrective measures may be taken during voice training more intelligently.'

Types of Phonic Respiration

According to which muscle movements predominate, various types of breathing are recognised as variants of the normal breathing pattern during which costal and abdominal movements occur simultaneously and regularly. There is evidence that breathing for speech varies according to body type. The normal breathing pattern of the tall, thin ectomorph will show differences from that of the rotund endomorph (Hixon, 1987). Hixon's investigations also show that most normal individuals use rib-cage movements predominantly although at times they use rib-cage and abdominal movements. Some speakers may use a predominantly abdominal movement but the pattern is consistent in each individual.

Abdominal breathing

In this type of breathing there is very little costal movement but movement of the abdominal wall is evident as the diaphragm moves up and down. This may follow pregnancy when the muscles are weak and the stomach muscles sag. It is common in middle-aged and corpulent men with pronounced girth (the 'beer and spaghetti tummy') who take no exercise and are constantly short of breath. Excessive fat deposits impair lung function (Cotes, 1979).

Clavicular breathing (costal breathing)

This is the reverse of abdominal breathing and is an habitual breathing disorder associated with anxiety and tension. It also occurs in individuals who suffer from asthma. The external intercostal muscles and the accessory muscles elevate the shoulder girdle and the upper portion of the chest. Tension and effort radiate into the infrahyoid muscles (see p. 23).

Breath support in singing

This is a breathing technique used in singing and very different from that used in speech. The technique greatly increases vocal volume, pitch range and a swelling tone. It is generally agreed to be essential for producing all the aesthetic features of artistic performance. There is much disagreement concerning how it is achieved and what exactly is the nature of the control exerted over the respiratory muscles. Luchsinger (1965c) reviews the conflicting theories which endeavour to explain this support to the singing voice, called 'appoggio' by the Italians, 'appui' by the French, 'Stütze' by the Germans and 'rib reserve' by the British.

Isshiki (1964) has contributed a scientific investigation into the relationship between the intensity, subglottic pressure, glottal resistance and airflow rate in trained singers. However, this was related to vocal cord behaviour and not in conjunction with that of the respiratory muscles. A study of respiratory function by Gould and Okamura (1973) showed that total lung volumes are not significantly larger in the trained singer when compared with those of the untrained singer. The most obvious difference is the increase in vital capacity and decrease in residual volume in the trained singer.

The support given to the voice is felt subjectively as a great increase in the mastery of performance and power. This is accompanied by a feeling of tension in the chest. Last (1984) suggests that this is evoked by the opposing actions of the external intercostals and the diaphragmatic movement. Inhalation is accompanied by elevation of the ribs in which the diaphragm is lifted up. At the same time the diaphragm is pulled down by the central tendon and the internal intercostals, and the pull against the external intercostals is felt. Expiration is then controlled by the contraction of the abdominal muscles with the rib cage still held in its elevated position. Air pressure is raised below the glottis and air is used under great control very sparingly, with vocal fold vibrations adjusted for intensity and pitch by the ear. The importance of abdominal muscle support in singing is clearly illustrated by Sataloff, Reinhardt and O'Connor (1984). A professional singer, unable to sing after becoming quadriplegic, was given a device to provide abdominal support which restored his singing ability and substantially improved respiratory function.

It is interesting to note that in order to enhance the tension of the abdominal wall and to provide support for the action of the diaphragm some traditional Japanese singers bind the abdomen while performing (Kirikae, 1981).

When the diaphragm has achieved its resting elevated position, the ribs can be lowered and the 'rib reserve' of air is useful for extending the phonation time for a phrase or exacting aria.

During pregnancy breathing is hampered by the accommodation of the baby. The diaphragm is pushed up and the chest wall is expanded by pressure from the uterus. As a result there is a diminution in residual volume of air and functional and residual capacity. A certain degree of breathlessness may be experienced and the singing voice will suffer.

Although speech therapists will have ill-trained and untrained singers in all types of music referred for treatment, it is outside the province of the speech therapist (unless a trained singer) to teach rib reserve breathing. The fundamental principles of natural voice production will set the artist on the right path but the competent singing teacher, unblinded by science, is the appropriate instructor in the art of singing and its aesthetic qualities.

Chapter 3 The Larynx and the Organs of Articulation and Resonance - Anatomy and Physiology

The Larynx

The larynx is situated in the neck at the level of the third to sixth cervical vertebrae. It is continuous with the trachea (windpipe) below and the pharynx above. It consists of a framework of cartilages bound together by ligaments, membrane and muscles. The larynx is suspended from the hyoid bone and it follows its vertical movements in deglutition and in the production of high and low notes. Housed within the laryngeal frame or 'voice box' are the vocal folds which constitute the vibrator that generates the voice.

The primal function of the larynx is to protect the lungs from the entry of foreign particles. It is situated in front of the oesophagus (gullet) and is attached to the oesophagus by the cricopharyngeal sphincter muscle which controls the oesophageal entrance at the level of the fifth vertebra.

Cartilages of the Larynx

The principal cartilages are the cricoid, thyroid and arytenoid cartilages.

Cricoid cartilage

This forms an inflexible ring at the top of the trachea. It is shaped like a signet ring - narrow in front and broad behind.

Arytenoid cartilages

There are two of these. They are pyramidal in shape and their bases articulate with the cricoid shoulders on either side of the mid-line. Their articulation is by a synovial joint which allows rotation and swivelling movements.

Thyroid cartilage

This is a large cartilage shaped like an open book with the spine in front, the angle of which forms the thyroid angle (Adam's apple). The sides are quadilateral in shape with inferior and superior horns to the posterior corners.

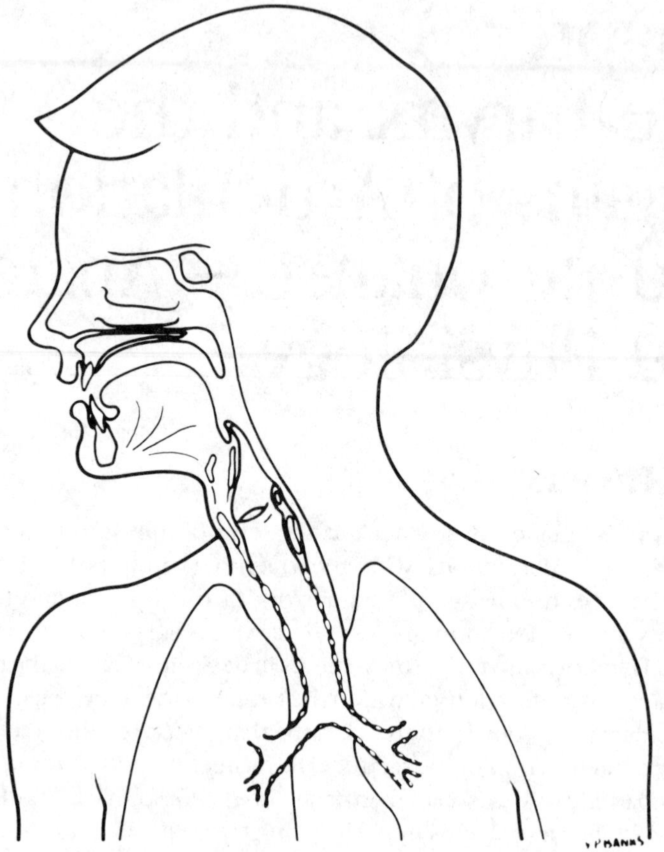

Figure 3.1. The vocal instrument.

The vocal folds extend from the interior thyroid angle to the arytenoids across the laryngeal cavity.

Epiglottis

The epiglottis is a large leaf-like cartilage which figures conspicuously in most diagrams of the larynx. It is not considered important in phonation and certainly does not participate in generation of the fundamental note. It is attached to the posterior cricoid elevation and the root of the tongue. It funnels food into the oesophagus and away from the laryngeal inlet, and yet deglutition can proceed perfectly well minus an epiglottis. It is thought to be the vestige of a primitive olfactory system associated with sniffing and monitoring scent in animals, possibly while eating (Negus, 1949; Perkins and Kent, 1986). As regards voice, it must have a not negligible influence upon vocal tone because it changes position with tongue movements and alters the shape and size of the pharyngeal cavity.

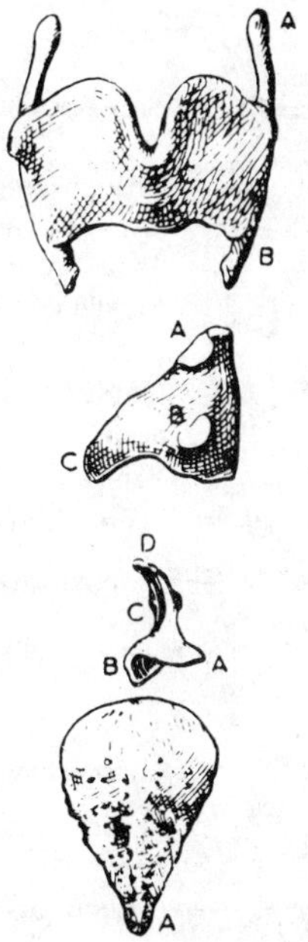

1

Thyroid:
(A) superior horn;
(B) inferior horn;
(C) laryngeal prominence.

2

Cricoid left lateral aspect:
(A) facet articulates with arytenoid;
(B) facet articulates with inferior horn of thyroid;
(C) anterior narrow portion of cricoid.

3

Left arytenoid, medial aspect:
(A) vocal process;
(B) articulates with cricoid;
(C) lateral surface;
(D) corniculate cartilage.

4

Epiglottis:
(A) attached to inner angle of thyroid.

Figure 3.2. The laryngeal cartilages.

The Extrinsic Laryngeal Muscles

The extrinsic muscles are classified as suprahyoid and infrahyoid and alter the position of the larynx in the neck via their attachment to the hyoid bone from which the thyroid cartilage is suspended.

The suprahyoid muscles elevate the hyoid bone and thereby the larynx. They are the stylohyoid, mylohyoid, geniohyoid and the digastric.

The infrahyoid muscles, or strap muscles, are the sternothyroid, sternohyoid, thyrohyoid and omohyoid. They serve as anchorage to the larynx and as depressors in sounds of low pitch.

Although not traditionally considered as extrinsic laryngeal muscles, the pharyngeal constrictor muscles (superior pharyngeal constrictor, hypopharyngeal, thyropharyngeal, cricopharyngeal) and the extrinsic tongue muscles (styloglossus, genioglossus, hypoglossus) certainly affect laryngeal position and spatial relations. They should, perhaps, be included in the category of extrinsic laryngeal musculature.

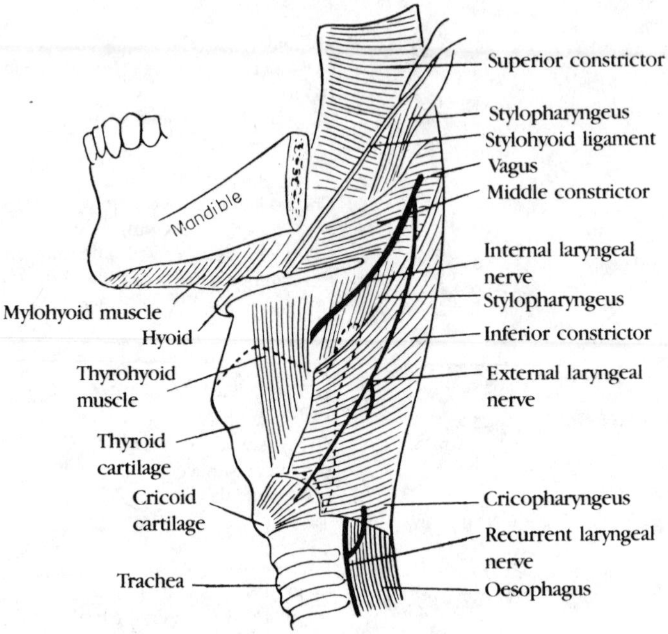

Figure 3.3. Some extrinsic muscles of the larynx and the nerve supply.

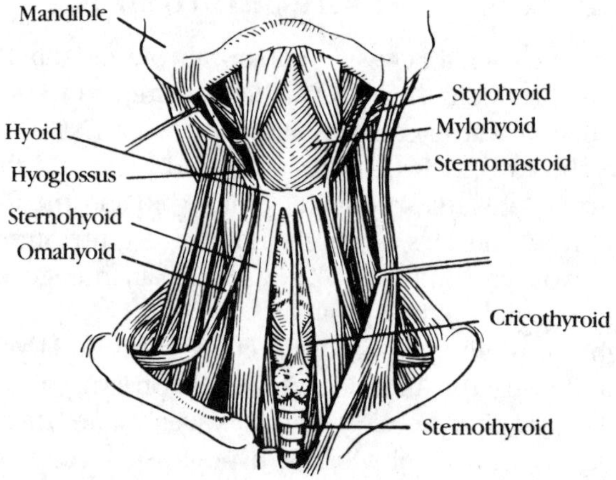

Figure 3.4. Suprahyoid and infrahyoid muscles (anterior view).

The Intrinsic Laryngeal Muscles

The intrinsic laryngeal muscles are named according to their attachment to the laryngeal cartilages. They do not affect the spatial relations of the larynx in the neck but constitute the vocal folds and control phonation. The muscles are all paired except the transverse arytenoid muscle which is a single muscle.

Thyroarytenoid muscle

This constitutes the body of the vocal fold. It is of unique and complex structure as has been shown by Hirano's investigations using high speed photography and morphological dissection of the muscle (Hirano, 1974). He revised the traditional concept of vocal fold architecture which had been restricted to the cricovocal membrane, conus elasticus and vocalis muscle (Negus, 1949, 1957; Luchsinger and Arnold, 1965).

The thyroarytenoid muscles are attached to the interior angle of the thyroid cartilage where they are fixed adjacent to each other. They extend back to the anterior surfaces of the arytenoids and their vocal processes. Their free margins confront each other across a triangular space called the glottis, glottic aperture or rima glottidis. Each thyroarytenoid muscle has superior and inferior portions: the ventricular and vocal folds.

Ventricular folds

The superior portion forms the false, ventricular or vestibular fold which under normal circumstances does not participate directly in phonation. The folds approximate in swallowing making a firm valve or seal. There is a space between the false fold and the vocal fold below which is known as the laryngeal ventricle, sinus or vestibule. The cavity is well supplied with mucous glands so that the vocal folds are lubricated by mucus which protects them from the effects of friction.

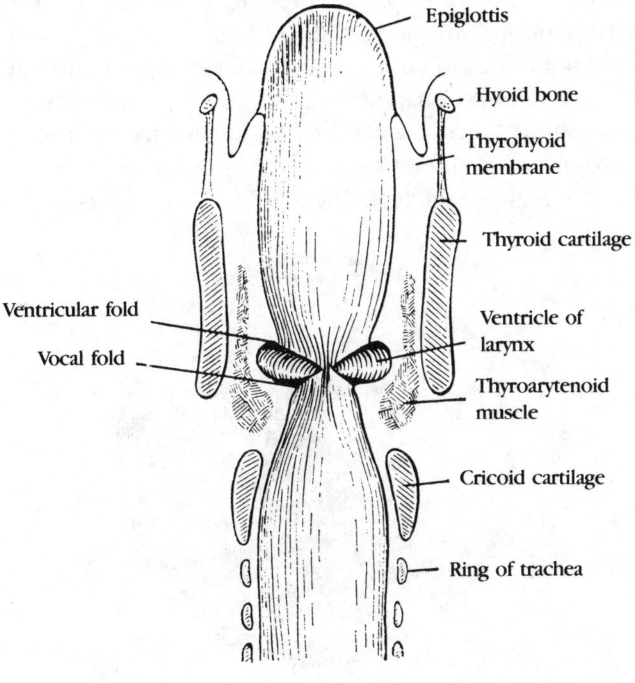

Figure 3.5. Coronal section of the larynx, the anterior section being viewed from behind.

Vocal folds

The lower portion of the thyroarytenoid muscle forms the true vocal fold. The free edges of these two folds are covered with a superficial membranous layer of squamous epithelium and interwoven in the layers below are elastic and collagenous fibres of the vocal ligaments (see details below). The folds are white in appearance and contrast with the red false folds when viewed from above in a laryngoscopic mirror.

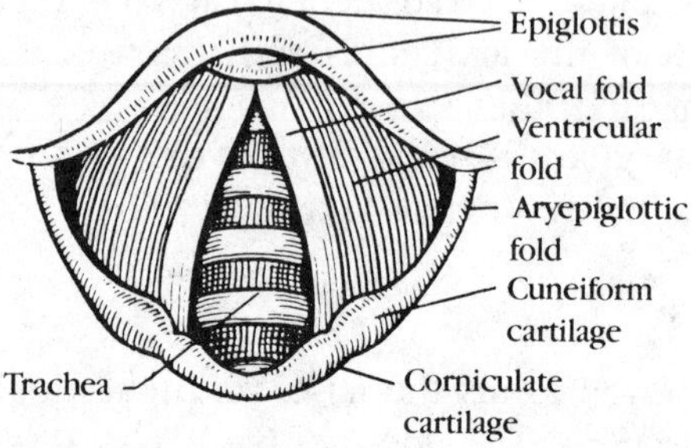

Figure 3.6. Laryngoscopic view of the interior of the larynx.

Structure of the vocal folds

The true vocal folds are highly elastic and have a complex histological structure which accounts for the extraordinary versatility of the voice and the wide range of pitch, volume and quality of which the instrument is capable. The thyroarytenoid muscle coat of squamous cell epithelium gives it a thin cover which maintains the shape of the vocal fold. Beneath this membranous cover there are three layers of connective tissue which compose what is called the lamina propria. The superficial or top layer of the lamina propria consists of a loose fibrous matrix which Hirano (1974, 1981) likens to gelatin. This is

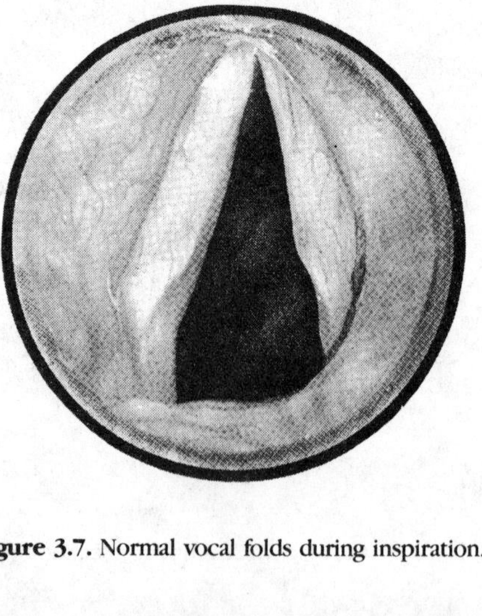

Figure 3.7. Normal vocal folds during inspiration.

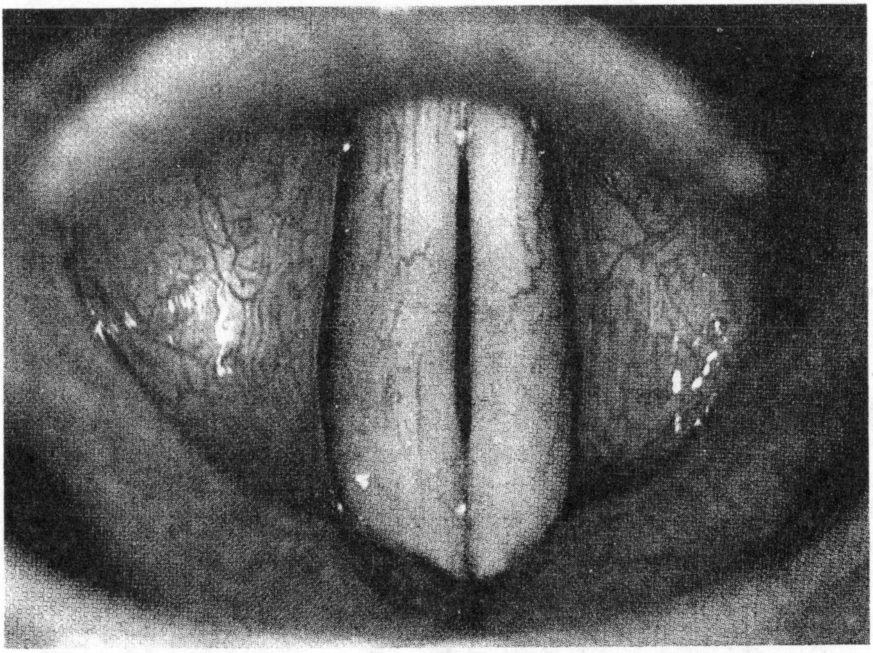

Figure 3.8. Normal vocal folds during phonation.

Reinke's space which can fill with oedema in pathological conditions such as laryngitis or vocal abuse.

The second, or intermediate, layer of the lamina propria consists of elastic fibres. Finally, the third, or deep, layer consists of collagenous fibres. The intermediate and deep layers are known as the 'transition' (Kahane, 1986) and these layers form the vocal ligament. The layer structure varies in thickness throughout the vocal fold length and is constructed in a way that reduces any mechanical damage which might be caused by vibration at the ends of the folds. The body of the thyroarytenoid muscle over which the epithelial cover and lamina propria lie is the vocalis muscle (see below).

The four layers described above fill in the detail of the cricovocal mucous membrane and conus elasticus. Each layer of the vocal fold has different mechanical properties important in vibration. The layers are passive, not containing muscle fibre, but controlled actively by the vocalis and responding to air pressure.

Divisions of the vocal folds

The anterior two-thirds of the vocal fold constitute the membranous portion which is known traditionally as the pars vocalis. It is highly elastic, mobile and active in phonation and it is in the middle of this portion that the greatest excursions occur because of position and structure.

The posterior third is that part into which the vocal process of the arytenoid

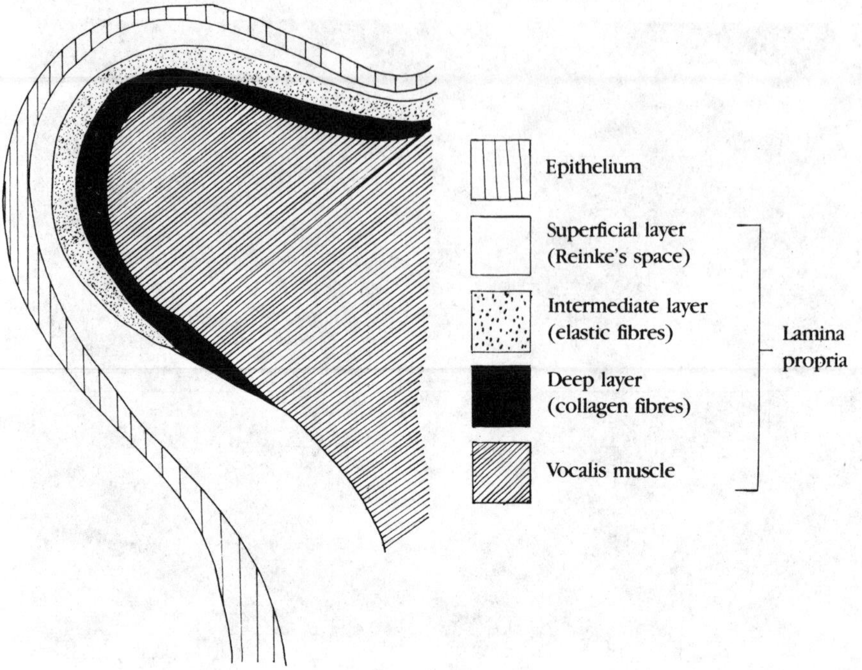

Figure 3.9. Histological structure of the vocal folds.

cartilage penetrates. This is the cartilaginous part of the 'pars respiratus' which does not participate in phonatory vibration except in deepest notes when the whole fold enacts a rolling motion.

Vocalis muscle

The vocalis muscle aids adduction of the vocal folds and controls their thin-edged membrous length. It can shorten and thicken the fold and effect rounding of the lips of the glottis by contraction while the cover and lamina propria are slack. Contraction also stiffens the vocal folds in an action which is independent of the vocal fold length. In high speed photography undulations are visible passing over the vocal folds and involving their thin cover (Hirano, 1981).

Cricothyroid muscle

The cricothyroid muscle originates in the anterior and lateral surface of the cricoid cartilage and is inserted in the inferior border of the thyroid cartilage. On contraction, the cricoid is tilted up anteriorly and down posteriorly. It brings the vocal fold into a paramedian position and stretches, lengthens and thins the vocal fold. The free edges of the folds become sharp as their four layers are stiffened while, at the same time, the posterior cricoarytenoid braces back the arytenoid. It is the most important muscle for raising pitch and

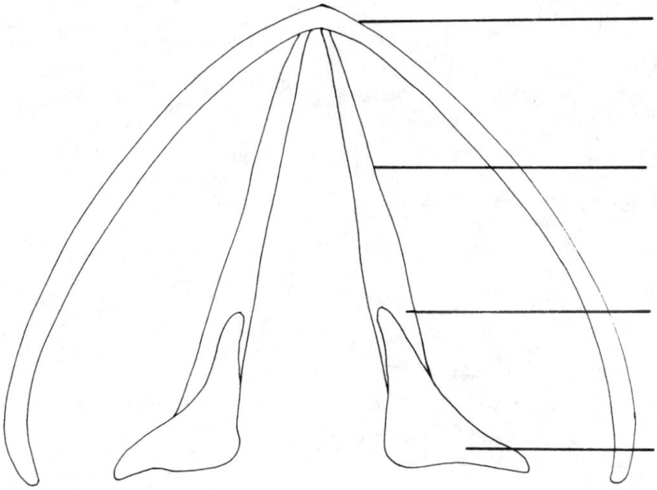

Figure 3.10. Vocal folds: membranes and cartilaginous portions.

achieves this in conjunction with the lateral cricoarytenoid and the thyroarytenoid (Hirose and Sawashima, 1981).

Posterior cricoarytenoid muscle

This originates in the broad outer surface of the cricoid cartilage and is inserted in the base of the arytenoid cartilage. It abducts and pulls upwards and backwards the vocal process of the arytenoid and thus elongates the vocal fold. It is the major abductor of the vocal folds (Last, 1984).

Zemlin, Davis and Gaza (1984), in a study of the fine morphology of the posterior cricoarytenoid, have resolved a long-standing disagreement of the exact function of the muscle and contradictions in the electromyographic results of many researchers. There are two separate bundles of muscle which have separate tendons. Therefore there are two muscles, not one, forming the posterior cricoarytenoid. One muscle has oblique fibres and the other is composed of vertical and lateral fibres. The horizontal fibres rotate the arytenoids on their axes and swing the vocal processes outwards. The vertical fibres draw the arytenoids away from each other by pulling down, laterally on the sloping upper border of the cricoid lamina. The net result of the action of the whole muscle is rotation and separation of the arytenoids. The existence of a dual muscle action is of particular relevance in the variable positions assumed by the vocal folds in paralysis of the recurrent laryngeal nerve (see p. 298).

Lateral cricoarytenoid muscle

This originates along the superior and lateral borders of the cricoid cartilage and passes back obliquely to the outside corner of the arytenoid cartilage. It

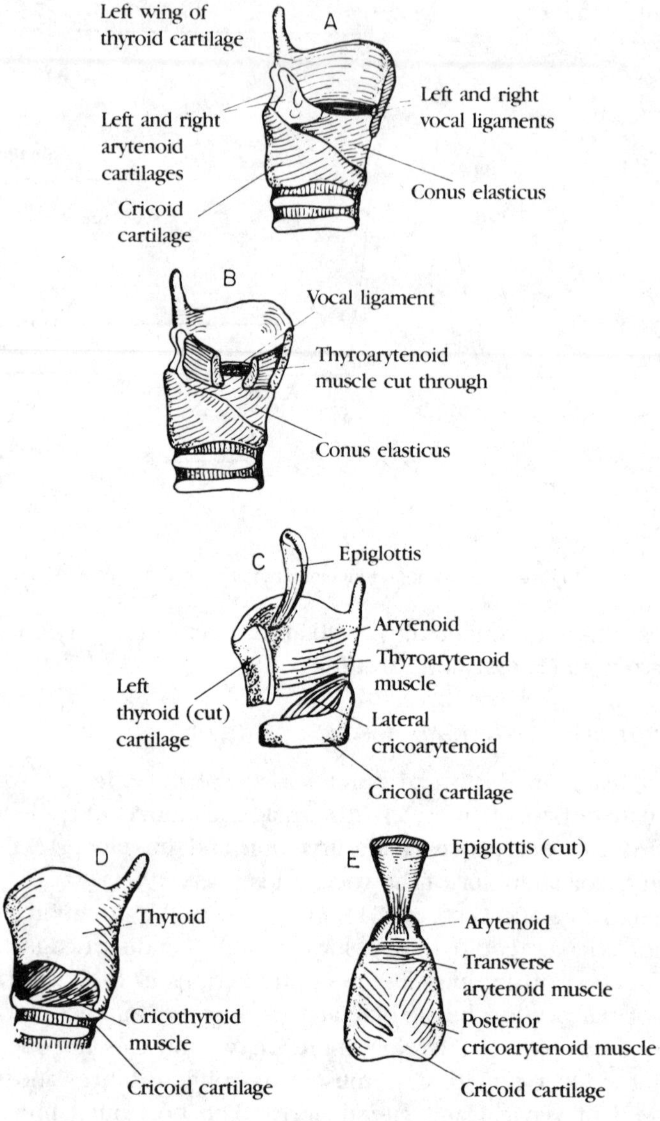

Figure 3.11. Intrinsic laryngeal muscles.

rotates the arytenoid forwards and slightly inwards acting as an antagonist to the posterior cricoarytenoid muscle and an adductor of the vocal folds.

Interarytenoid muscles

The interarytenoids are composed of the transverse arytenoid, a single muscle, and the oblique arytenoids, which are a crossed pair of muscles. They pull the posterior medial borders of the arytenoids together.

A cautionary remark is appropriate here, however. Attempts at delegation of specific functions to individual laryngeal muscle pairs is really little more than an academic exercise in phonic physiology. In reality the intrinsic laryngeal muscles participate together in a fairly coordinated harmonious and rhythmical mechanical system which controls muscle energy and posture in relation to subglottic air pressure.

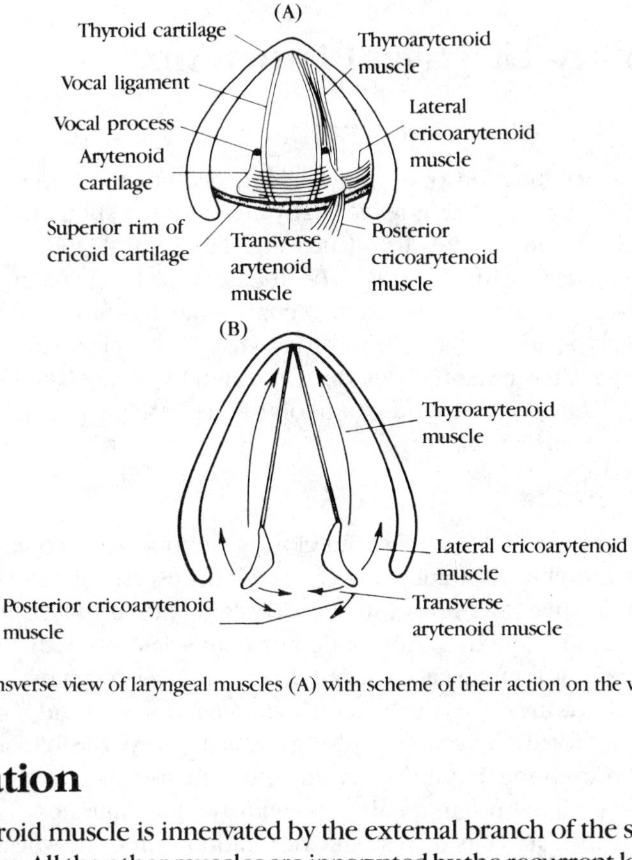

Figure 3.12. Transverse view of laryngeal muscles (A) with scheme of their action on the vocal folds (B).

Innervation

The cricothyroid muscle is innervated by the external branch of the superior laryngeal nerve. All the other muscles are innervated by the recurrent laryngeal nerve. The superior and recurrent laryngeal nerves are branches of the vagus nerve.

Blood Supply

The larynx is supplied by the superior laryngeal, cricothyroid and inferior laryngeal arteries. The vascular network of the vocal folds is adapted for a vibrating structure; there is a marked decrease in volume of blood in the vocal fold while it is vibrating so that circulation and metabolism are not disturbed (Mihashi *et al.*, 1981). There is no blood supply to the vocal ligaments, hence their white appearance in laryngoscopy.

Lubrication

The mucous membrane lining the normal, healthy larynx and vocal tract is always moist. This lubrication is provided by the mucous gland in the ventricle. The dryness and irritation which is caused by infection, atmospheric changes and certain emotions are uncomfortable and have noticeable effects on the voice. In a dry atmosphere the mucous membrane overlying the vocal folds becomes dry and its normal undulations are reduced (Hiroto, 1981).

Primary Laryngeal Functions

Swallowing (deglutition)

The primary function of the larynx is to prevent food entering the airway during swallowing. This is achieved by means of the sphincteric action of the aryepiglottic folds and the true and false vocal folds, which occurs simultaneously with elevation of the larynx (Logemann, 1983a). The importance of laryngeal elevation in controlling pressures and function of the cricopharyngeal sphincter, in order that the bolus can pass into the oesophagus, has recently been demonstrated by Mendelsohn and McConnel (1987). The protective function of the larynx results in suspension of respiration during swallowing.

Coughing

Coughing is preceded by forceful closure of both true and false folds which follows a quick inspiration due to sudden descent of the diaphragm. Air pressure is then built up below the adducted folds as the diaphragm ascends spasmodically, aided by the abdominal muscles, until the folds separate explosively and mucus is expelled. Expiratory effort against a closed glottis such as this is known as the Valsalva manoeuvre (Slonim and Hamilton, 1976). During any form of exertion involving use of the arms, the folds are again firmly closed preventing expulsion of air and collapse of the chest walls, thus providing a fixed origin for the arm and shoulder muscles.

When the larynx is at rest and respiration quiet, the vocal folds remain abducted and move up and down slightly in sympathy with the outflow and inflow of respiratory air. The folds are drawn wide apart to a position of full abduction in forceful inspiration.

Vocal Fold Vibration

Immediately prior to phonation the vocal folds rapidly abduct to allow the intake of air. This has been termed the 'pre-phonatory inspiratory phase' by Wyke (1983). The pre-phonatory expiratory phase begins as the diaphragm and other muscles of respiration relax. The vocal folds rapidly adduct before the exhaled air reaches them.

In production of notes of middle pitch, the interarytenoid muscles adduct the cartilaginous posterior third of both vocal folds and hold them together while the anterior two-thirds of each fold are gently adducted but free to vibrate in the outflowing breath stream. As pressure builds up below the folds they are blown apart and upwards which sets in motion sound waves. The release of air results in a simultaneous drop in pressure below the folds so that they are sucked down again. This is known as the Bernoulli effect. Separation and recoil constitute one cycle of vibration. Each cycle consists of three phases: pre-setting, adduction, aerodynamic separation and recoil.

Body cover theory

Studies show that an undulating wave of movement of the mucous membrane travels from the lower to the upper surface of the vocal fold during each cycle of vibration. The mucous membrane vibrates more than the vocalis muscle

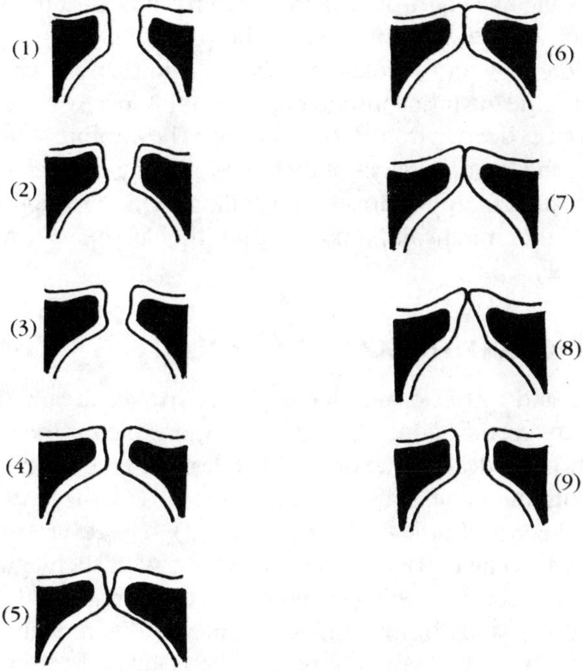

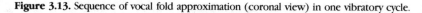

Figure 3.13. Sequence of vocal fold approximation (coronal view) in one vibratory cycle.

during phonation. The chief role of the vocalis then is to control the shape of the fold and to provide the appropriate degree of tonicity to allow normal vibration to take place (Hiroto, 1981; Perkins and Kent, 1986). The complexity of the simultaneous patterns of vibration during phonation, and their inter-relationship, is the subject of extensive research (Bless and Abbs, 1983). The developing field of computer simulation is making a significant contribution in this area.

Vocal pitch and volume

The time one vibratory cycle takes determines the frequency (pitch) of the fundamental note which is measured in number of cycles per second or hertz

(Hz). The size of the excursions executed by the vocal folds determines the size of the air waves generated and the volume of sound. Insufficient approximation of the folds results in air wastage and production of breathy voice. The folds fail to approximate completely along their membranous portion, with a slightly increased aperture in the cartilaginous section. As a result, turbulent air escapes and is audible in the voice.

The rate of the vibration of the vocal folds is controlled by the changes in vocal fold length, tension and bulk and resistance to subglottic air pressure. As pitch rises from the middle range the length of the vocal folds increases by action of the internal muscles while at the same time the vocalis thins and stiffens them. In falsetto the posterior two-thirds of the folds are approximated and only the knife-like edges of the anterior third vibrate. At the same time the suprahyoid muscles elevate the larynx (Shipp, 1975).

In the middle register the folds are triangular in shape in cross-section. In low chest notes the intrinsic muscles relax, the folds increase in bulk, and their opposing surfaces deepen from 3 mm to 5 mm. They vibrate slowly along their whole length, the lower surfaces of their 'lips' making contact and separating as the upper surfaces approximate in a rolling motion or figure of eight. In lowest notes the infrahyoid muscles pull the larynx down (Shipp and McGlone, 1971).

Wyke's Neuromuscular Control System Theory

The extrinsic and intrinsic muscles of the larynx as already described are under voluntary cortical control. They are responsible for the pre-phonatory tuning which precedes phonation and is followed by the phasic, tonic and volitional contractions and also maintenance of length, tension, bulk and position of the vocal folds (Bowden, 1972). However, the phonatory modulations which take place in speech happen with such lightening speed that it seems that such fine tuning cannot be cortically regulated (Wyke, 1983). The linguistic demands of intonation, phonemic differentiations and emotional nuances in quality would appear to be regulated by an independent subcortical reflex neural system.

Free fibrils and terminal filaments enclosed in capsules constitute the receptor end organs (the mechanoreceptors) embedded in the laryngeal tissues at sites sensitive to muscle stretch and airflow pressures. Wyke (1967, 1969, 1972) has postulated that mechanoreceptors are found in three sites as follows:

1. The mucosal lining of the larynx (subglottic mucosal mechanoreceptors).
2. The capsules of the articulatory joints (articular mechanoreceptors).
3. The extrinsic and laryngeal muscles (myotatic mechanoreceptors).

The corpuscular nerve endings in the subglottic mucous membrane covering the inferior surface of the vocal folds are particularly numerous and sensitive to the stimuli of muscle stretch and air pressure levels. They discharge impulses into the afferent fibres of the vagus. The myotatic mechanoreceptors in each extrinsic and intrinsic laryngeal muscle respond to the upward stretching of the vocal folds caused by the expiratory air stream.

Stimulation of all categories of laryngeal mechanoreceptors initiates activity in the larynx which ensures that the vocal folds are stabilised and return to their pre-set pattern following displacement by the expiratory air stream. This process, by monitoring the tonicity and position of the vocal folds, enables necessary adjustments to be made instantaneously and accurately. Although it would seem inevitable that there must ultimately be integration of this servo-system with other control systems during phonation, Wyke states that this process is independent of auditory feedback. The action of the reflexogenic system can account for the otherwise inexplicable instantaneous fluctuations in pitch and also explains the range of phonatory symptoms in cases of vocal misuse.

The hypothesis concerning the reflex mechanoreceptor system has been chiefly promoted by the researches of Wyke who has applied the concept to voice pathology. However, although other researchers in the field affirm the histological proof regarding the presence of mechanoreceptors in the larynx, their precise function remains a matter of controversy. Whether stimuli in the laryngeal mucosa, muscles and joints can operate in isolation and control aspects of laryngeal motor activity remains open to question (Kirchner, 1983). It seems to us a feasible proposition which does not conflict with the complex structure of the lamina propria and the mucous membrane body cover theory.

Organs of Articulation and Resonance

The fundamental laryngeal note has separate properties of pitch and volume only in theory. In actual fact this note is not a pure note (sine wave) but in the moment of generation creates subsidiary sound waves. Thus the laryngeal note instantly acquires quality. The sound waves become increasingly more complex as they travel up the vocal tract. Besides the vocal tone engendered, specific resonance frequencies passing through the pharyngeal, nasal and oral resonators form the vowels and diphthongs of speech. A laryngeal note in fact cannot be made without uttering a vowel of some nature.

The articulators are the lips, tongue, jaws and soft palate enclosed in the oral cavity. The lips form the inlet and the faucial arches form the outlet posteriorly to the oropharynx. Between the faucial arches the tonsils are housed in the tonsillar sinuses. The adenoidal pad is in the nasopharynx. The roof of the oral cavity is composed of the hard and soft palates. The enlargement of this resonator, which is so important to the quality of the fundamental note, is achieved by the temporomandibular joint which enables the mandible to be lowered and raised. The articulators are responsible for alterations in the dimensions of the oral cavity. In addition they perform the necessary phonetic gestures for pronunciaton of vowels and consonants.

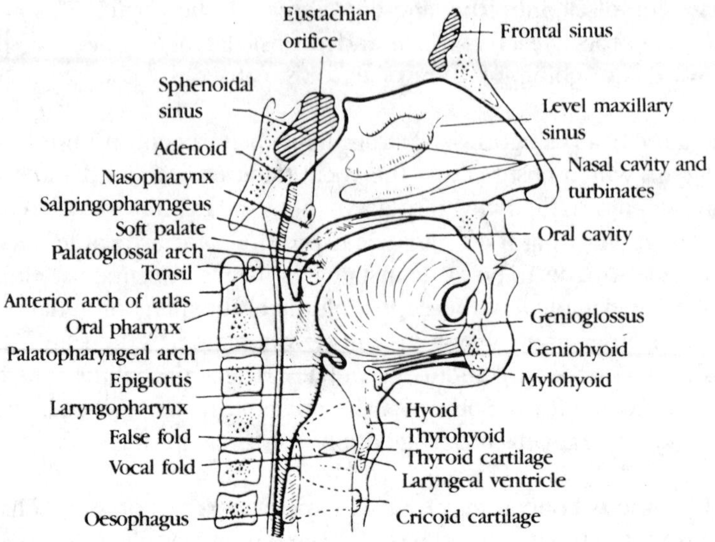

Figure 3.14. Sagittal section through nose, mouth, pharynx and larynx to show relative positions of organs of articulation, resonance and phonation.

Lips

The lips are formed by the orbicularis oris which is a sphincteric muscle encircling the mouth opening. A number of paired muscles account for the extreme mobility of the lips. The risoris retracts the mouth and according to Gray's anatomy (1949) produces 'an unpleasant grinning expression' – overlooking its pleasing risible potential. The buccinator (buccina = trumpet) compresses and protrudes the lips. The lips are important in pronunciation of bilabial /p.b.m.w/ and labiodental /f,v/ phonemes. Varying degrees of lip-rounding, protruding and spreading achieve vowel distinctions as for example: /u:, i: ɑ:/.

Tongue

The tongue's primary function is in swallowing but it is also the most important articulator of consonants and vowels. The intrinsic muscles form an intricate network of superior and inferior, transverse, vertical and longitudinal fibres (genioglossus, geniohyoid and mylohyoid). These muscles anchor the tongue to the hyoid but otherwise the tongue is free to move in the oral cavity. Tongue movements are closely related to vertical movements of the larynx because of their common attachment to the hyoid bone. The tongue is able to assume a vast number of shapes. It is divided down the centre by a fibrous septum (raphe) and is attached to the floor of the mouth by the frenum.

The movements of the back of the tongue change the shape and patency of the oropharynx which, besides being essential in the articulation of vowels and diphthongs, also affects quality of the voice. A relaxed tongue opens up the oropharyngeal outlet and retraction of the tongue narrows it. Separation of the jaws and lowering of the tongue increase the volume of the oral cavity.

Historically, it is interesting to note that the 'tongue' has been regarded as synonymous with language. Biblical examples are 'the confusion of tongues' and Moses explaining to the Lord he is 'slow of tongue'. Shakespeare is strewn with references. Hamlet tells the players to speak 'trippingly on the tongue', not to 'mouth'. Celia chides 'Cry holla to thy tongue, I prithee, it curvets unseasonably'.

The word tongue is no longer used in this way, but the French still make the distinction between 'la langue' and 'la parole'. The English use such expressions as 'shut your mouth', 'tongue-tied', 'hold your tongue', 'lost your tongue'. These expressions are now becoming anachronistic. Even putting out the tongue is not so frequent a component of defiant body language, possibly because through the media epithets come more readily to the tongue.

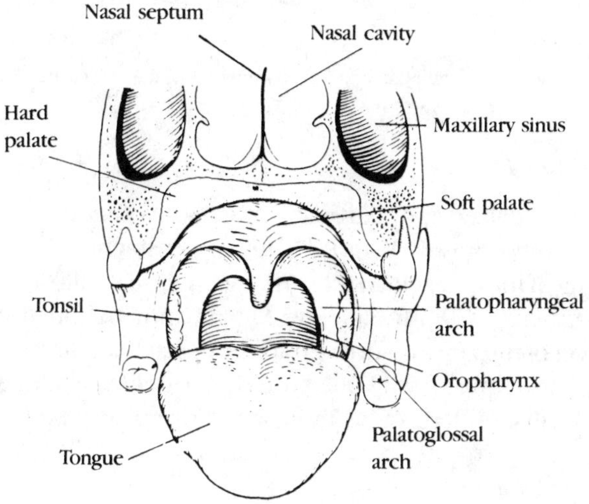

Figure 3.15. Oral view of palate and pillars of fauces.

Soft palate (velum) and the palatopharyngeal sphincter

The soft palate is primarily designed to prevent regurgitation of food down the nose. In swallowing, it is elevated as the tongue passes the food bolus into the pharynx. When the mouth is shut, the palate is lowered and closes the oropharyngeal outlet permitting nasal breathing at rest. The palate is elevated in the articulation of vowels and consonants except in the case of nasal consonants /m, n, ŋ/.

The soft palate, in conjunction with the posterior and lateral walls of the pharynx, forms the palatopharyngeal sphincter. It is an entirely muscular flap attached to the hard palate anteriorly and hanging free posteriorly, terminating in the uvula. The rise and fall of the velum can be inspected in a mirror as the vowel /ɑː/ is articulated.

The soft palate is composed of several paired muscles, some fibres of which are inserted in the tongue and others in the pharynx.

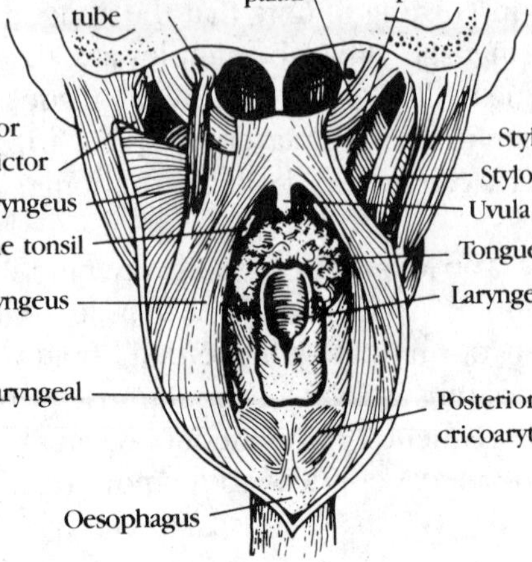

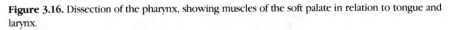

Figure 3.16. Dissection of the pharynx, showing muscles of the soft palate in relation to tongue and larynx.

Tensor palati

This forms the palatal aponeurosis to which the other muscles are attached. It arises in the anterior wall of the cartilaginous eustachian tube and is involved in the opening of the eustachian tube in yawning and swallowing (Hanjo, Okazaki and Kumazawa, 1979; McWilliams, Morris and Shelton, 1984). It maintains equalisation of the air pressure within the eustachian tube and the external air pressure. This explains why one swallows to relieve feelings of pressure and deafness in lifts, underground trains and during air travel.

Musculus uvulae

Fibres of the musculus uvulae descend from the palatal aponeurosis and meet

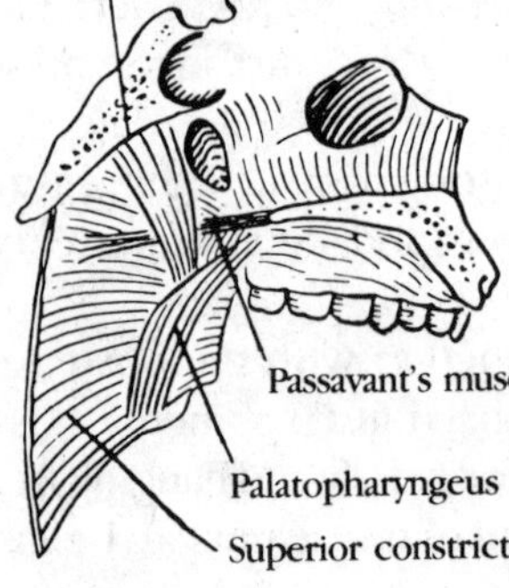

Figure 3.17. The muscles of the nasopharyngeal isthmus and Passavant's muscle. (After Calnan.)

in the uvula. On contraction, the paired muscles raise the ridge on the nasal surface of the palate which Pigott (1977) believes to be significant in assisting sphincteric closure of the nasopharyngeal isthmus (Pigott and Makepeace, 1975). This ridge, commonly called Passavant's ridge (see below), is observable in fibreoptic examinations in cases of palatopharyngeal incompetence (cleft palate).

Palatoglossus

Fibres of the palatoglossus originate in the sides of the tongue and ascend into the palate in the form of an arch, the palatoglossal arch, which is known as the first faucial arch. Fritzell (1969) maintains that the soft palate does not descend by force of gravity alone but is pulled down by the palatoglossus. The muscle is antagonistic to the levator palati and assists in the quick flickering movements of the palate in articulation. Calnan (1973) noted that throughout speech the velum is raised and at the ready to make pharyngeal contact.

Levator palati

Fibres arise in the petrous portion of the temporal bone, descend along the route of the eustachian tube and are inserted in the aponeurosis. It elevates the palate and is the most important muscle in obtaining competent palatopharyngeal closure. Degree of elevation of the palate varies during speech and at times may be above or below the level of the hard palate. The soft palate 'kneels' against the posterior pharyngeal wall but often fails to make a complete seal (Calnan, 1957) even during normal speech which shows no sign of hypernasality.

Palatopharyngeus

This muscle forms the second faucial arch. Fibres arise in the palatal aponeurosis and enter the lateral walls of the pharynx. It forms the palatal arch or posterior pillar of fauces. Specialised fibres of the palatopharyngeus form a sphincter muscle, at the level of the hard palate, which enters the superior tube of the superior constrictor of the pharynx (Fritzell, 1969). These specialised fibres of the palatopharyngeus compose Passavant's muscle or ridge.

The palatopharyngeus assists in the sphincteric closure of the nasopharynx in swallowing, causing bunching of the lateral pharyngeal walls. Passavant's muscle at the same time raises a ridge or ring encircling the superior wall of the pharynx at the level of the atlas vertebra. This action is not present in normal speakers but appears as a compensatory mechanism with elevation of the velum in cases of repaired cleft palate suffering from palatopharyngeal incompetence (Calnan, 1953).

McWilliams, Morris and Shelton (1984) have provided a comprehensive survey of the research findings concerning the mechanism of the velopharyngeal sphincter. They point out that interest in the 1950s and 1960s focused on elevation of the palate. With improved instrumentation, movement of the lateral walls of the pharynx has engaged the interest of researchers in the last 20 years (Pigott, 1977). Hirschsberg (1986) has written a more recent review of velopharyngeal insufficiency.

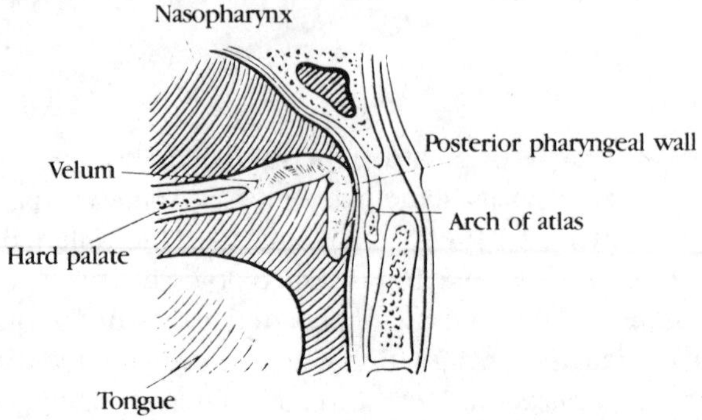

Figure 3.18. Site of contact of the elevated velum with the posterior pharyngeal wall in speech. (After Calnan.)

Superior pharyngeal constrictor

This muscle forms the uppermost section of the pharynx and on contraction assists sphincteric closure of the nasopharyngeal port in conjunction with the levator palati. Fritzell (1969) found both muscles to be consistently active in speech. The superior constrictor also assists lateral movement of the pharyngeal walls medially.

Pharynx

This is a muscular tube extending from the lower border of the cricoid cartilage to the under-surface of the skull. It varies in length as do the necks of different individuals but is generally estimated at between 13 cm and 14 cm long. Above, it is continuous with the nasal cavity and opens laterally into the oral cavity. Below, it leads into the laryngeal inlet anteriorly and the oesophagus posteriorly.

The pharynx consists of the nasal, oral and laryngeal parts which are formed by the superior, middle and inferior constrictors respectively. The fibres of the cricopharyngeus muscle, which form the most inferior part of the pharynx, are in tonic contraction at rest. This prevents reflux of the stomach contents into the pharynx and ensures that air does not enter the oesophagus during respiration (Logemann, 1983a). These muscles decrease the circumference of the pharynx on contraction and assist in swallowing. The dimensions of the pharynx also change according to the prevailing emotional state. The constrictor muscles may tighten sufficiently for the individual to be 'choked with emotion' or to feel a 'lump in the throat' when near to tears. These involuntary pharyngeal responses have a marked effect on voice quality (Julian, MacCurtain and Noscoe, 1981). The importance of the pharynx to voice quality is acknowledged by singers who stress the importance of an 'open

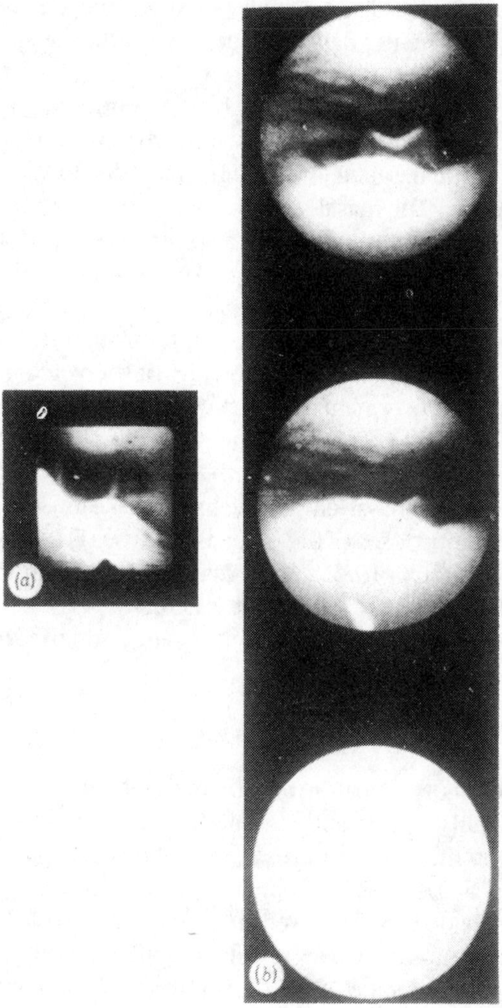

Figure 3.19. Fibreoptic nasendoscopic view of the palatopharyngeal isthmus (normal palate) (a) The segment of the isthmus viewed through the Olympus 3 mm bronchoscope can be compared with the view at a similar moment in closure using the Storz–Hopkins telescope. The curve of the cartilage of the epiglottis gives positive identification of the site in this single frame. (b) Three frames from 16 mm Ektachrome EF 1742 colour film at 25 frames/s. Recorded direct. Normal closure in three frames. (By courtesy of R.W. Pigott (1977) *Proc. R. Soc.*, **195**, 269.)

throat'. A short and capacious pharynx is possibly advantageous in singing (Van den Berg, 1962; Sundberg, 1974). Henderson (1954), in a description of Kathleen Ferrier's pharyngeal cavity, stated that it was so capacious it could easily accommodate a moderately sized apple.

Nasal cavity

The original function of the nose was olfaction and this is still so among animals. In humans the sense of smell is far less sensitive but we savour the taste of food by smell. The tongue distinguishes between sweet, sour, bitter and salt but we do not really taste the flavours of food with the tongue but by smelling their fragrance.

The nasal cavity is divided into two chambers by the central nasal septum and communicates with the nasopharynx posteriorly. The frontal and paranasal sinuses drain into the nasal chambers which are divided laterally by three turbinates or conchae. The nasal chambers are lined with ciliated mucous membrane for shunting mucus and also warming and filtering inspired air – a necessary form of air-conditioning, as Negus (1957) described it. The paranasal sinuses lead off from the choanae.

The nasal cavity endows weak sound waves passing through it with nasal tone and is therefore important in shaping the quality of the voice generally and the articulation of nasal consonants in particular as explained above. Although the importance of certain supraglottic air spaces as resonators of the fundamental note is generally acknowledged, there is disagreement concerning the contribution of the nasal cavity and paranasal sinuses. Proctor (1980) states that one of the purposes of the paranasal sinuses is the provision of resonators for the voice. Bunch (1982), however, believes that 'the sinuses play little or no part in the vocal resonance that is actually perceived by the audience'. She does agree that vibration will be felt by singers in the air spaces and bones of the head.

Thorax

Finally, the role of the chest as a resonator must be remembered. Its structure has been described in detail (p. 10) and its role in voice production with regard to breathing. It is of importance in resonance of low notes, especially baritone and bass. It acts as a sounding board and is a universal resonator. Vibrations can be felt if the hand is placed over the clavicles as a prolonged low note is maintained. It contributes necessary resonances in male voices and less in female. Evidence of the importance of the thorax and subglottic airways as resonators is questioned by Proctor (1980), nevertheless the difference between tenor and soprano in producing notes of the same pitch is due in large part to chest resonance in the male.

Chapter 4 Normal Voice Production

The simplest definition of normal voice is that it is 'ordinary': it is inconspicuous with nothing out of the ordinary in its sound. To achieve this standard of acceptibility the voice must be loud enough to be heard, and appropriate for the age and sex of the speaker. It must be reasonably pleasing to the ear of the listener, modulated and clear, not droning and flat or hoarse and breathy. It must be appropriate to the context and not too loud and assertive. The quality of voice should not have pronounced imbalance of resonance.

Acoustic analysis is complex but basic concepts governing the generation and behaviour of sound waves can be presented simply. In the physical world energy is required for any event to occur. The event will not stop until all the energy has been converted into another form. The propagation of a musical note requires energy to activate a vibrator and a resonator to enhance the fundamental note. The note generated has characteristics of pitch, loudness and quality (or timbre) if we use perceptual terms. The physical correlates of these are frequency, intensity and resonance. Expired air provides the energy required to activate the laryngeal vibrator and produce sound waves which pass through the vocal tract (the resonator) conforming to the laws of acoustics.

Properties of Sound Waves

The sound waves generated by a vibrator can pass through gases, solids and liquids, and therefore create subsidiary vibrations in adjacent structures and enclosed spaces. Sound waves travel in a longitudinal waveform composed of a succession of compressions and rarefactions of the medium's molecules. Each cycle of compression and rarefaction is an oscillation. Frequency (F) is dependent upon the number of oscillations per second and is perceived as pitch. Loudness is the perceptual correlate of the amplitude of a sound wave. The characteristics of a sound wave can be demonstrated with a tuning fork.

Frequency (pitch)

A tuning fork is tuned to vibrate at a certain pitch. When struck, the prong will pass back and forth past the mid-line at a set speed. One complete journey from side to side is called a cycle. In the case of the tuning fork tuned to middle C this will be 264 oscillations per second. The frequency of the tuning fork remains constant. As the prong travels from side to side the air particles are compressed in the direction in which the prong is travelling, leaving a drop in pressure behind. The vacuum immediately fills with air particles. This disturbance generates the periodic air waves which travel as pulses of compression and rarefaction radiating in all directions from the point of origin. The perceived pitch of a sound increases in proportion to its frequency of oscillation.

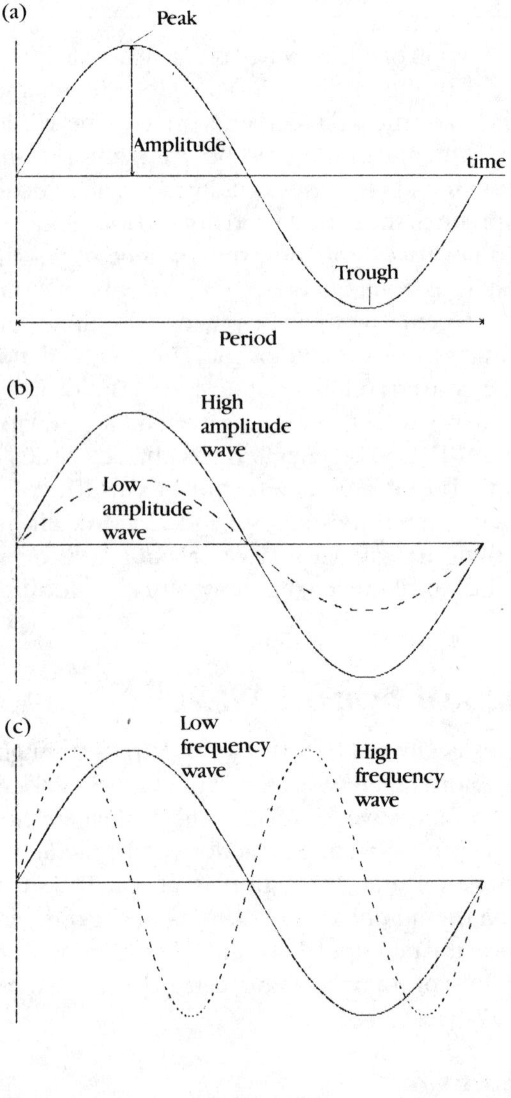

Figure 4.1. (a) Sound wave; (b) sound waves of different amplitude (frequency equal); (c) sound waves of different frequency (amplitude equal).

Intensity (loudness)

The energy with which the tuning fork is struck determines the distance the prong travels from side to side past the mid-point. A small blow produces a small movement and a hard blow, one of greater amplitude. The larger the wave generated, the louder the sound. As the waves travel away from the source, energy is converted into other forms by impact with air particles and other molecules, the waves become smaller and the sound fades but always retains the same fundamental pitch. The intensity of sound is measured on a logarithmic scale in units known as decibels (dB) which are measured in relation to the threshold of audibility.

Characteristics of the vibrator

The pitch of a vibrator, i.e. the number of oscillations per second it can execute, is dependent upon its size, shape, elasticity and mass. As long as these factors remain constant the pitch never varies, however strongly the vibrator is set in motion. The vibrating force, whether it be a blast of air or a blow, only changes the volume of the sound. For instance, a pendulum keeps up the same number of movements to one side and then the other of the mid-line and so does a swing, however strongly or lightly it is pushed and however far it travels in these excursions. A straight spring or tuning fork tuned to the pitch of middle C will always pass back and forth past the mid-line at a rate of 264 Hz whatever the amplitude of the vibration and therefore size of the sound waves generated.

Noise

All musical sounds are characterised by sound waves of recurring patterns at regular intervals and are said to be periodic. Noises are aperiodic, consisting of a mix of sound waves having no regularity or mathematical relation to each other. Such noises are bangs, hisses, squeaks and shrieks.

Resonance (quality or timbre)

A single regular waveform as produced by a tuning fork is known as a pure tone or sine wave. This is the simplest form of oscillation. In nature, vibrators do not produce pure notes but create many sympathetic vibrations as well which are dependent upon the mode of vibration generated by the vibrator which produces the fundamental frequency (F_0). A string of a violin when bowed executes figures of eight, different lengths of it vibrating at different frequencies. In the case of vocal folds, different modes of vibration have already been described (see Chapter 3). The frequencies of these complementary waves are always multiples of the fundamental pitch and harmonise with it, forming the harmonics of any musical note. A tuning fork produces a sine wave, but if its base is placed on a table this will act as a resonator – a 'sounding board'. For example, if the fundamental frequency is 100 Hz then the harmonics multiplied by 2, 3, 4 etc. will be 200 Hz, 300 Hz, 400 Hz. If the

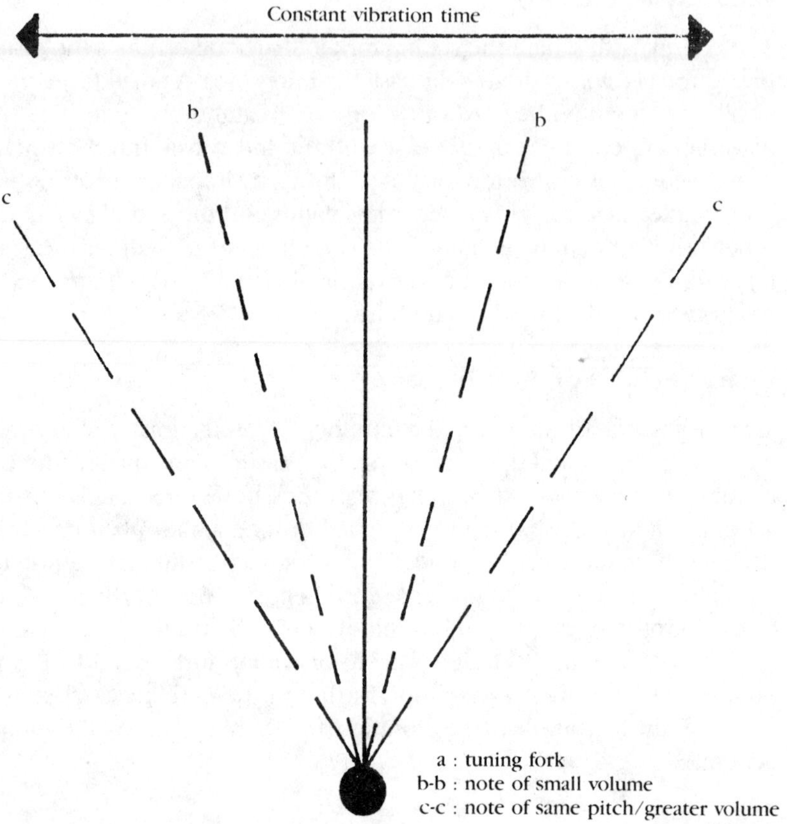

Figure 4.2. Tuning fork.

fundamental frequency is 264 Hz (middle C) the harmonic series is 528 Hz, 792 Hz, 1056 Hz.

Fry (1979) stresses that this simple rule of multiplication of the fundamental frequency, which is the essence of a harmonic, is not a theoretical but a mathematical fact. It is the different combinations of harmonics which provide the individual quality or timbre of a sound. When a trumpet and piano play a note of the same loudness and pitch each instrument is recognisable by its timbre, quality or resonance.

Vowels and diphthongs are musical sounds and are distinguished by their specific harmonic structures. Figure 4.3 shows the difference in mode of sound waves for vowels and noises when translated into visual form on a cathode-ray oscilloscope.

The fundamental pitch of a musical note always predominates over the subsidiary sound waves of resonance on account of its greater energy. Thus a note of certain pitch does not change pitch when harmonics which are weaker in energy are added to it.

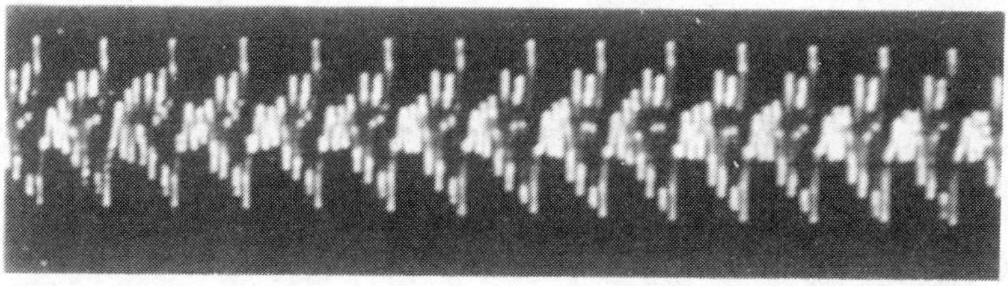

A: /ɑ/

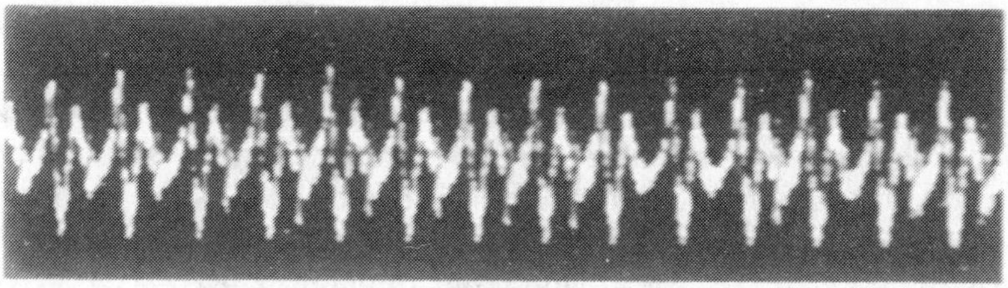

B: /i/

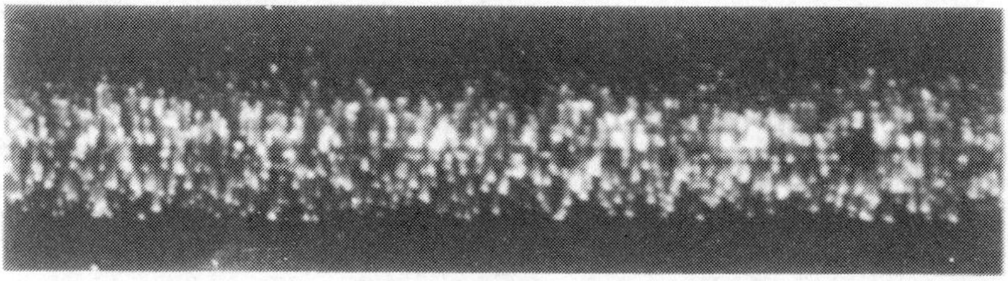

C: /s/

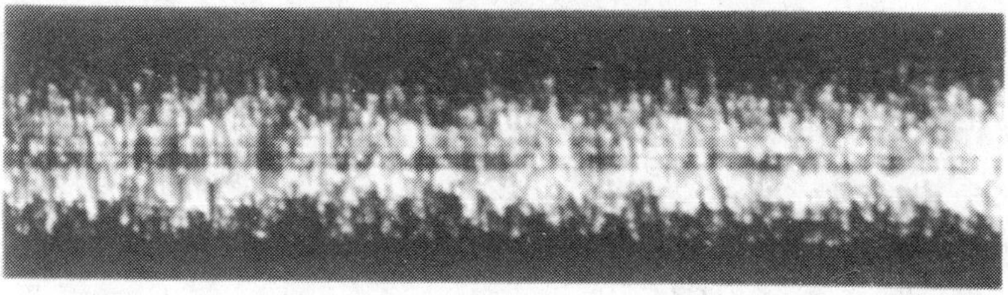

D: /ʃ/

Figure 4.3. Sound waves in visual form shown by a cathode-ray oscilloscope.

Vocal Characteristics

Vocal fundamental frequency

The fundamental frequency of the voice is determined by vocal fold length, tension and mass in combination with subglottic pressure. Vocal fold vibration increases as vocal fold tension is increased and mass is reduced, thus producing a note of higher pitch than when the folds are relaxed, bulky and vibrating more slowly.

Pitch perturbation (jitter)

When consecutive vibratory cycles of the vocal folds vary in frequency so that there is pitch variation in a short-term speech signal, the phenomenon is referred to as pitch perturbation or jitter. These terms are applied to frequency variability due to involuntary changes in the fundamental frequency. Although jitter occurs in the normal voice, there is a marked increase in dysphonic patients. Jitter measurements are important in the evaluation of dysphonia and laryngeal abnormality (Hartman and Von Cramon, 1984; Zyski *et al.*, 1984).

Speaking fundamental frequency

On average the habitual pitch level, which is variable according to the individual and circumstances, is estimated to be roughly as follows (Boone, 1977):

Men	128 Hz
Women	225 Hz
Children	265 Hz

Luchsinger and Arnold (1965) estimate that a child's and a small woman's (i.e. soprano) modal speaking fundamental frequency will be in the region of 300 Hz, whereas a bass will be in the range of 100 Hz. These authors give the following estimates:

1. Men: median speaking range

Bass	98–110 Hz
Baritone	117–133 Hz
Tenor	147–165 Hz

2. Women: median speaking range (one octave higher than men)

Contralto	220 Hz
Mezzo-soprano	226 Hz
Soprano	262 Hz

In singing, the pitch range is much more extensive although there is some disparity between the measurements given by various writers arising from different assessment methods. Luchsinger and Arnold (1965) suggest a singing range of 147–349 Hz for men and 249–698 Hz for women while Perkins and

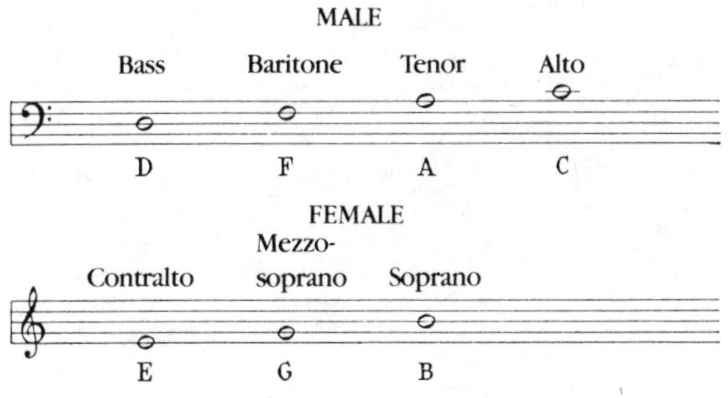

Figure 4.4. Middle notes of singing range in male and female voices.

Kent (1986) give ranges of 80–700 Hz and 140–1000 Hz respectively.

Maximum frequency range can extend from a lowest F_0 of 77 Hz to a highest F_0 of 567 Hz in a young man. The voices of women of a similar age can range from 134 Hz to 895 Hz (Baken, 1987).

Fundamental frequency and its variation with gender and age has been the subject of many studies. These are comprehensively reviewed, and the results tabulated, by Baken (1987). Habitual pitch levels vary according to the individual and the prevailing circumstances.

Vocal registers

As already described the shape, length, density and elasticity of the vocal folds alter constantly in production of notes of different frequency. Traditionally, voice registers have been classified as head, middle and chest. Voice scientists have observed the vibrator in action with high speed motion photography and stroboscopic flash while monitoring airflow pressure, pitch and volume, and spectrography. As a result, they find traditional terminology unsatisfactory and now categorise three main vocal registers as vocal fry, modal and falsetto. Baken (1987) uses pulse, modal and loft registers as equivalent terms. This classification is related to the vibratory pattern of the vocal folds and the acoustic parameters being produced (Hirano, 1981).

Vocal fry, also referred to as creak, is characterised by a long closed phase in the vibratory cycle. It is apparently a fairly common occurrence in everyday speech (Fry, 1979) and is frequent in vocal strain and abuse. The frequency involved is within the range of 20–60 Hz.

The modal register can be divided into chest, middle and head as of yore and encompasses the range of notes employed in speech. The membranous portions of the vocal folds approximate and make complete contact in each closed phase. This is the register used for speech.

Falsetto is achieved by closure of the posterior two-thirds of the vocal folds with only the anterior one-third knife-thin edges vibrating. Under high subglottic pressure, and with folds so short and tense that no vibration is visible, a laryngeal whistle is produced. In such high notes the larynx is lifted and the pharynx shortened. The suprahyoid muscles assist the manoeuvre.

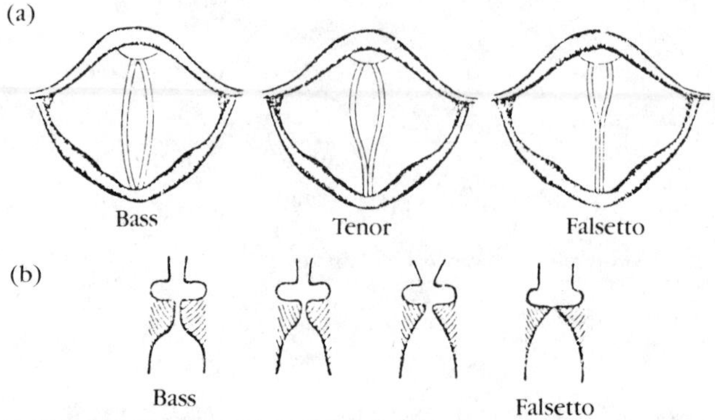

Figure 4.5. (a) Laryngoscopic view of vocal folds in phonation, open phase; (b) coronal view of vocal folds in phonation, closed phase showing change of bulk of vocal folds (from tomographs).

Vocal intensity

Vocal loudness varies according to respiratory airflow and subglottic pressure which affects the size of the excursions executed by the vocal folds. Increased loudness can only be achieved by increasing vocal fold resistance to increased airflow.

Fry's (1979) decibel scale of speech, records the average intensity of conversational speech, three feet from the speaker, as 60 dB. During quiet voiced speech the average level is approximately 35–40 dB; during shouting it is 75 dB.

Amplitude perturbation (shimmer)

Amplitude perturbation is instability of the intensity of a short-term vocal signal and is comparable to frequency perturbation (see p. 48). Measurements of shimmer quantify the variability of the intensity of the fundamental note. Baken (1987) cites research which demonstrates the importance of shimmer to the perception of hoarseness.

Harmonics-to-noise ratio (H/N ratio)

The voice is composed of periodic waves and random noise (aperiodic waves). Noise is a sound which is not a harmonic of the fundamental note. If the noise component increases and replaces the harmonic structure, the quality of hoarseness is perceived. The more severe the hoarseness, the greater the increase in aperiodic sound, i.e. a high noise-to-harmonics ratio.

The H/N ratio has therefore been investigated by researchers as a potential means of measuring hoarseness (Yanagihara, 1967a; Yumoto, Sasaki and Okamura, 1984) and microcomputer analysis of H/N ratio will be available to voice clinicians in the near future (Baken, 1987). Although it cannot be used diagnostically in relation to laryngeal abnormality, the H/N ratio will be an important factor in the assessment of hoarseness (Yumoto, 1983).

Vocal resonance

Maximum resonance occurs when the frequency of the excitor is within the same range as the natural frequency of the resonator. This natural frequency is dependent on the physical features of the resonator.

The body of a musical instrument forms its resonator and determines its characteristic tone whether composed of wood, metal or plastic. The resonator system of the human musical instrument is composed of the structures and air-filled cavities below and above the larynx, including the laryngeal cavity and ventricle. The chest and vocal tract act as a universal resonator which gives every voice its unique character, but the tract embraces a number of specific resonators such as the nasal, oral and oropharyngeal cavities which can be manipulated to produce specific harmonics and the vowel characteristics.

The vibrating column of air, when it passes up the vocal tract, reverberates with sound waves reflected from the walls of the resonators. The pitch of resonant sound waves depends upon the size and shape of its resonator, the size of its orifices and the tension, density and mass of its walls. If surfaces are tense the waves reflected will be higher in pitch than those generated by relaxed muscular surfaces which absorb or damp sound waves. The surrounding structures will pulsate in time with the fundamental frequency (note) and also impart vibrations, though weakened, to cavities behind. The velum serves this purpose in a way comparable to the diaphragm of a drum.

Resonance pitch and 'optimum resonance'

Resonators have a natural vibrating frequency of their own. This means that when a sound of a frequency which complements that of the resonator is produced, the resonator will resound, speak and amplify that note. At the same time unsuitably pitched sound waves will be damped or filtered out. The contribution of the resonator is to enrich the sound played on it. If a tuning fork is struck and held at the mouth of a glass cylinder into which water is poured gradually, a moment will come when the column of air remaining has the right resonance pitch to match the fundamental pitch of the fork. Then the resonant note leaps into prominence and optimum resonance is achieved (see Chapter 9, p. 151). A note resonated in this way is commonly said to be amplified and this is how it sounds psychologically to the listener. However, in physical terms this is not strictly accurate. Resonators are not amplifiers and the energy they express is less than the source of energy put into the system by the fundamental note. The perception of resonant pitch is crucial to voice production. The laryngeal note is insignificant without its system of resonators. The principal feature to stress is that the resonance frequencies are always weaker (have less intensity) than the fundamental pitch of the vibrator which always predominates.

Vowel formants

In considering vocal resonance all unobstructed sounds coming from the larynx and through the vocal tract are vowel sounds. In the production of good voice in speech, therefore, concentration is upon vowels and their articulation.

The resonant pitches of the vocal tract are primarily altered by the tongue gestures in vowel articulation. The many positions assumed by the tongue and jaws in speech alter the size of the oral cavity, the width and length of the pharynx and the size and shape of their orifices. The resonant pitches of vowels are known as formants. Although formants are recognised in all musical sounds, since they are harmonics, the term is usually confined to the harmonics of vowels.

The varying shapes of the oral and pharyngeal cavities in articulation of the vowels /iː. ɪ, aː, ʌ/ are shown in Figure 4.6. Note the elevation of the soft palate which alters position and is most tensed for /iː/. The diaphragm of the velum will reflect sound waves but acts also as a sounding board with sound waves passing into the nasal cavity. These are too weak to cause nasal tone but impart head resonance which would be missed if a cold in the head obstructed the nasal cavities.

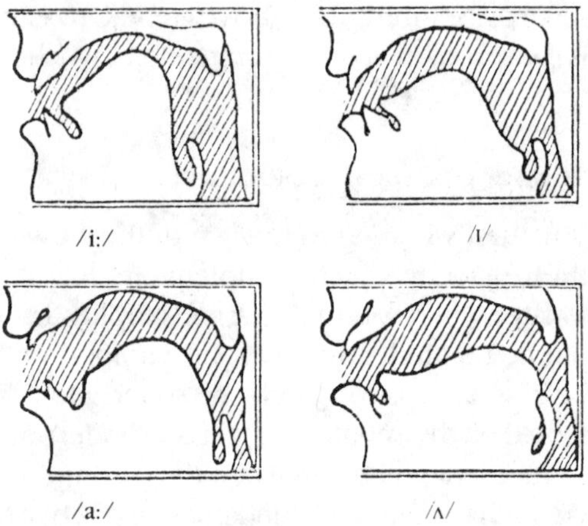

Figure 4.6. Changes in oral and pharyngeal cavities as seen in lateral photographs, in articulation of vowels /iː/, /ɪ/, /aː/ and /ʌ/.

The vowels are distinguished by a number of formants of which two are recognised as being the most conspicuous in contributing to vowel differentiation. The spectrograms of vowels show their formants and incidentally how they differ from time to time in the pronunciation of the same speaker as well as from speaker to speaker. The harmonics change constantly as vowel articulation is affected by the preceding and following consonants which they are said to 'resemble' (Gimson, 1962). The formants also change with child, male and female pitch ranges but the vowels remain recognisable. This is because of the contrastivity of the linguistic system and the ability of the language centres of the brain to discard redundant information and fit an individual's peculiar resonance system into the linguistic system.

The mean frequencies of first and second formants of pure English vowels /iː, ɪ, æ, ʌ/ are (Fry, 1979):

		F_1 (Hz)	F_2 (Hz)
/iː/	(eel)	300	2300
/ɪ/	(bit)	360	2100
/æ/	(hat)	750	1750
/ʌ/	(cut)	720	1240

It is tempting to speculate that F_1 and F_2 are related to the linked oral and pharyngeal resonators respectively. However, the vocal tract resonance system works as a whole and it is impossible to isolate the resonant pitch of the linked resonators.

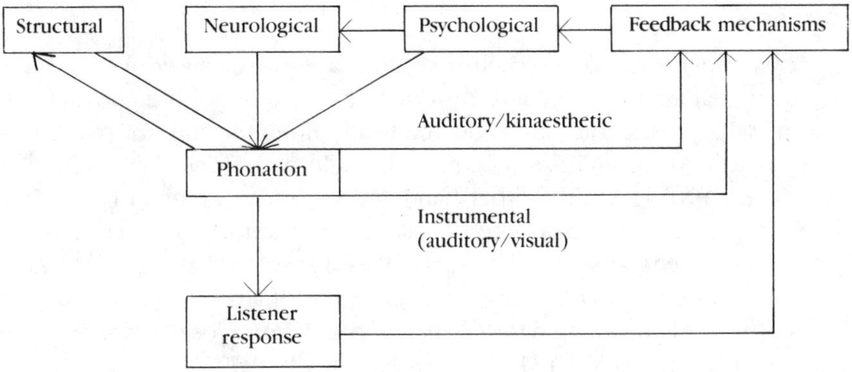

Figure 4.7. Determinants of phonation.

Normal Vocal Variants

Glottal attack

Hard attack

The hard attack occurs at the onset of phonation when, instead of their usual gentle approximation, the vocal folds make abrupt contact for an instant so that the breath stream is interrupted and then released explosively. This device is used normally for emphasis in words with an initial vowel and in some English dialects, such as Cockney, the glottal plosive replaces certain oral plosive consonants. It is also the normal mode of articulation in German for vowels at the beginning of words.

When its use is linguistic it is innocuous but, when it is a physiological symptom of laryngeal tension and incorrect methods of voice production, it can be harmful and result in mucosal changes of the vocal folds. The singer who mistakenly develops this method of initiating phonation, thinking that it will increase articulatory clarity, risks producing an unpleasant sound in addition to damaging the vocal folds (Bunch, 1982). Its use is apparent in moods of fear, anger and impatience (Luchsinger and Arnold, 1965). Hard attack rapidly reaches its maximum amplitude and shows greater air consumption than soft attack (Koike, Hirano and Von Leden, 1967).

Soft attack (breathy attack)

The vocal folds do not fully adduct at the onset of phonation, when soft attack is used, and some unvibrated air passes through the glottal chink. Such phonation can be associated with emotions of joy and pleasure. Soft attack is totally inappropriate for the singer who is aiming at a clear vocal note because the breathy quality will be apparent at onset and volume and projection radically reduced. Classical singing requires coordination of a 'precise momentary closure of the vocal folds' (Bunch, 1982) with a gentle breath stream.

Whisper

In quiet whisper the folds are slightly separated along the anterior two-thirds and a triangular aperture remains posteriorly as the arytenoids do not adduct. In strong whisper the folds are adducted firmly along the anterior two-thirds and air is forced through the posterior triangle with considerable friction (Luchsinger, 1965a). On the other hand, Monoson and Zemlin (1984), in a quantitative study of whisper, note that the position of the vocal folds is variable in different subjects. The edges may be separated along their whole length and more so in faint whisper. The degree of airflow is important. In some cases the anterior two-thirds may approximate closely leaving a gap between the arytenoids. The fold edges do not vibrate.

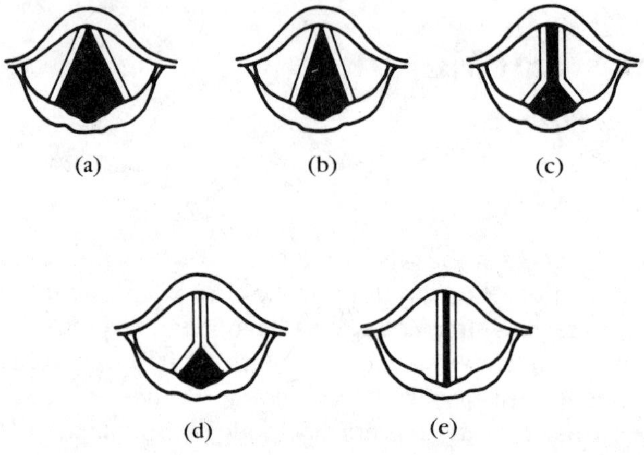

Figure 4.8. Positions of vocal folds in action (laryngoscope view). (a) Full abduction; (b) gentle abduction; (c) gentle whisper; (d) stage whisper; (e) phonation.

Vibrato

The management of vibrato in singing is a necessary skill which adds emotion and beauty to the voice. It involves a frequency modulation superimposed upon the pitch frequency of the note sung. It also requires small intensity modulation of a few decibels. The hub frequency swing varies but is in the region of a quarter tone. There are individual differences in frequency and intensity changes among singers. Enrico Caruso produced a frequency modulation of 6.3 Hz. Lily Pons had 'quaver' and frequency modulation of 7.5 Hz. Maria Callas had a modulation (messa di voce) of 6.5 Hz. On average, the vibrato range is 5–8 Hz and the intensity increase is 9 dB.

The vibrato adds great attractiveness to the singing voice when properly controlled. If absent the voice sounds metallic. An excessively high number of pulsations gives rise to the unpleasant quality known as tremolo. Slow pulsations give an impression that the voice is wobbling.

Trill

Trill is achieved by rapid variation of pitch by one semi-tone (Proctor, 1980). Vennard and Von Leden (1967) submitted the trills of four outstanding sopranos to spectrographic analysis. They concluded that the rate of pitch fluctuation in a trill is very little faster than that of a vibrato, but the extent of the pitch variation is increased so that the ear can perceive the two pitches involved. Rhythmic contractions of the whole laryngeal structure accompany a trill, but the visible movement of the larynx has no connection with the 'wobble' voice quality resulting from excessively slow vibrato.

Yodel

Yodelling is a particular style of singing peculiar to the Swiss Alps and has occasionally been used by popular singers. It is thought to have originated in imitation of the alpenhorn and the shawm, an ancient wind instrument similar to the clarinet and common to all pastoral people (Luchsinger, 1965c). The yodel consists of sudden jumps in pitch from chest register to head register on vowel sounds only, not words. Good air support is necessary and this is provided by activity of the diaphragm. The yodel has great carrying power and is an effective means of calling the attention of a neighbour on another mountain top and is not, as might be expected, for rounding up lost sheep and goats.

The Singing Voice

'Covered' voice

In the teaching of singing the mastery of special singing techniques is essential, especially for the opera singer. The means of increasing strength, a swelling tone, and beauty to the voice is agreed to be that of producing the 'covered' voice. How this is actually achieved has long been a bone of contention among singing professors. The Italian school advocates the open singing technique with open mouth and smiling lips, a wide open and relaxed throat being apparently the chief aim. For dramatic singing, the 'covered' voice is advocated mainly by the German school because it gives added power and emotional tension to the voice. The technique necessitates descent of the larynx, simultaneous widening of the pharyngeal cavity and increased air pressure. Luchsinger (1965c) says that 'covering' the voice means a slight darkening of the vowels on higher pitch levels to avoid excessively bright timbre in singing. Covering is also used to facilitate changes from one register to another.

The singing formant

Sundberg (1974, 1977) has made a valuable contribution to understanding the nature of the covered voice in his acoustic studies of what he terms the singing formant. This is formed by a fusion of the third and fourth formants of the resonance frequencies. The combination of these peaks of resonance results in a band of maximum energy in the region of 2500–3000 Hz. The singer's formant is most likely to occur at high frequency and intensity (Hollien, 1983). This optimal frequency occurs at a bandwidth in which orchestral energy is low. As use is being made of optimal resonance the operatic singer is able to be heard without using excessive effort, above the apparently much greater volume of the orchestra.

Sundberg (1974) has also provided an articulatory interpretation of the singing formant. In male singers the peak envelope is in the region of 2.8 kHz and in order to achieve this three conditions have to be met:

1. The cross-sectional area must be at least six times wider than the laryngeal tube orifice. If mismatched an extra formant is added.
2. The sinus of Morgagni (laryngeal ventricle) must be wide in relation to the larynx tube and if mismatched an extra formant may be added between the third and fourth formants of normal speech.
3. The piriform fossa must be wide, which reduces the fifth formant to about 3 kHz.

These three conditions can be fulfilled when the larynx is lowered. The two linked resonators of larynx and pharynx produce the resonance characteristics of voice. Sundberg avers that there is no case for the terms 'head', 'chest' and 'mask' resonance currently used in vocal pedagogy, but such terms are undoubtedly useful in teaching students.

Bunch (1976), in a cephalometric study of the structure of head and neck during sustained phonation of covered and open singing, confirmed that enlargement of the pharyngeal cavity is a major factor in production of 'covered' voice.

Achievement of the singing formant is dependent, therefore, upon lowering the larynx and lengthening and widening the pharynx while relaxing the tongue and mandible. It is important that the pharyngeal muscles are relaxed and the voice is produced effortlessly. This will not occur if the larynx is forced down in the vocal tract and if the supraglottic resonators are tense. Perfect technique in a singer will greatly improve a mediocre voice and further enhance an excellent voice. However, perfection depends upon the singer's musical talent coupled with the genetic anatomical endowment. It is this which accounts for a Caruso, Ferrier, Callas or Pavarotti.

A comparative study by Burns (1986) of the singing voices of opera singers and 'country and western' singers illustrates the importance of the use of the singing formant as a protective mechanism in addition to its aesthetic function. His hypothesis was that country and western singers use faulty singing technique which does not incorporate the singing formant and that this accounts for the vocal abuse frequently occurring in this group. Acoustic analysis of the speaking and singing voices of both groups revealed that, as expected, the opera singers used the singing formant but the country and western singers used formants almost identical to those of speech when they were singing. Unfortunately, for country and western singers, and for rock and many pop singers, attempts to use the singing formant would destroy the vocal quality which is highly popular and an integral part of a particular style of singing.

Emotional Expression

Every change in vocal pitch sparks off a whole new spectrum of harmonics. Fry (1979) attributes the emotional colouring of the voice to changes in fundamental pitch due to changes in tension of the vocal folds matched to anxiety or content. Pitch is an easily measurable quantity in physics, but the weaker harmonic background to vowel formants is difficult to assess. The personal characteristics of a voice which we readily recognise as being that of a particular person and no other, cannot be pin-pointed reliably by instruments (Tosi, 1979). As slight changes in pitch take place in the inflections of speech conveying such feelings as hate, love, anger and sorrow, the whole vocal tract resounds with emotion and is detected by the ear. These shades of meaning are as elusive and fleeting as light and shade reflected on water and perceived by the eye as real but yet immeasurable. The intuitive interpretation of tones of voice is of enormous importance in human relationships and the establishment of rapport or antipathy.

Chapter 5
Voice Mutation: Infancy to Senescence

Infancy

The infant larynx

It is not possible to examine the larynges of neonates with any invasive techniques. Information has to be acquired by examination of excised larynges which is in many ways unsatisfactory compared to examination of living organs. There is some difference of opinion therefore concerning the exact length of the vocal folds at birth but the most notable feature is the minute size of the laryngeal sphincter. Negus (1949) reported that the folds are 3 mm long at 14 days, 5.5 mm at 1 year, 7.5 mm at 5 years, 8.0 mm at 6 years 6 months and 9.5 mm at 15 years. Hirano, Kurita and Nakashima (1983), in the examination of 88 Japanese infants, calculated that the length of vocal folds in the newborn varied from 2.5 mm to 3.0 mm. Variance in size and weight of infants influences laryngeal size.

The fibres of the vocalis muscle are incomplete at birth and develop alongside the thyroarytenoid muscle which increases considerably in size from the ninth month. Von Leden (1961) and Hollien (1980) reported that the length of the vocal folds increases by about 80% from birth to 12 months of age.

The mucosal cover of the vocal folds is very thick in relation to the length and there is no vocal ligament observable in early infancy. This develops between 1 and 4 years. The intermediate and deep layers of the lamina propria are not differentiated into collagenous and elastic fibres. Hirano, Kurita and Nakashima (1983) provide an excellent set of histological pictures illustrating the differences in structure of the vocal folds at birth, in the child and in the adult.

The thick loose layer of the lamina propria is prone to develop acute oedema which is the cause of croup. Although the airway is constricted, total obstruction does not occur because the membranous length is almost the equivalent of the cartilaginous length of the fold (Hirano, 1981; Hirano, Kurita and Nakashima, 1983; Kahane and Kahn, 1984; Kahane, 1986).

Respiration

The glottis is sphincteric and opens and closes reflexly in concert with inspiration and expiration (Terracol, Guerrier and Camps, 1956). The pharynx is hypersensitive which ensures instant spasmodic closure of the glottis at the slightest excitation from saliva or milk. This is followed by immediate expulsion by coughing and spluttering accompanied by poorly coordinated inspiratory and expiratory action which, however, proves effective.

Before birth the lungs are yellowish and solid, tucked away in the back of the chest. Immediately the child is delivered, 'the tissues of the lungs expand like the petals of a flower and the colour changes to rose red' (Thomson, 1976). This is because of the in-rush of blood and air into the expanding lung tissues. From the dramatic moment of the birth cry, the infant is launched into automatic life-supporting respiration. During the first year control over vegetative respiration gradually develops. The infant acquires the ability to change from quiet breathing to the changed rhythm and volume necessary in vocalisation, in babbling and eventually speech.

Study of respiratory movements can be registered by magnetometry which tracks the anteroposterior diameter of the rib cage and abdominal wall. Impedance pneumography measures the circumference of the same structures. Such measurements are non-intrusive but accurate and have revealed that breathing in infants is extremely variable. At one month, breaths may be taken at a rate of 87 per minute and irregularity is not uncommon (Perkins and Kent, 1986). The rate decreases gradually to 61 breaths per minute at 6 months, and 42 per minute at 12 months (Langlois, Baken and Wilder, 1980).

The diaphragm is the chief muscle involved in respiration in infancy. The ribs are relatively perpendicular to the spine and do not contribute to thoracic movement until the child is able to sit and assume upright posture. The act of crying necessitates changes in respiratory patterns and provides essential preliminary exercise for phonic respiration.

Vocal signals

The voice is used to signal distress and discomfort and to emit cries for help. The first cry at birth is probably the most dramatic use of voice an individual will ever make. It signals that the infant is alive and respiration has commenced.

The primitive nature of the baby's vocal apparatus means that comparison with a musical instrument at this stage is invalid. The sounds emitted are aperiodic noises which encompass a considerable range of frequencies and an amazing volume of sound considering the tiny instrument. The larynx with its sphincter mechanism works in much the same way as a siren emitting pulses of air, and not at all like a string vibrator.

The vocal tract above the larynx is also primitive in development and restricted in resonance potential. In the neonate the epiglottis is at the level of the first cervical vertebra (C1) and the inferior border of the cricoid cartilage is at the level of C4. (These positions descend to C3 and C6 in the adult.) As the thyroid cartilage and hyoid bone are adjoining at birth the epiglottis is near the velum and the root of the tongue is in the oral cavity. During the first 4 years the root of the tongue and the larynx descend into the pharynx. The vocal tract of the newborn is incapable of producing the full range of speech sounds although the formants of vowels /æ/ and /ʌ/ are apparent in sound spectrographic analysis (Ringel and Kluppel, 1964). The formants produced inevitably reflect the characteristics of a vocal tract which, at birth, resembles that of non-human primates more than that of human adults (Lieberman, 1967). The larynx moves up during crying.

The cries of the newborn have been studied extensively with spectrographic recordings and acoustic analysis (Murry, Hoit Dalgaad and Gracco, 1983). An early study was carried out by Fairbanks (1942) on his son from the age of 1 month to 9 months. He recorded the fundamental frequency of hunger wails. At 1 month the mean fundamental frequency was 373 Hz and subsequently increased to a mean 814 Hz at 5 months, and then stabilised at a decreased mean of 640 Hz at 9 months. He attributed the regular and rapid rise in frequency up to 5 months to increased neuromuscular development and not to increasing length of the vocal folds. The plateau was thought to be due to conditioning to the speech environment. This has been confirmed by Siegel (1969) with infants of 3 months of age, besides Osgood (1953) and Lenneberg, Rebelsky and Nichols (1965) who studied vocalisations of infants in their first year.

Wasz-Höckert *et al.* (1968) carried out a spectrographic and acoustic analysis of the infant cry. The subjects were 39 boys and 4 girls of age range 1-30 days, and 87 infants age range 1-7 months. They distinguished four characteristic signals produced by babies: birth, hunger, pain and pleasure cries. The birth cry is tense, raucous and short, about 1.5 seconds in duration or less. The pain cry is tense, the longest signal and the best identified. Maximum mean pitch recorded was 740 Hz and minimum pitch 460 Hz and this cry has a mostly falling or flat melody. The hunger cry mean ranges from 500 Hz to 320 Hz and has a rising falling melody. The pleasure cry which does not emerge until around 3 months has a rising falling melody with mean pitch ranges from 650 Hz to 360 Hz. It is never tense but lax and is often nasal and contains no glottal plosives, vocal fry or subharmonic breaks.

A study of a male and female for the first 141 days of life, by Sheppard and Lane (1968), showed that the fundamental frequency for the male baby's cry was 443 Hz with a range of 404-481 Hz. The mean for the female baby was 414 Hz with a range of 384-481 Hz. Ostwald (1963) emphasised that the fundamental frequency of a newborn infant's cry may fluctuate from 400 Hz to 600 Hz. Other studies have shown that a pitch range from 300 Hz to 800 Hz is possible. This accounts for the heart-rending and ear-splitting potential of the infant cry. The amplitude of these wails appears not to have engaged the interest of most researchers in the field. Langlois, Baken and Wilder (1980) comment on the fact that scant attention has been paid to the infant's development of respiratory control despite its relevance to the understanding of speech development.

It is generally believed that a mother is able to identify the cause of her baby's crying, whether hunger or pain, by its acoustic quality. However, research shows that mothers cannot identify cry samples correctly according to the cause of the cry. In a review of studies of perceptual identification of cry types, Hollien (1980) concluded that cries actually contain insufficient perceptual information to identify the reason for crying. The cry attracts the mother's attention and is subsequently identified by environmental clues. Increases in amplitude and duration of wails provide information regarding the degree of distress. However, a mother can identify the voice of her own infant crying. Valanne *et al.* (1967) examined the ability of mothers to identify the hunger cry of their own newborn infants during the lying-in period. They found that mothers were successful in identifying their own babies from an audiotape recording which included various other infants. Formby (1967) and Murry (1980) reported similar findings. The baby's cry has individual and personal characteristics as one would expect from the fact that they have different physiognomies.

Vegetative sounds

Infants produce a range of non-crying sounds described as 'vegetative'. These include coughs, burps, hiccups, lip smacking and sucking, spitting etc. accompanied by ingressive as well as egressive breathing. The study of vegetative sounds is naturally less interesting than that of infant cries. The gradual emergence of 'comfort sounds' as Lewis (1936) described them, as distinct from discomfort cries, is the first step in the acquisition of speech. Vocal play and babbling are an important transitional stage of development leading into the prosodic features of speech.

Pathological and diagnostic aspects

The early cries clearly detectable by ear in infants with neurological disorders have been studied extensively and their relevance in diagnosis is stressed. Wasz-Höckert *et al.* (1968) studied infant cries in babies with pathological conditions. Such studies are of value in diagnostic paediatrics. In babies suffering from kernicterus it is well known that the level of serum bilirubin does not always reflect the presence or absence of neurological damage but acoustic analysis of the babies' cries can. Down's syndrome babies have characteristic cries and the cri-du-chat of the chromosome 5 deficiency is unmistakable. Colton and Steinschneider's (1980), and Michelsson and Wasz-Höckert's (1980) reviews of cry analysis in early infancy are recommended for further study. Michelson, Raes and Rinnie (1984) have also used a cry score as an aid in infant diagnoses.

There is also evidence that the cry of the baby at risk from sudden infant death syndrome (SIDS) has acoustic characteristics which could help to identify the vulnerable infant. Stark and Nathanson (1975) found that in addition to these cries exhibiting higher fundamental frequency levels than normal, there was evidence of sudden shifts or breaks in pitch level and voiced inspiratory sounds. Their acoustic studies showed more instances of vocal tract constriction and this was thought to be due to the back of the tongue touching the soft palate and therefore obstructing the airway intermittently. Steinschneider (1972) concluded that SIDS infants have a high degree of respiratory instability and that the unusual features of the cry may be another sign of poor respiratory control. Premature infants have incoordinated muscular activity especially during sleep. The thoracic muscles may try to inspire while abdominal muscles expire (West, 1979).

Pre-linguistic tonal development

Lewis (1936), in his classic study of infant speech, distinguished both discomfort and comfort sounds. He stressed the pleasure evinced by the baby in making and experimenting with musical vowel-like sounds, also the pleasure shared by the mother and her response in encouraging these first elements of vocal communication.

At 6 weeks a forward baby's response to a strange face and voice is negative but mother's face and voice evoke pleasure. The baby will respond with pleasure to the mother's voice even when she is out of sight. The first smile appears a couple of weeks later and coos, gurgles and little shrieks are produced, especially when the baby is spoken to and caressed (Stark, 1979; Illingworth, 1980). Mother and responsive minders reinforce social reactions, especially by talking to the baby, all of which is crucial for normal emotional and speech development. The child therefore needs to be caressed and talked to when handled.

The comfort sounds increase steadily. A healthy sign is the variability and pitch range of the musical glides which are emitted. This tallies with maturation of the vocal folds and improved muscular coordination. Expiration is matched to phonation and control of breath groups subserve vocal expression (Lieberman, 1967). Throughout the developmental sequence cortical and neuromuscular maturation keep pace.

Green and Conway (1963) in collecting material for their audio-recording of infant speech development evaluated recordings of dozens of infants. They were interested in the earliest appearance of musical sounds as distinct from crying and scolding noises. The progressive development of inflectional glides in cooing and babbling was noted. The earliest appearance of an upward glide from C_3 to C# was in a girl 2 weeks old, and in the same child the range increased from C_3 to E_3 at 7 weeks (Table 5.1). A baby boy ranged from C# to F# in glides of a semitone on one breath at 5 weeks and achieved an inspiratory crow at G_4#. This child had varied vowels and diphthongs and varied musical inflection at 16 weeks, rising and falling between C_2# and E_2. He produced these delightful musical glides up and down the scale within the range of C_2# and E_2# and as a social response at 18 weeks when rhythmic syllables and babbling were developing rapidly. This child spoke early and was followed up until 2 years of age.

Upward glides appeared in these babies first, then rising and falling glides which increased in quantity and range progressively covering approximately an octave at 6–7 months. The influence of heard speech is obviously strong in

Table 5.1. Frequency (Hz) to musical note conversion table

	Frequency for octaves							
Musical note	C_{-3}	C_{-2}	C_{-1}	C_0	C_1	C_2	C_3	C_4
C	16.35	32.70	65.41	130.81	261.63	523.25	1046.50	2093.00
C# and D*b*	17.32	34.65	69.30	138.59	277.18	554.37	1108.73	2217.46
D	18.35	36.71	73.42	146.83	293.66	587.33	1174.66	2349.32
D# and E*b*	19.45	38.89	77.78	155.56	311.13	622.25	1244.51	2489.02
E	20.60	41.20	82.41	164.81	329.63	659.26	1318.51	2637.02
F	21.83	43.65	87.31	174.61	349.23	689.46	1396.91	2793.83
F# and G*b*	23.12	46.25	92.50	185.00	369.99	739.99	1479.98	2959.96
G# and A*b*	25.96	51.91	103.83	207.65	415.30	830.61	1661.22	3322.44
A	27.50	55.00	110.00	220.00	440.00	880.00	1760.00	3520.00
A# and B*b*	29.14	58.27	116.54	233.08	466.16	932.33	1864.66	3729.31
B	30.87	61.74	123.47	246.96	493.88	987.77	1975.53	3951.07

After Baken, 1987.

this development and is present as what Piaget (1952) described as 'contagion' as early as 1 month old.

The great versatility in vocal behaviour is confirmed by Murry *et al.* (1983) in their study of one child's hunger, discomfort and non-distress cries from 2 weeks to 12 weeks of age. They distinguished clearly seven melody types in each of the three categories of vocalisation. The rapid shifts and wide frequency range reflected increasing respiratory and phonatory control, exhibiting early communication behaviour. The emergence of cooing was studied by Stark (1978), and features of infant vocalisation by Stark, Rose and McLagan (1975) in the first 8 weeks of life.

Predictions of speech development

Greene and Conway also observed several male children whose 'singing' was very limited in range and also duration and were late in speech development. Speech therapists have in these inflectional melodies sufficient clues to predict late or normal speech development. Absence of pre-linguistic vocalisation may, however, signify general retardation, socioeconomic deprivation or neglect in which the child is not encouraged with loving speech and attention (Winitz, 1969).

Between 3 months and 6 months babbling of syllables develops. This is common to all races and is a biologically determined human trend. Wasz-Höckert *et al.* (1968) found no difference between Swedish and Finnish babies. Deaf babies babble in the same way as hearing children but this soon dies away without the stimulation of heard speech. Between 6 months and 12 months, vocalisation begins to assume the characteristics of communicative speech. The child is said to be 'talking scribble' or jargon and the inflections of speech are so real and well organised by rhythm, intonation and breath group that 'pretend' conversations can be held. That is to say they are pretend for the adult but so animated that they must be real for the child in that the intention to convey meaning is there. This is the origin of prosody which precedes words and provides whole tonal patterns into which segmented features will come to be fitted during the second year. The 'first word' becomes stable and identifiable at 12-14 months. The linguistic, segmental and grammatical stage of speech has begun (Crystal, 1976).

Childhood

Vocal range

The fundamental frequency continues to decrease with age and by 5 years the child's speaking voice settles under the influence of the environment at a median pitch in the region of middle C, or maybe two or three semitones higher. The child's singing range, which varies very little in boys and girls, covers the middle octave at the age of 7 years according to Tarneaud (1961). At 8 years the lower range is only slightly extended and the voice ranges from B_2 to B_3. At 9 years the range extends a little further in both directions from B_2 to D_4. The range of voice in both girls is similar despite the vocal folds of boys being 8% larger (Cotes, 1979). In brief, the voice range for both sexes remains constant at about two and a half octaves between 6 and 16 years (Aronson, 1980).

Respiration

Before puberty lung function is almost identical in boys and girls of equal size. Boys' chests, however, grow in lateral and longitudinal dimensions more than girls. It is interesting to note that a low level of activity in childhood affects size of the lungs. Cotes (1979) found that children living in high blocks of flats, where opportunity for exercise was limited, had 7% less vital capacity than physically active children. This is a factor which must not be overlooked in measurements of airflow and phonation time in children.

Adolescence

Respiration

The young adult has approximately four times the lung volume of the 5 year old. Vital capacity is at its peak during the late teens and early twenties after which it gradually deteriorates with reduced diaphragmatic action. Breathing rate is between 10 and 22 breaths per minute (Perkins and Kent, 1986).

The larynx

During the period 10-14 years there is a sudden increase in rate of growth and size. Hormonal changes take place and male and female characteristics emerge. The mutational period may be complete at 14 years in boys but in girls it continues on average until 15 years. The voices of girls mature due to enlargement of the larynx consistent with general body growth. The voices of boys drop a pitch due to rapid growth of the larynx. The voice drops an octave and the vocal folds double in length. The internal angle of the thyroid cartilage decreases so that the Adam's apple develops.

In girls the mean length of the vocal folds is 15 mm before puberty and this may increase to 17 mm in a contralto. During the mutational period a boy's vocal folds may increase to a maximum of 23 mm in the bass voice. The minimum vocal fold length for the male is 17 mm, so it can be seen that a tenor and a contralto may have much the same pitch range, but it is the larger resonators of the larynx, pharynx and the chest which distinguish the male voice from the female.

The layer structure of the lamina propria of the vocal fold matures in adolescence and by 16 years it resembles the structure of the adult vocal fold. Prior to this the layers are less well defined. This change in the inner structure of the vocal fold mucosa is a significant factor in voice mutation besides the increase in length of the vocal folds.

Vocal pitch

Voice mutation and vocal pitch are unquestionably tied to growth of the larynx and lengthening of the vocal cords. McGlone and Hollien (1963) found that the girl's vocal pitch is at its highest at 7–8 years, drops 2.4 semitones between 11 and 15 years, and remains at much the same level throughout life.

Michel, Hollien and Moore (1966) recorded the speaking fundamental pitch of 15-, 16- and 17-year-old girls and found that this was 207.5 Hz, 207.3 Hz and 207.8 Hz respectively. This indicates that fundamental frequency is established at 15 years in girls and pubertal mutation is over although body growth continues up to 20 years of age and over.

Vocal shifts and breaks

The pitch breaks which occur in children's voices over the age of 7 years have received much attention on account of the need to understand and manage the voice mutation difficulties of adolescence in singing. Weiss (1950) in his comprehensive survey of the literature cites 334 sources. We are indebted to him also for his clarification of the problems involved. Weiss defines 'break of voice' as a sudden and involuntary change in the pitch and quality. 'Voice break' therefore should be properly confined to the characteristic fluctuations in pitch and quality in adolescence during the period of voice mutation. The voice may rise or fall an octave and change register, rising to falsetto or falling to the bass register. The voice 'breaks' analysed in the work of American workers described below either refer to the mutational period of voice break in adolescence or to 'shifts' in pitch during childhood. These shifts consist of abrupt and uncontrolled rises and falls in vocal pitch due to poor coordination of the laryngeal musculature associated with general bodily growth. In pre-pubertal boys these shifts do not have the masculine quality which is so conspicuous and bizarre a feature of the real break of voice in adolescence.

The young boy's resonator system naturally cannot produce the necessary resonance characteristics of the adult male voice.

The vocal shifts would appear to be a perfectly normal physiological feature of juvenile laryngeal function. These shifts may also be aggravated by vocal strain imposed by vocal abuse in children who shout and scream at football matches and in the playground. Vocal shifts and subharmonic breaks were recorded in infants by Wasz-Höckert *et al.* (1968).

Fairbanks, Wiley and Lassman (1949) and Fairbanks, Herbert and Hammond (1949) studied the voice breaks in voices of 7- and 8-year-old boys and girls. They concluded that the pitch changes recorded occurred as frequently in girls as in boys and were not sex linked or confined to adolesence.

Luchsinger (1962) states that the real voice break or 'stormy' mutation occurring in male adolescence is not the general rule and is encountered in only a minority of boys due to vocal or psychogenic strain. Weiss (1950) suggested that the sudden drop or rise in the voice, changing momentarily from the childish treble to the adult male voice or vice versa, is so conspicuous that it has accordingly been considered the main characteristic of the pubertal voice change by speech pathologists, whereas it is actually uncharacteristic.

Singing in adolescence

Dawson (1919) in his book *The Voice of the Boy* attributed pitch breaks to collapse of the voice due to misuse and vocal strain. None of his pupils suffered from 'breaking' of the speaking or singing voice. The boys' voices just slid down the scale. He evaluated the pitch of their singing voices at frequent intervals and shifted them after 12.5 years from soprano to alto and gradually to tenor or baritone by 15 years as their voices dropped with growth of the larynx. Failure to sing well he attributed to vocal abuse in early childhood and advocated early training in breathing technique. The majority of experts stress the dangers for both boys and girls of singing in the mutation period and will not permit serious voice training to begin until 17 years with girls and 18–19 years with boys. Weiss points out that very few choirboys, possibly a mere 2%, ever turn into good adult singers and this he attributed to the irreparable damage contracted in adolescence. Few singing teachers or choirmasters instruct their pupils in the fundamentals of good voice production and many fail to appreciate the dangers of the pubertal period.

The mutational period of the singing voice lasts much longer than that of the speaking voice and this also is not often understood and recognised by singing teachers. Growth in height may continue long after the voice has broken and during this time the voice is vulnerable and cannot achieve its adult potential on account of physiological immaturity. The vocal folds may continue to increase in length as late as 20 or 24 years of age.

Middle Age to Senescence

Respiration

The lungs deteriorate with increasing age (Cotes, 1979) due to changes in the tissues. These changes are more marked in men than in women and result in gradual reduction in strength of the respiratory muscles. Reduction in the mobility of the thoracic cage also occurs due to stiffness in the costovertebral joints. In advanced age the lungs and bronchi shrink and sink to a lower position in the thorax. The sensitivity of the airway is reduced with increasing age and coughing is less likely to occur (Slonim and Hamilton, 1976).

Changes vary greatly with different individuals and their lifestyles. Physical activity will prevent noticeable deterioration in respiration. Exposure to pollutants, especialy smoking, reduces the elastic recoil of the lungs. The correlation between smoking and carcinoma of the larynx and lungs is generally acknowledged but its effects on the airway prior to these diseases becoming established is relevant when considering phonation. Cotes (1979) notes the substances in cigarette smoke and their effects on the body. Particles of dust in the smoke cause irritation, and the tar deposit damages the bronchial epithelium and contributes ultimately to emphysema. The oxygenation of the blood is impaired by the carbon monoxide while the nicotine increases cardiac frequency and systemic blood pressure. Inhalation of tobacco smoke results in an immediate rise in airway resistance because of the smoke dust particles which are being deposited. The adverse effect lasts many hours. The vocal folds are likely to be abused if the smoker has a frequent, forceful cough. Comparable symptoms are thought to occur in the 'passive smoker', meaning the non-smoker who inhales another's smoke.

As age advances, closure of the respiratory bronchioles is increased during expiration and the residual volume increases. At 20 years the residual volume in the male is on average 1.5 litres but at age 60 years it is 2.2 litres. The expendable expiratory volume of air for phonation will grow less, and can be maintained by exercise and conscious control. The respiratory aspect of ageing voice may have little noticeable effect on speech but will prove to be an obstacle in maintaining the singing voice.

Laryngeal calcification

The cartilages of the larynx may begin to calcify and lose their elasticity after the age of 25 years although this is not necessarily the case. Zenker (1964) says that the thyroid cartilage may still be elastic at the age of 70 years and yet be rigid in much younger individuals. In Kahane's (1983) study of excised larynges, the laryngeal cartilages showed signs of ossification from the third decade in men and the fourth decade in women. Pantoja (1968) examined the cartilages of 100 normal adults. He found that ossification in the thyroid cartilage begins in the inferior horns and progresses along the inferior and posterior borders and then along the anterior border and angle. He confirmed that calcification is not constant and may be absent even in the oldest patients.

In singers and dramatic actors who preserve their voices into old age, the calcification presumably has not taken place. It is generally agreed that female laryngeal cartilages change more slowly, and that these changes progress less far, than in males (Kahane, 1983).

Vocal fold histological changes

Another aspect of ageing is the atrophy of the laryngeal muscles. Luchsinger (1962) described the false folds as narrower and the vocal folds more visible in the laryngoscopic mirror so that the opening into the laryngeal ventricle appears very wide. The vocal folds are visibly less tense and may exhibit bowing. The mucous membrane can be reddish or show yellow or brownish pigmentation. In these circumstances the voice will become unsteady and lack resonance.

Honjo and Isshiki (1980) studied a number of individuals, of mean age 75 years, and attributed changes in colour of the vocal folds to fat degeneration or keratosis of the mucous membrane. The age changes differed significantly between men and women. Vocal fold atrophy and glottic gap was frequently seen in aged men, while in women oedema of the vocal folds was a predominant characteristic. The changes in the male vocal folds were judged to be due to senescent change of muscle and mucous membrane. The hormonal imbalance during the menopause may account for the ingested appearance of the female vocal folds. Changes in mass of the vocal folds have been described by many writers (Honjo and Isshiki, 1980; Mueller, Sweeney and Baribeau, 1985). The reduction of glottal efficiency accompanied by bowing of the vocal folds occurs in some individuals. The voices of Sir Georg Solti (75 years) and Lord Denning (80 years) give evidence of such deterioration although both men are physically and intellectually active.

Vocal health

The physical changes associated with physiological ageing naturally contribute to changes in the acoustic characteristics of voice (Ramig and Ringel, 1983; Ringel and Chodzko-Zajko, 1987). There is a general belief that the old have stereotypical voices as exemplified by actors in the role of elderly characters, especially in men. Shakespeare describes the sixth stage of man with the shrunken shank and the big manly voice turning towards childish treble which 'pipes and whistles in his sound'. However, this is not so in real life as a general rule. With improved health and longevity vocal deterioration is greatly delayed. Physiological age can be totally unrelated to chronological age. That 'you are as old as you feel' is a fact and the vigour experienced in the prime of life may be extended into the seventies and even eighties. Women, however, have the advantage over men and remain younger and live longer.

The degree of deterioration of the voice is less noticeable in people who have naturally well-produced voices and especially in professionals with training in voice production who know how to breathe, project and resonate the voice and maintain good posture. Dame Sybil Thorndike, when over 80 years of age, still had a fine acting voice although of a rich and mature quality belying her age. Martinelli, the Italian tenor, was still singing and recording at the age of 76 years at the Metropolitan Opera House and sang part of Terandotte at 82 years. Amado (1953) reminds us that several other male singers have preserved their voices at concert level over the age of 70 years. He names Malfia Battistini and Leon Melchissedec but no female singers of comparable age. More recently one can cite the case of Salvation Army Commissioner, Catherine Bramwell-Booth who, at the age of 100 years, had an extraordinary youthful and delightful voice.

Nevertheless, it has been found that listener judgement can detect age changes in the voice and speech of the ordinary elderly (Ptacek *et al.*, 1966; Shipp and Hollien, 1969; Oyer and Deal, 1985). Judgement is not entirely related to vocal clues but various other features of delivery. Ptacek *et al.*'s study involved 72 healthy subjects none of whom had a hearing loss greater than 35 dB. The 10 listener judges were student graduates in speech pathology. They were told only the sex of each subject and had to judge whether the recorded samples of voice and speech were from people under 35 years or over 60 years. Each subject had recorded a prolonged vowel (4 seconds) and Fairbank's Rainbow Passage (played forwards and backwards). There was correct age recognition judgement at a 75% mean for the vowel, an 87% mean for the 'reverse' reading and a 99% mean for the 'forward' reading. The judges listed phrasing, speed, hesitancy, voice breaks and vitality as being the features which had indicated vocal age to them and which had influenced their judgement. This study showed that even inexperienced listeners can identify the aged voice and that correct listener judgement increases with the advancing age of the speakers.

Pitch changes

The literature concerning pitch changes from adult life to old age is extensive but not in total agreement. Mysak (1959a) and Mysak and Hanley (1959) in their studies of adult males found that voice pitch falls in middle age from that of early adulthood but thereafter rises with increasing age. In middle age the fundamental pitch was 110 Hz but had risen to 124.9 Hz in the 65–79 year group and to 142.6 Hz in the 80–92 year group. In another study of pitch in the adult male by Hollien and Shipp (1972), similar results were described. The mean frequency level was found to fall progressively to age 40 years; there was a progressive rise from 60 to 80 years. The elderly women studied by McGlone and Hollien (1963) also exhibited raised pitch with increasing age with a mean fundamental pitch of 196.6 Hz in the 65–79 year group and a mean fundamental pitch of 199.8 Hz in the 80–94 year group.

Honjo and Isshiki (1980) found that, as expected, the differences in vocal characteristics in elderly men and women reflect the differences they found in the vocal folds. As a result of vocal fold atrophy, elderly men tend to have a higher fundamental frequency than younger men. In contrast, aged women frequently have a lower fundamental frequency and more restricted pitch range than young women because of vocal fold oedema.

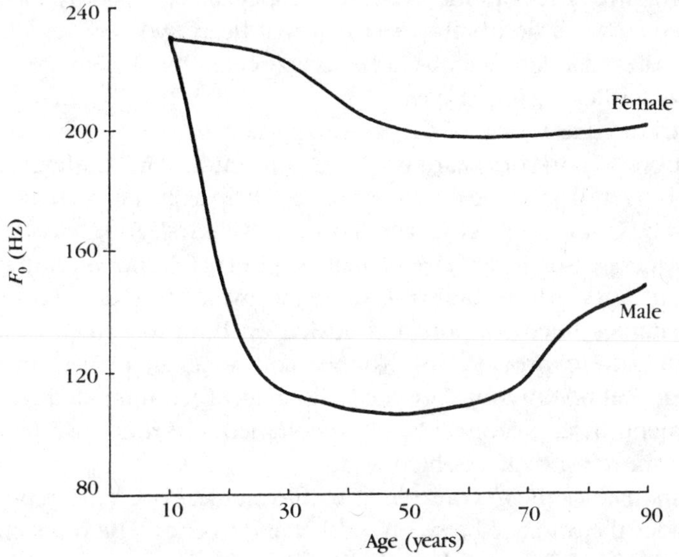

Figure 5.1. Graphic illustration of differential trends in male and female age-related changes in speaking fundamental frequency.

Table 5.2. Age-related changes in speaking fundamental frequency

Age (years)	*Mean SFo (Hz)*	
	Males	*Females*
20–29	120	224
30–39	112	213
40–49	107	221
50–59	118	199
60–69	112	199
70–79	132	202
80–89	146	

Data sources:
Males: Shipp and Hollien (1969).
Hollien and Shipp (1972).
Females: Stoicheff (1981).

Vocal amplitude

The reduction of expiratory volume due to the lung changes already described reduces the intensity of the voice in some cases. On the other hand an increase in the loudness of speech is observed by Greene (1982) and attributed to hearing loss. Ryan (1972) studying the acoustic aspects of the ageing voice draws attention to the fact that all the sensorimotor processes slowly deteriorate and adversely affect articulation and the resonance of the voice. Hearing loss is of great significance in control of vocal volume and the hard-of-hearing need to raise the voice to hear themselves, especially against a background noise. Schow and Nerbonne (1980) tested the hearing of 202 elderly residents of a nursing home with age range 65–98 years. There was evident progressive deterioration in hearing, especially for high frequencies. This was predictable, whereas the discovery that hearing deteriorated more seriously in males than females was rather unexpected but is consistent with the pattern of earlier ageing in males.

Deafness in old age is one of the most common threats to psychosocial communication. Wearing of a hearing aid and instruction in lip-reading is often rejected but by tactful handling from relatives and help from a speech therapist the voice can be maintained. As Takano-Stone (1987) says, 'The goal of care is to assist the older person to achieve the highest level of functioning and to live the remaining years in a meaningful, satisfying manner' as defined by the individual. Families need support and advice on how to care for elderly relations. The advice provided by Skinner and Vaughan (1983) in their excellent practical book *Enjoy Old Age* is a strongly recommended guide to self-management. Takano-Stone (1987) recommends various psychosocial remedies for the sensorially disabled.

Vision is another factor in controlling vocal volume. Poor sight renders it difficult to judge the distance between speaker and listener. The voice may be deliberately reduced in intensity when not wishing a tête-à-tête to be overheard, as may be the case in hospital or residential home (Greene, 1982).

The elderly themselves are often aware that their voices are deteriorating. Mueller (1978) reported that many elderly people complained of changes in vocal pitch, reduced pitch range, control and vocal quality. It is important to recognise that gross vocal change is unusual rather than common, except in those of very advanced years. Since adequate communication is of vital importance in maintaining social contacts as physical possibilities diminish, preservation of voice must not be overlooked in therapy which principally concentrates on the linguistic failures of old age. A well-preserved voice helps maintain self-respect and self-image. At a time when so much attention is paid to hair replacement, cosmetic surgery (Brennan, 1979), cosmetics and dress by both males and females in the fight against old age, preservation of the voice and its prosodic and paralinguistic features is essential.

Part II
Voice Disorders

Chapter 6
Dysphonia: Classification and Perceptual Assessment

The causes of voice disorder are many and encompass a wide range of behavioural conditions besides diseases which adversely affect phonation. The aetiological classification in Table 6.1 demonstrates the diversity of conditions which can produce dysphonia.

Table 6.1. Classification of voice disorder

Behavioural	*Organic*
1. *Excessive muscular tension* No changes in laryngeal mucosa	1. *Structural abnormalities* Laryngeal web Cleft palate Nasal obstruction Trauma
2. *Excessive muscular tension - changes in laryngeal mucosa* Vocal nodules Chronic laryngitis Oedema Polyps Contact ulcers	2. *Neurologial conditions* Recurrent laryngeal nerve paralysis Pseudobulbar palsy Bulbar palsy Cerebellar ataxia Tremor Parkinsonism Chorea Athetosis Apraxia Multiple lesions, e.g. motor neurone disease, multiple scerosis
3. *Psychogenic* Anxiety state Neurosis Conversion symptoms Delayed pubertal voice change (puberphonia) Trans-sexual conflict	3. *Endocrinological disorders* Thyrotoxicosis Myxoedema Male sexual mutational retardation Female virilisation due to adverse hormone therapy Adverse drug therapy
	4. *Laryngeal disease* Tumour - benign/malignant Hyperkeratosis Papillomatosis Cyst Laryngitis - acute/chronic Cricoarytenoid arthritis Granuloma Fungal infection

Although classifications such as the one in Table 6.1 are conveniently tidy, the clinical reality is likely to be more complex. The emotional stress involved in an organically based voice disorder may introduce a psychogenic factor to the original problem. The physical effort used to produce a forced whisper in some conversion symptoms can result in a true laryngitis.

Diagnosis

Diagnosis and assessment of voice disorder (dysphonia) requires collaboration between all the professional specialists who can contribute information concerning the patient's problems. Voice clinics are being established in an increasing number of centres so that the patient benefits from the coordinated approach of a professional team. This consists of the laryngologist and speech therapist and may include many others, such as a social worker, psychiatrist, audiologist, physiotherapist and medical electronics engineer.

The laryngologist

In the UK the dysphonic patient is initially referred by a general practitioner to the laryngologist who is responsible for medical and surgical treatment. It is imperative that malignancy should be excluded before other illnesses. It is generally accepted that dysphonia which persists for more than 2–3 weeks after onset should be fully investigated. As hoarseness can be 'the danger signal' of so many disorders and diseases, thorough investigations are needed. These will include indirect or direct laryngoscopy, X-ray examination of the upper respiratory tract including the nasal sinuses, chest and neck, examination of the ears and a hearing test, and possibly blood and sputum tests.

An important role of the laryngologist, besides heading the team, is to reassure the patient, when possible, that there is no malignancy and thus allay fears of cancer. Anxieties naturally develop before or after attending hospital and the rather alarming examinations, especially direct laryngoscopy under general anaesthesia which often leaves the throat sore and the neck stiff. Anxious patients focus on the discomfort felt and when told that there is nothing wrong may feel resentment and assert that their throats are worse than when they were admitted to hospital.

The patient who is a heavy smoker will be warned by the laryngologist of the dangers of contracting cancer at a future date. In some instances of excessive anxiety tranquillisers may be prescribed although this course of action is avoided if possible.

If the laryngologist explains the need for speech therapy and clearly indicates its importance the patient will embark on remediation appropriately motivated and with confidence. Voice therapy is sometimes considered unnecessary and too time consuming by the patient, especially if the voice recovers completely after surgery. In the long run avoidance of therapy does not save time but frequently leads to recurrence of the problem.

The speech therapist

In any setting, the speech therapist must regard a laryngological examination and report as mandatory before accepting a patient for treatment. There is grave danger to the patient in treating even the mildest case of hoarseness without first obtaining a laryngological examination and diagnosis. This applies to both children and adults. Seemingly mild symptoms of vocal misuse with huskiness and deterioration in vocal efficiency can be the first signs of neurological disorder or systemic disease, especially carcinoma. Any pressure upon the speech therapist to begin treatment without the laryngologist's report must be resisted because of the possibility of serious disease being overlooked. In addition, a valid remeditation programme cannot be evolved without clear information concerning laryngeal function and the type and site of mucosal changes.

> Case note
> A hospital secretary asked a speech therapist to see her husband who had a persistent hoarseness following 'flu. He was scared of hospitals but he could have easily visited the speech therapist on his way home from work in order to be given some helpful advice and thus avoid the Ear, Nose and Throat Department. This request was refused on the grounds that a laryngological report was essential initially. The couple rather resented this response and regarded it as uncooperative professionalism. Eventually the husband agreed to see the laryngologist and cancer of the larynx was diagnosed. He underwent a course of radiotherapy and a lasting cure was achieved. If diagnosis had been delayed a laryngectomy would probably have been necessary.

Throughout rehabilitation the speech therapist needs to remain in close contact with other members of the team, such as medical and nursing staff, and especially with the laryngologist in charge of the dysphonic patient. In addition, reports should be sent to the laryngologist following the therapist's first interview with the patient, prior to each review appointment the patient has with the laryngologist, and on completion of the course of voice therapy. The ideal is to hold the therapy session in the same premises and at the same time as the ENT out-patients clinic. This is not always possible but the therapist should aim to be present when a patient undergoing a course of voice therapy is reviewed. The therapist may view the larynx during indirect laryngoscopy and the patient's progress, and possible changes in remediation strategy, can be discussed. The reciprocal exchange of information and discussion is helpful and instructive to all members of the team and proves highly beneficial to the patient.

The Case History

Data relating to each case are advisedly assembled on a standard form. The case sheet can be short and concise as chosen by Boone (1977) or in great detail in

Case Information Sheet

Name: **Diagnosis:**

Date of birth:

Hospital number:

Address:
Home: Consultant:

Work: General Practitioner:

Telephone numbers:

Occupation/school:

Referral source: **Date referred:**

Date first seen:

Laryngological reports:

Laryngeal symptoms:

Diagnosis:

Hearing test result:

Medical reports:
(paediatric, neurological, psychiatric, etc.)

Paramedical reports:
(physio-, occupational therapist etc.)

Case Information Sheet (contd)

Medical history:

Previous illnesses: Date:

Investigations: Date:

Drugs prescribed (past and present): Date:

Present health:

Patient's (or carer's) information:

Domestic situation:

Housing conditions:

Working conditions:

Socioeconomic factors:

Hobbies and interests:

Health (weight, energy, fatigue, sleep, appetite etc.):

Patient's attitude (content, resentful etc.):

Smoking:

Alcohol:

Diet:

Patient's account of voice problem:

Onset:

Remissions and recurrences:

Reaction to dysphonia:

Opinion re. cause:

Throat sensations (irritable/sore/aching etc.):

Understanding of laryngologist's explanations:

Diagnostic listening and observation:

General impression of personality and relationships:

Paralinguistic features:

posture –

gesture –

eye contact –

Tense/relaxed:

Case Information Sheet (contd)

VOCAL ASSESSMENT

Vocal note:

Habitual pitch:

Intonation:

Vocal range:

Loudness:

Resonance:

Voice onset

Breathy/hard attack:

Delayed/correctly timed:

Maxmimum phonation time (MPT):

Rate of utterance:

Articulation:

Focal tensions -

Regional accent -

Respiration:

Type -

Rhythm -

Rate -

Vocal profile results:
(Laver (VPA); Crystal etc.)

Acoustic analysis results:
(SonoGraph; Visispeech etc.)

Respirometry results:

Recordings:

Audio (date):

Patient's reaction to playback -

Video (date):

Patient's reaction to playback -

a research-orientated voice clinic, as used by Gordon (1986) at the Victoria Infirmary, Glasgow. A scheme followed routinely ensures that all the information needed is recorded and that nothing is forgotten. It sets a standard guide for assistants and students so that the details relating to any patient are complete. A computer database (complying with data protection laws) or a card index recording each patients' name, hospital number, age, address, telephone number and diagnosis is also useful.

First Interview

The goals to be achieved during the patient's first interview with the speech therapist are broadly the same whatever the aetiology of the voice disorder. The compilation of a comprehensive account of the patient and the voice disorder is a priority but it is only one aspect of a meeting during which the rapport is established, explanations are given and a course of action is proposed. To concentrate entirely upon asking questions and making perceptual and instrumental evaluation of the voice at this stage may overwhelm and discourage a patient who is already anxious and probably has little idea of the speech therapist's role in the treatment schedule.

Eliciting information

The type of information required is listed on pp. 78–80 but some consideration should be given to the most efficient way in which it can be collected. A straightforward question and answer approach may, in fact, inhibit a patient and possibly reduce the information given. Relevant facts may be omitted and the opportunity to assess the voice in conversation is reduced. In many cases, the most productive approach is to tell the patient that although there is a laryngoscopic report it is helpful to hear the details of the voice problem from its inception. Any diffidence on the patient's part may be overcome by the speech therapist asking open-ended questions and prompting with encouraging remarks and questions which explore a new area where information is required. In order to enable the patient to speak freely the therapist has to appear relaxed and interested. It is during this interview that the therapist's own voice quality and communication skills will be particularly influential in affecting the amount and type of information acquired. The therapist's attitude should be friendly and sympathetic but at no time should professional distance be lost.

Recording data

Thought also has to be given to the method of recording data. Writing down every fact that is given will certainly reduce the flow of information and an audio-tape recording is intimidating and must not be made without the patient's agreement. A combination of careful listening and writing down factual details, such as dates, during the interview is best. Immediately writing up the case details after the interview is appropriate in most instances.

Clinical conditions

Ideally this interview should take place in a quiet room without interruption from other colleagues or the telephone and where the patient knows that there is no likelihood of being overheard. The patient's previous contacts, unless attending a private office, will have been in the limited privacy of an ENT clinic or a general ward. In the privacy of the first interview patients will frequently divulge significant information, previously unrevealed, and admit to not understanding aspects of their condition which are fundamental to treatment.

Does the patient understand?

The diagnosis

Once the case history has been thoroughly documented as outlined above, the first need is to verify that the patient understands the diagnosis and the results of any tests. It is a common experience among professionals to encounter patients who emphatically deny that they have been given explanations concerning their condition and the treatment which has been planned for them so far. There are a number of reasons for this. In some cases the patient has not actually received explanations, sometimes because assumptions are made that another member of the team has covered this aspect. More frequently, when an explanation has been given it is not meaningful to the patient. This may be because the language used is inappropriate. Professional people sometimes fail to realise that the jargon which they use with each other is incomprehensible to those who have no knowledge of anatomy and physiology. Patients can soon become lost in a linguistic limbo. The simple term 'vocal abuse' is not understood but sounds threatening, while attempts at colloquialisms such as 'corns in the voice box' can conjure up bewildering pedestrian images. Language may also be inappropriate because of the speaker's sociolinguistic and cultural assumptions. In general, the patient's anxiety and apprehension has prevented explanations being understood and there are fears that asking for the information to be repeated runs the risk of looking foolish.

Speech therapy

It should be established whether or not the patient understands why a referral to the speech therapist has been made. As a result of misconceptions concerning the speech therapist's role, reactions may include willing compliance purely because the laryngologist has made the referral or surprise because 'I speak alright, it's just my voice'. The dysphonic patient who has no mucosal changes in the larynx and who has been told by the laryngologist that the larynx is normal, may be fearful that the speech therapist 'is a shrink'. In order for the therapist to gain the patient's confidence any such misunderstandings must be discussed. It should be made clear that the purpose of the initial interview is assessment of the voice problem in the light of the laryngological findings and that this is the basis for planning suitable treatment.

Normal voice production

While not wanting to be patronisingly simple in explanations of how the patient's laryngeal function differs from normal, the therapist must discover the extent of the patient's knowledge. The individual who visualises the larynx as a harp-like structure with several vibrating 'cords' in a vertical position is not well equipped to have insight into the condition.

The patient's account of the problem

Development of the voice disorder

A chronological account of the development of the dysphonia is necessary in order to establish the history of the disorder. The patient will have opinions as to the cause, and provide information concerning the onset and related events. The voice may have deteriorated steadily or there may have been periods of varying length when the voice was normal or markedly improved.

Usual daily pattern

It is helpful to know whether there is any daily consistency concerning the pattern of the dysphonia. In some disorders there is a noticeable tendency for the voice to be less efficient by the end of the day; in others the opposite applies or there is no apparent consistency. Any correlation of increased dysphonia with certain activities is noted as are periods of normal voice.

The voice at interview

The patient's own evaluation of the voice is important, how it is during the interview and whether it is much worse or better under interview conditions. Reported sensations such as soreness or aching in the throat should be noted.

Patient's view of the problem

The speech therapist's opinion of the severity of the dysphonia may not agree with the patient's opinions. The actor whose voice becomes mildly breathy by the end of a performance may be very concerned by the symptom. A market trader whose voice is severely hoarse at the end of a day's trading will only consider that he has a problem when he has no voice. The obvious anxiety of the professional voice user and all those whose ability to communicate effectively depends on an efficient voice, making maximum use of paralinguistic features, should not be dismissed as neurotic. The fears may be well founded in a particular situation for that particular person.

Occupation

Vocal strain occurs frequently in those whose occupations make severe demands upon the voice, such as teachers, lecturers, preachers, singers, actors and salesmen. People who work in the noisy surroundings of shops, factories and restaurants are also prone to vocal strain. Environmental conditions in the place of work may include irritants which aggravate the mild chronic laryngeal inflammation. A smoky, dusty or over-dry atmosphere with non-humidified central heating can be harmful. The sensitive mucous membrane of the larynx becomes dry and irritants provoke coughing which, in turn, further aggravates the condition.

The importance of voice to the patient's job, and whether or not employment is in jeopardy because of the dysphonia, must be established. 'Rationalisation' of staff as a result of increasing technology and financial pressures means that redundancy hangs over the heads of many people. The individual who anticipates being made redundant, or who is in a career backwater because of a take-over, can experience the same level of anxiety as someone who is unemployed. These stresses will affect treatment.

Home environment

Information is required concerning the patient's home life, encompassing the physical environment and other members of the family or those with whom the home is shared. Shouting at a dog can have a traumatising effect on the larynx but is frequently less forceful than shouting at a difficult child when frustration and anger are powerful components. The laryngeal effect of shouting at a deaf relation is aggravated by irritation and the guilt with which it is frequently associated. In any relationship which is unsatisfactory the effect of severe dysphonia on communication can increase the existing problems. More detailed information concerning domestic relationships is usually acquired during later sessions.

Social life

The patient's social life may be vocally demanding, with activities such as choral singing and amateur dramatics, or considerable time being spent in the smokey and noisy atmosphere of a pub, or shouting at football matches. Some households talk against the constant background noise of television or radio. In addition, a more complete profile of the individual is compiled by discovering interests and hobbies.

Diagnostic listening and observation

From the moment of first meeting and throughout the patient's account considerable information can be collected by the therapist through observing non-verbal communication and listening to vocal features. Levels of motivation and potential cooperation become apparent and influence the therapeutic approach.

Posture reflects tension both generally in the body and specifically in the neck and face. It will also provide information about the individual's personality and feelings of self-worth. Eye contact, facial expression and hand movements give clues as to the emotional state. The therapist should be alert to the patient who gives out ambiguous messages; an assurance that all is well at home may be accompanied by a facial expression that 'says' the opposite and with eye avoidance. Minimal facial expression can signal a negative response to the therapist or it may be indicative of depression or hide intense emotion. The mask-like face of the patient with Parkinson's disease, which is neurologically based, conceals emotions which must not be overlooked.

Aspects of Voice Production

Respiration

Habitual breathing patterns at rest and during connected speech are observed. These may be clavicular and shallow or the speaker may use particularly long phrases during very rapid speech with minimal breath support. The control of the airflow may be poor. Noisy, rapid or effortful breathing at rest will have considerable significance for therapy.

Phonation

The following features should be noted:

1. Pitch, resonance, volume, range and flexibility including intonation patterns and prosody. The severity of impairment of these individual parameters and the overall impression of the severity of the dysphonia.
2. Laryngeal note: the voice may be breathy, harsh, hoarse, exhibit vocal fry, sound effortful or have a 'wet' quality.
3. Vocal attack: the extremes of hard glottal attack or breathy onset are not mutually exclusive and may be apparent in one individual.
4. Vocal habits: throat clearing and various types of coughing are common vocal habits which can be either a contributory factor or a result of the dysphonia, but in both cases harmful to the vocal folds.
5. Observation of the neck during phonation will reveal whether the strap muscles are tense and visible. Pronounced vertical excursions of the larynx during speech should be noted.
6. Maxmimum phonation time (MPT): this is the time in seconds for which a vowel can be maintained at a comfortable pitch and volume after taking a deep breath. MPT is greater in males than females; in males it falls within limits of 25–35 seconds and in females within 15–25 seconds. It is markedly less in certain cases of laryngeal pathology (Hirano, 1981).
7. Vocal fatigue: onset of vocal fatigue may occur during conversation or reading aloud with all, or some, vocal parameters being affected.

Articulation

Articulation reflects excessive muscular tension when there is marked mouth-closure during speech, a pattern which may give a hypernasal quality to the voice. The speaker may also clench the teeth when at rest. Marked tongue bunching in these individuals can lead to supraglottic tension and raised larynx. The individual with aspirations to higher social status may assume an accent which is accompanied by considerable tension. In any case, different accents require different articulatory movements, such as more or less lip-rounding, which affect vocal quality.

Audio-tape Record

An audio-tape recording should be made in order to monitor progress as treatment advances. The voice should be recorded in the following contexts.

1. Conversation.
2. Reading aloud: a standard passage should be used for all recording so that comparisons can be made. A commonly used text for this purpose is 'The Rainbow Passage' (Fairbanks, 1960).
3. Prolonged vowels: these are phonated in 'normal' speaking voice and as vocal glides to demonstrate vocal range. The vowel sounds used to measure MPT can also be recorded.

This recording should be played to the patient and reaction to hearing the voice noted. Although video-recording can be a useful tool during treatment most patients would find it intolerable in the early stages of treatment.

The Patient's Immediate Needs

The interview should terminate with the knowledge that the patient has been given a clear idea of the aetiology of the dysphonia and the outline of the treatment proposed. The patient must leave the session with some positive advice and knowing that the initial stages of treatment have begun. If the therapist regards this session as one in which assessment material alone is amassed without any immediate gains obvious to the patient, there is a high risk of losing the patient's confidence and jeopardising future treatment.

Clear explanations from the therapist concerning the normal anatomy and physiology of respiration and phonation, the reasons for the dysphonia, and possible courses of action to improve the situation are what most patients require at this stage. Opportunities for questions to be asked and answered will help to improve the patient's insight into the condition and therefore provide a sound basis for therapy. Therapist–patient rapport is improved if the therapist gives some indication of understanding the practical and emotional effects of dysphonia.

Recommendations concerning voice conservation, relaxation and therapeutic procedures, which can be practised until the next appointment, give the patient the opportunity to participate actively in the treatment programme from the beginning. The patient's immediate needs are paramount and the session should recognise this throughout. The speech therapist must avoid becoming immersed in taking case history details and conducting a battery of tests which can be postponed until later.

Perceptual Vocal Assessment

The assessment of dysphonia which relies upon auditory perception ('the ear') of the therapist is, in the final analysis, the most telling evaluation possible. How a voice sounds and how far the voice meets the speaker's needs is the ultimate dictum in the rehabilitation programme. The clinician needs intensive training in the vocal dimensions which identify pathology most effectively. Rating voice quality perceptually is universally acknowledged as a difficult task and one which requires long experience (Bassich and Ludlow, 1986; Wendler and Anders, 1986).

It is generally recognised that no electronic instrument can replace 'the ear'. Instruments can nevertheless provide accurate measurement of specific parameters in voice production such as volume, pitch and airflow. The therapist has to assemble such information and form a cohesive whole with other psychological and physical factors which will influence the assessment. Subjective and instrumental assessment results form the baseline upon which progress is evaluated.

The great difficulty regarding vocal evaluation is the problem of description. There are no reliable verbal terms defining vocal characteristics although there is a continuous struggle to produce a definitive descriptive terminology. Adjectives may have different meanings for different people. Renfrew, Mitchell and Wallace (1957) had assessed cleft palate cases for 4 years. They completed a standard assessment form routinely and found that they were not always in agreement. Eventually, Renfrew set up a project to evaluate the validity of their completed forms. The three experienced therapists listened to recordings of cleft palate cases and completed forms independently. When assessments were compared, it was found that there was considerable divergence in their ratings relating to factors such as slight, moderate and excessive nasality, audible nasal escape and mixed resonance although they were in agreement concerning the type of dysphonia. Similar difficulties are described in profiling voice by Wilson and Rice (Shanks, 1979) and Wynter and Martin (1981).

Fairbanks (1960) thought the great variety of vocal symptoms perceptible could be classified under three headings: harshness, breathiness and hoarseness, and given ratings on a scale of 0 to 5. Few experts can agree with this: hoarseness is breathy, and harshness may mean metallic (Aronson, 1980). One is reminded of the dilemma in which wine experts find themselves when attempting to describe the subtle flavours of vintage wines and their elusive qualities. For example, Johnson (1987) describes a great burgundy, the Domaine Romanee Conti as:

> Overwhelmingly high-toned smell of violets to start with, changing within twenty minutes to a more deep and fruity bouquet which seemed at first like oranges, then more like blackcurrants. The flavour was best half an hour after opening - exotically rich and warm.

Actors voices have been described as rich and fruity also.

A universally acceptable and understood nomenclature would be of great value in writing reports, assessing treatment and progress and comparing research results of other workers in the field. There is as yet no reliable means of recording the individual's vocal fingerprint and the possibility of it ever becoming available appears remote. One has only to listen to computerised speech to appreciate the difficulties involved in producing normal voice by electronic voice encoding and synthesis (Parsons, 1987).

Nevertheless, researchers endeavour to overcome the difficulties of compiling an accurate verbal profile which is universally acceptable. Wynter and Martin (1981) spent 5 years in an attempt at training students in speech therapy to remember and identify characters of dysphonia by listening to sample recordings. A team of experienced speech therapists had classified and agreed on the description of 100 recordings. The categories were: creaky, husky, hoarse, harsh, disordered pitch, disordered resonance and 'others'. The 'others' included voices that 'defied any attempt to be categorised under present terminology'. This admission of course caused complications from the outset but the final admission of defeat took 5 years to materialise. The results of the research were disappointing since the auditory perception of the trained students failed to match closely the perception of the researchers.

Case (1984) lists over 40 vocal misuse and abuse characteristics and what amounts in reality to 40 bones of contention.

The 'GRBAS' scale

Similar problems have been noted by the Committee of Phonatory Function Tests of the Japan Society of Logopedics and Phoniatrics. The 'GRBAS' scale for evaluating hoarseness on five scales - grade (i.e. degree of voice abnormality), rough, breathy, asthenic and strained - is accompanied by a standard tape of voice samples. As evaluation is subjective and requires training, as do other voice profiles, it is not necessarily a completely reliable method of evaluation (Hirano, 1981).

The Vocal Profile Analysis (Laver)

The search for a verbal blue-print was pursued by Laver (1980) who endeavoured to establish a phonetic description of voice quality. He charted the positions of labial, mandibular, lingual, velopharyngeal and laryngeal structures to which he gave tension ratings. Phonation types are classified as harshness, whispery, breathiness, creaky, falsetto and modal. Originally, Laver thought that writing a book and producing a cassette of illustrative phonation types would produce therapists who could complete the Vocal Profile Analysis (VPA) without further training (Laver, 1980). It became evident, however, that seminars and specific training in labelling of Laver's phonation types was essential and these 3-day courses produce a high learning rate in the participants. The VPA presents a formidable list of items and demonstrates the immense variety of vocal qualities and phonetic gestures possible. This list alone provides a useful indicator of vocal features to be considered during assessment of the dysphonic patient. The charting of phonetic positions are based on listening and visual observation of articulatory sets unsupported by lateral X-ray pictures. The emphasis upon articulatory gestures is valuable in alerting the speech therapist to these important aspects of phonation and sites of excessive tension described above. (The Vocal Profile Analysis Protocol form is reproduced in Appendix II.)

Buffalo Voice Profile

The Buffalo Voice Profile used by Wilson (1987) rates the following parameters: laryngeal tone, laryngeal tension, vocal abuse, loudness, pitch, vocal inflections, pitch breaks, diplophonia, resonance, nasal emission, rate and overall voice efficiency on a seven-point scale with appropriate descriptive terms listed for marking with each category. He recommends that speech samples should include connected speech, oral reading, individual phonemes and counting.

Perceptual–acoustic relationships

Research conducted by Hammarberg (1986) was directed at correlating perceptual vocal characteristics of vocal dysfunction and acoustic characteristics. Initial studies showed that speech pathologists who were experienced in the diagnosis and therapy of voice disorders could agree on 12 voice quality parameters:

- Aphonic/intermittent aphonic.
- Breathy.
- Hyperfunctional/tense.
- Hypofunctional/lax.
- Vocal fry/creaky.
- Rough.
- Grating.
- Diplophonic.
- Voice breaks.
- Instability.
- Register.
- Pitch.

Acoustic correlates were found for nine of these voice qualities. Hammarberg (1986) points out that perceptual voice evaluation by clinically well-trained listeners, can be reliable if based on standardised rating procedures. Also that training for voice therapists can be more effective if perceptual-acoustic relationships are identified.

In conclusion, we heartily agree with Aronson's sensible observation: 'Faced with a dysphonia, the clinician's chief concern is diagnosis and not aesthetic values.' It is incumbent upon the speech therapist to start treatment of a patient immediately and this 'faute de mieux' has to be on the basis of a perceptual assessment initially. The value of such assessment is heavily dependent upon experience. Instrumental testing follows and treatment is adapted, if necessary, when test results are available. The results of instrumental tests which are acquired later can be accommodated in the rehabilitation programme as deemed necessary and as suggested in the following chapter.

Chapter 7 Dysphonia: Objective Assessment and Biofeedback

In addition to the traditional instruments used in the examination of the larynx, electronic technology has produced a wide range of instruments to measure the various physiological functions involved in voice production: muscle movements, vocal fold vibration and acoustic parameters. Respiratory volumes, airflow, pitch and intensity can be registered accurately. Measurements of resonance remain unsatisfactory, hence the endeavours to devise vocal profiles as explained in the previous chapter. Instruments assess isolated features but do not provide an integrated picture of voice production. The human ear has to be relied on to diagnose aberrant vocal quality and in this the trained listener is highly successful.

Many of these instruments are also suitable for use during remediation in addition to their assessment function. This chapter therefore includes some instruments which have only an assessment role and others which can be used for both assessment and for biofeedback. The baseline information which instruments provide is available for comparison with later assessments as treatment progresses. The rate of progress can be charted and the efficacy of treatment procedures can be monitored. In addition, during treatment the screen display or dial response allows a patient to monitor performance and attempt realisation of a target set by the therapist. Biofeedback of this type is a useful adjunct to therapy but should not be regarded as a substitute for personal instruction, emotional support and encouragement by the therapist which all dysphonic patients need.

Some of the most commonly used instruments are described in the following pages, although it has to be admitted that most will never appear in the average speech clinic. Many are expensive to purchase and further expenditure is required for technicians to maintain if not operate them. However, it is necessary to be aware of their potential if opportunities do arise for use in the clinic during treatment and research, and also to evaluate reports emanating from research laboratories and well-equipped voice clinics.

Lack of hardware does not mean that speech therapists do not achieve considerable success in assessment and treatment using their professional knowledge and experience. Ideally, this expertise is supported by the appropriate instrumentation. There are few comparative studies concerning the effectiveness of biofeedback and traditional strategies but those available are far from producing conclusive evidence of the excellence of new techniques (Andrews, Warner and Stewart, 1986). In many instances the laryngologist and patient can confirm that improvements or a return to normal function is achieved without having recourse to instruments. The aim of therapy is to achieve the maximum improvement in the shortest period of time. If instruments are available for assessment and treatment they must be used if they accelerate the rate of improvement. Instruments are tools which supplement a therapist's pragmatic treatment.

Assessment of Vocal Fold Function

Laryngoscopy

Indirect laryngoscopy

Indirect laryngoscopy is the standard clinical procedure in use by laryngologists for examination of the interior larynx. It is a mandatory routine examination which provides instant information regarding the laryngeal mucosa and gross vocal fold movement.

The laryngoscope consists of a small laryngeal mirror on a handle. The mirror is placed against the elevated soft palate as the patient says 'ah' while the laryngologist holds the patient's tongue, wrapped in gauze. Light from an external source is reflected from the laryngologist's head-mirror onto the laryngeal mirror and subsequently into the pharynx and larynx. The reflection of the vocal folds in the laryngeal mirror enables them to be viewed at rest and in phonation so that their appearance and movement can be carefully examined. In the mirror image the right and left vocal folds are reversed and the anterior commissure appears in a posterior position. This image is the one

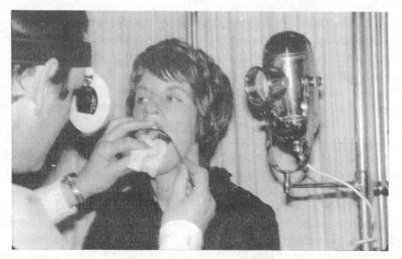

Figure 7.1. Indirect laryngoscopy.

which the laryngologist will use to illustrate his findings in the medical notes.

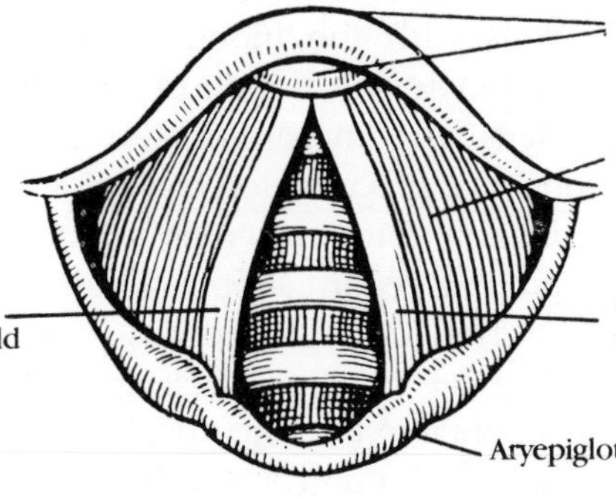

Figure 7.2. Mirror image of vocal folds on indirect laryngoscopy.

Direct laryngoscopy

Direct laryngoscopy is carried out under general anaesthetic. During this procedure the larynx is viewed by a magnifying microscope inserted through the oral cavity and into the pharynx. The larynx is viewed only at rest with the vocal folds moving towards the mid-line and away in a rhythmic movement generated by the respiratory cycle. A thorough examination of the vocal tract and the area below the folds is possible but the actual function of the larynx in phonation is not seen in the unconscious patient, of course.

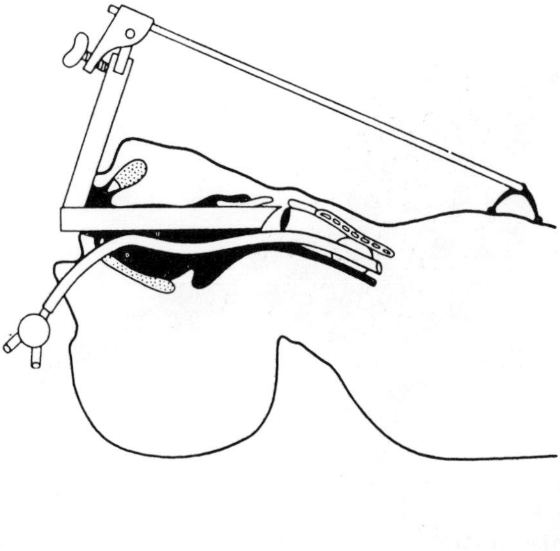

Figure 7.3. Direct laryngoscopy: laryngoscope and anaesthetic catheter in position.

Fibreoptic laryngoscopy

The mirror insertion in standard indirect laryngoscopy imposes considerable constraint upon the patient's potential phonation which is restricted to utterance of single vowels with the mouth wide open. The fibreoptic laryngoscope consists of a thin flexible bundle of glass fibres containing a light source and magnifying lens. The images are viewed through an eye piece. There is also an additional eye piece which enables a colleague to view the larynx during the examination. The otolaryngologist can examine the vocal tract and make a photographic record simultaneously (Lancer, 1986).

Before the cable is inserted through the nose and passed down to an appropriate position in the pharynx, a local anaesthetic spray is administered. An uninterrupted view is obtained of the vocal folds or palatopharyngeal valving as required. The hand control on the equipment enables the laryngologist to move the flexible end of the tube so that the vocal tract structures may be thoroughly examined. This procedure allows the patient to phonate and speak almost unimpeded. Some patients cannot tolerate the invasion and children especially may resist the procedure. Also, the anaesthetic has a very unpleasant taste. However, this examination is frequently a successful alternative for use with patients who are unable to cooperate with indirect laryngoscopy. The examiner needs much experience and skill. In patients with deflected septum, not uncommon in cleft palate, there may be obstruction to insertion of the scope (see 'Cleft palate').

We understand that American speech pathologists frequently carry out this examination and also use rigid endoscopes themselves. In the UK this is not so, but in other parts of Europe many phonologists are qualified doctors and competent to perform this investigation.

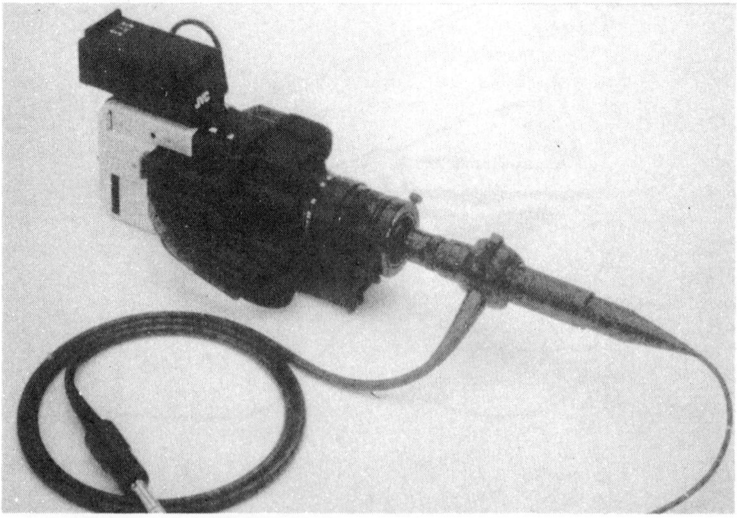

Figure 7.4. Flexible fibrescope and video camera. (Courtesy of Brüel and Kjaer, Denmark.)

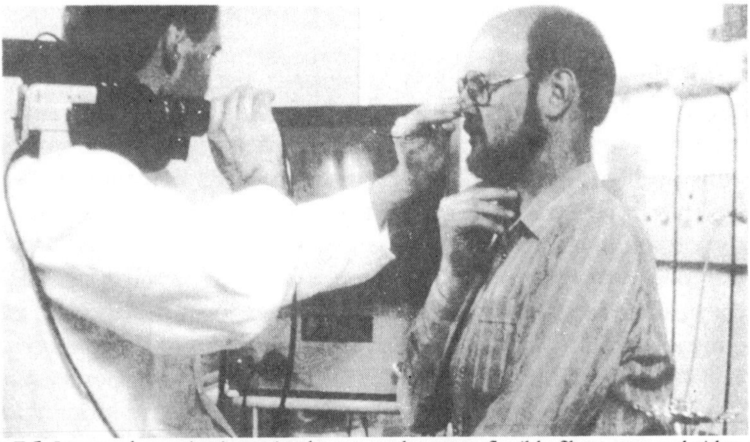

Figure 7.5. Laryngeal examination using larynx stroboscope, flexible fibrescope and video camera. (Courtesy of Brüel and Kjaer, Denmark)

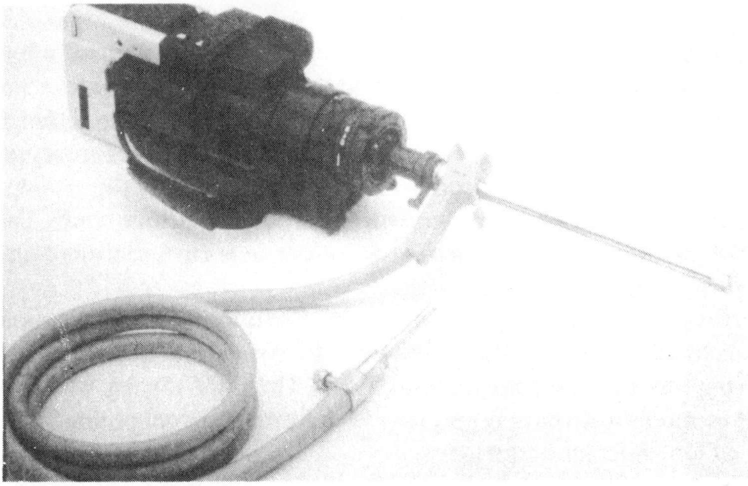

Figure 7.6. Rigid endoscope. (Courtesy of Brüel and Kjaer, Denmark.)

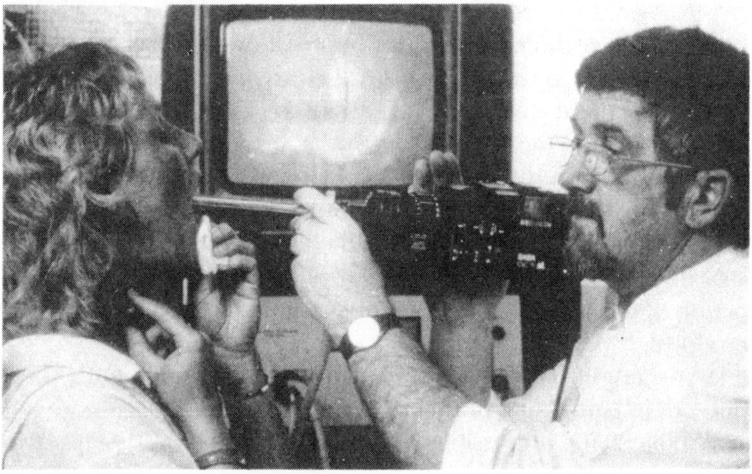

Figure 7.7. Laryngeal examination using larynx stroboscope, rigid endoscope and video camera. (Courtesy of Brüel and Kjaer, Denmark.)

Stroboscopy

Only gross disorders of vocal fold movement are discernible by indirect laryngoscopy and fibreoptic laryngoscopy because the vocal folds vibrate too rapidly for the eye to detect the individual vibratory cycles. The stroboscope solves this problem by providing a light source with intermittent flashes of light which can be synchronised with the vibratory cycles and is instantly responsive to the subject's vocal pitch changes. Flashes emitted at a slower rate than the phonation frequency produce a slow motion effect. The flash frequency can be so adjusted that the vocal folds appear to stand still and this can be manoeuvred to fix the image at different stages in the vibratory cycle (Baken, 1987). A rigid endoscope, flexible fibrescope or operation microscope is used to deliver stroboscopic illumination and to give magnification of the image so that minute lesions can be seen clearly.

Any asymmetry of movement can be detected. So visible is the detail that oedematous vocal fold membranes can be seen to meet in advance of the ligamentous portion or lamina propria. Vocal folds out of phase with each other may be a feature of incipient nodule or paresis. In cases of invasive carcinoma, absence of the mucosal wave is apparent. This wave is also absent in laryngeal paresis in which the paralysed fold shows a wide vibratory pattern (Kitzing, 1985). Videostroboscopy or high speed cine film of the moving vocal folds can be used to obtain a permanent record for further study. This is a useful facility which can be shown to the patient and help understanding of the condition.

Harris (1987) notes a further advantage of stroboscopic examination. It is possible to view the horizontal amplitude of the vocal fold beats in addition to observing the regularity of successive beats. The pitch display which can be linked to modern stroboscopes provides information concerning a patient's range of fundamental frequencies.

Laryngography (electrolaryngography, electroglottography)

This non-invasive technique provides information about vocal fold contact (Fourcin and Abberton, 1971). Two small electrodes are placed on the neck, one on each side of the thyroid cartilage. As a weak electrical current is passed from one electrode to the other across the larynx at the level of the vocal folds the instrument responds to changes in electrical impedance caused by their adduction and abduction. The waveform produced (*Lx* waveform) is dependent upon the degree of vocal fold contact. The apex of the waveform indicates the closed phase of the vibratory cycle, when there is maximum conduction of the current. The open phase of the cycle shows as a trough in the waveform.

The laryngograph only provides information concerning both vocal folds together, not impaired function of each fold. In some subjects with a double chin it is difficult or impossible to obtain an accurate response from the equipment.

Voiscope

Assessment and visual feedback is provided by the Voiscope manufactured by Laryngograph Ltd (Abberton and Fourcin, 1984). This instrument combines an electrolaryngograph with a display system consisting of two oscillopes. The *Lx* waveform is displayed on one and, on the other, the *Fx* display shows intonation patterns during speech. Displays can be fixed on the screen for as long as needed while a subject attempts to reproduce the same pattern in parallel and modify both prosodic and segmental aspects of speech (Fourcin and Abberton, 1977). Separate oscilloscope displays can also be produced by therapist and patient for comparison and targeting. Hard copies of these displays can be obtained when the Voiscope is interfaced with a microcomputer. Software has been developed for use in conjunction with a laryngograph for analysing the regularity of vocal fold vibration and various measures of fundamental frequency (Abberton, 1987).

Laryngograph Ltd also produce a portable, battery-operated laryngograph with an integral oscilloscope for *Lx* display. It can be interfaced to Kay Elemetric's Visi-Pitch (Baken, 1987).

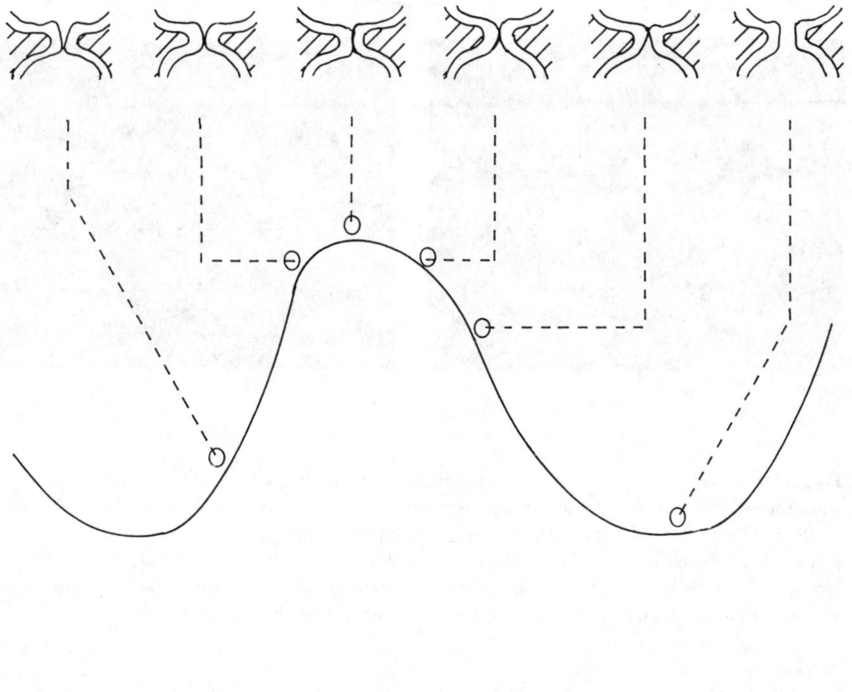

Figure 7.8. The laryngograph waveform and its relationship to vocal fold contact in one vibratory cycle. (After MacCurtain and Fourcin, 1982.)

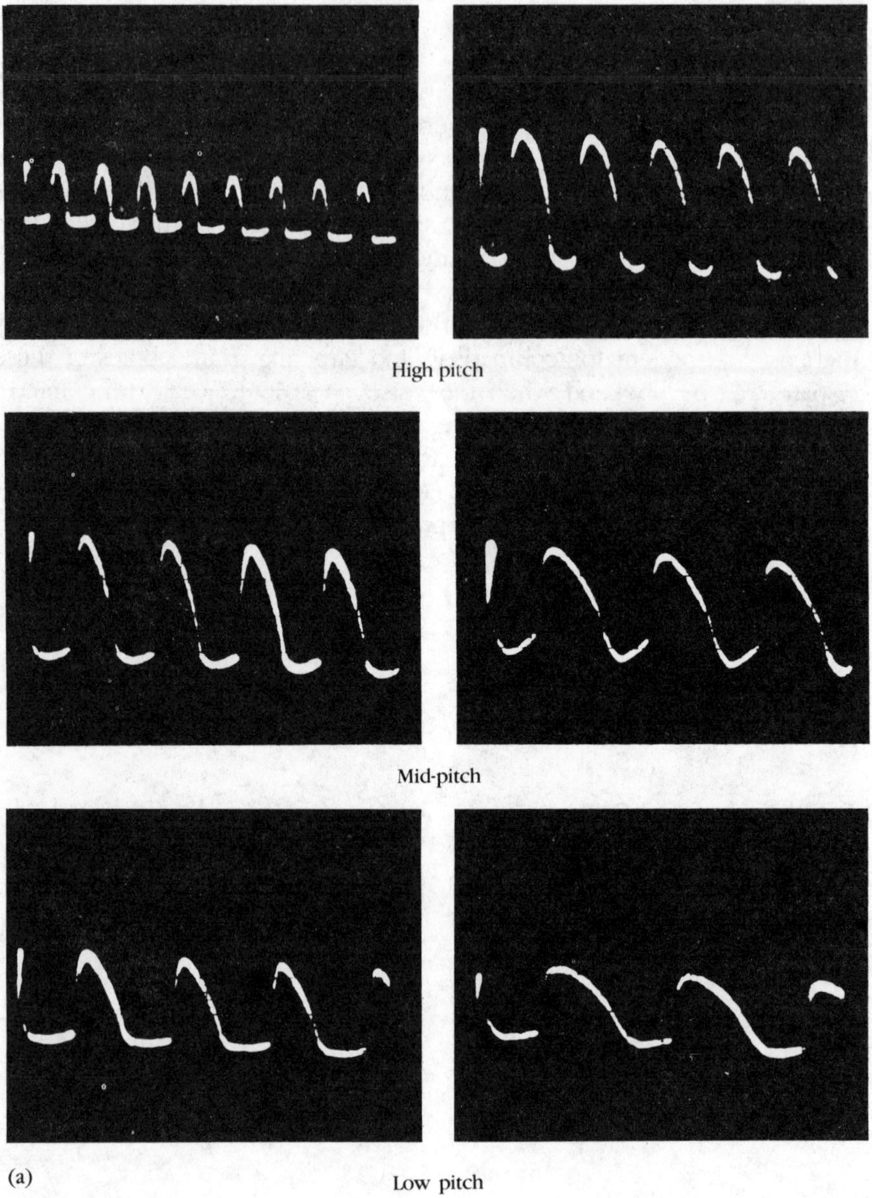

Figure 7.9. *Lx* used as a qualitative measure of vocal fold vibration patterns. (a) Normal *Lx*: female (left) and male (right) sustaining 'ee' at habitual high, mid and low pitch (from top to bottom). The higher number of frequencies produced by the female are shown by the greater number of 'waves'. The high amplitude of the waveform indicates deep vertical vocal fold contact, reduced at high pitch for the female as the vibrating edges of the cords become thinner. There is a well-defined closure in both samples, indicated by the almost vertical rise of the wave from the baseline.

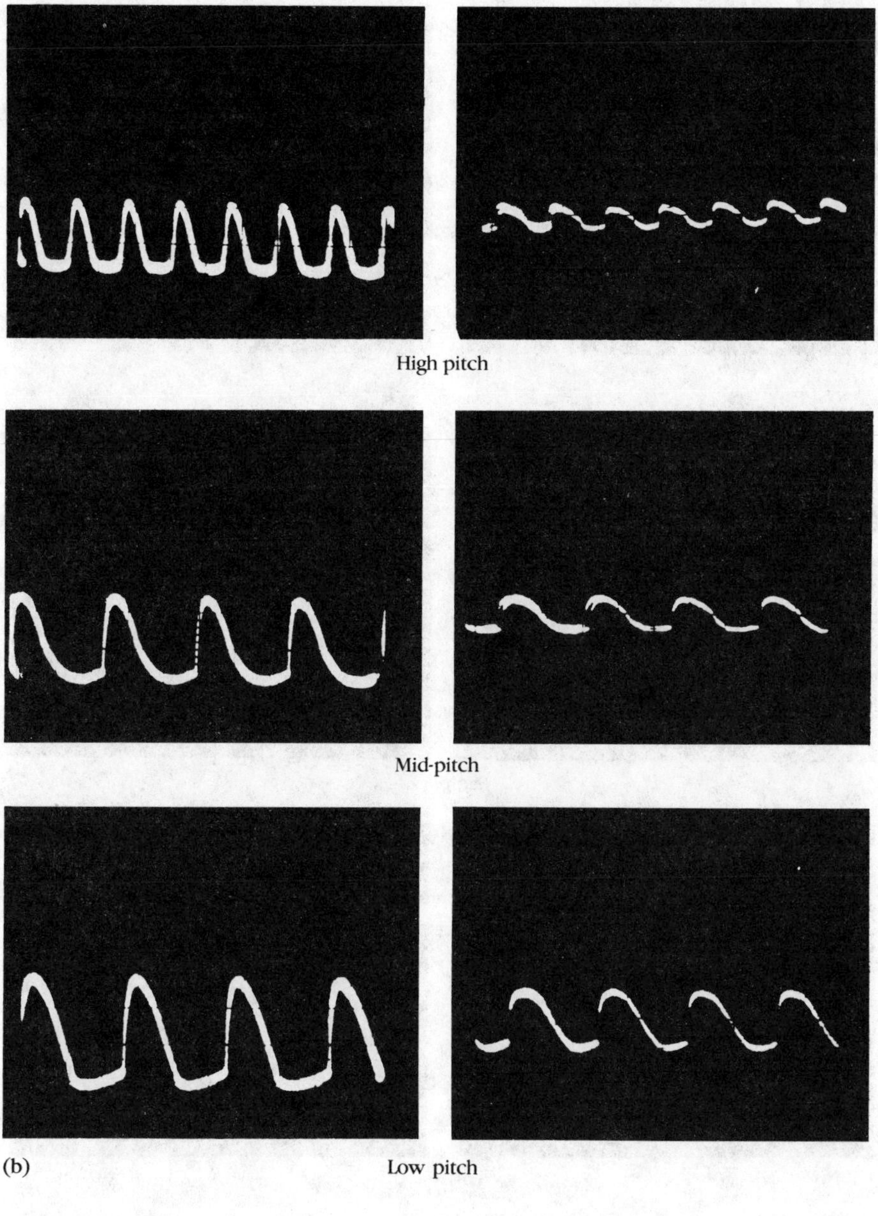

Figure 7.9 contd. (b) Contrast of the *Lx* from two females aged 28 years. The one on the left has normal vocal folds and the one on the right has oedematous vocal folds due to long-term use of inhalations to control asthma. *Lx* shows typical low amplitude, i.e. limited lateral vocal fold contact, a typical 'rounded top' to the wave and a long 'open phase'. This long open phase was confirmed auditorily by very whispery (breathy) voice quality.

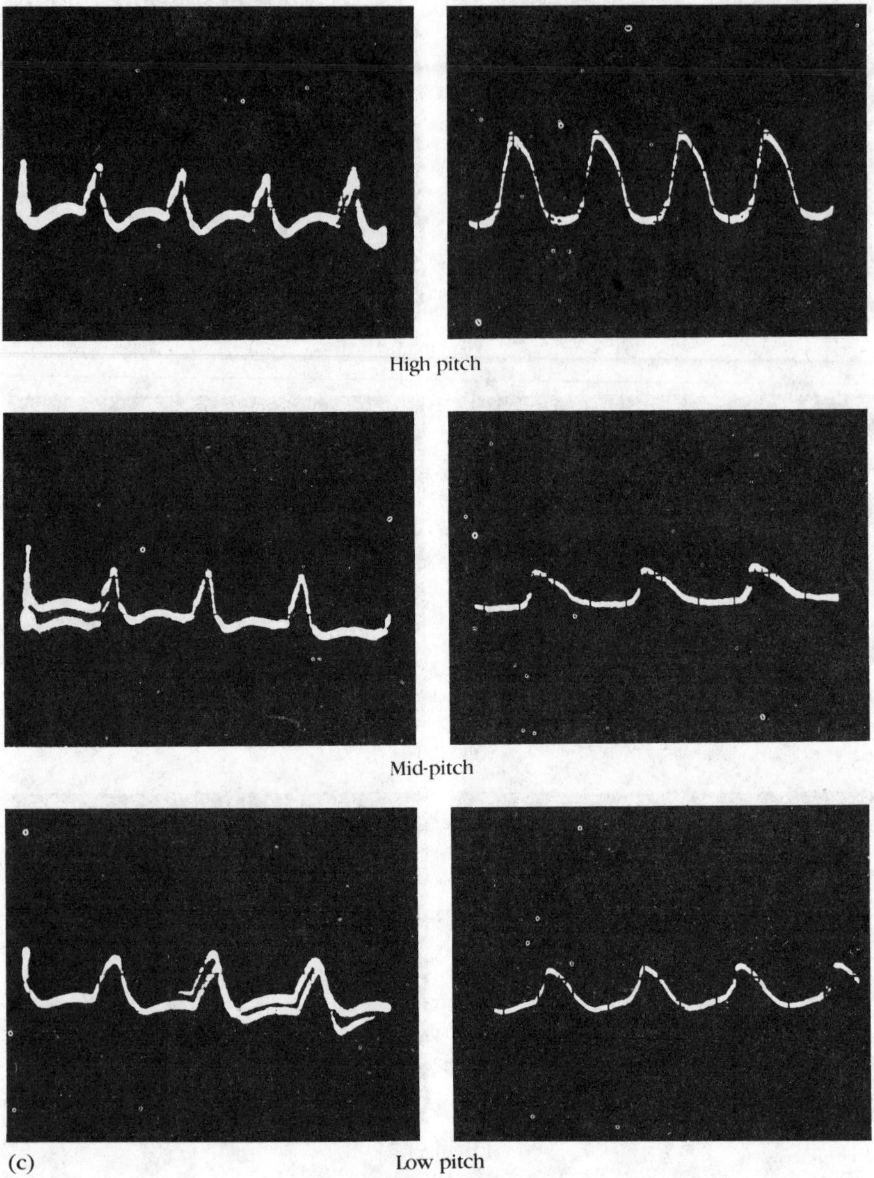

Figure 7.9. contd. (c) *Lx* waveforms before (left) and after (right) Teflon injection for long-standing left vocal fold palsy, since age 6, in a 24-year-old male. Trace on the left shows a very long open phase with gradual and extremely short duration closure, a very abrupt opening of the folds and poor ability to vary pitch. (Dual parts of the trace are due to the extreme effort involved in sustaining phonation which lead to excessive movement of the larynx.) Postoperative *Lx* on the right shows waveforms of more normal appearance, particularly at high pitch, which even shows deep vertical contact. Mid and low 'ee' show a less efficient mode of vibration (low amplitude and long open phase) but the waveforms show the more typical sudden closure and gradual opening, regular and periodic. Pitch control is still imperfect as evidenced by mid-pitch actually being of lower frequency than the attempted low pitch. (The authors are indebted to Eva Carlson, MSc, Chief Speech Therapist, St Thomas's Hospital, London for the analysis of laryngograph waveforms in Figures 7.9–7.12.)

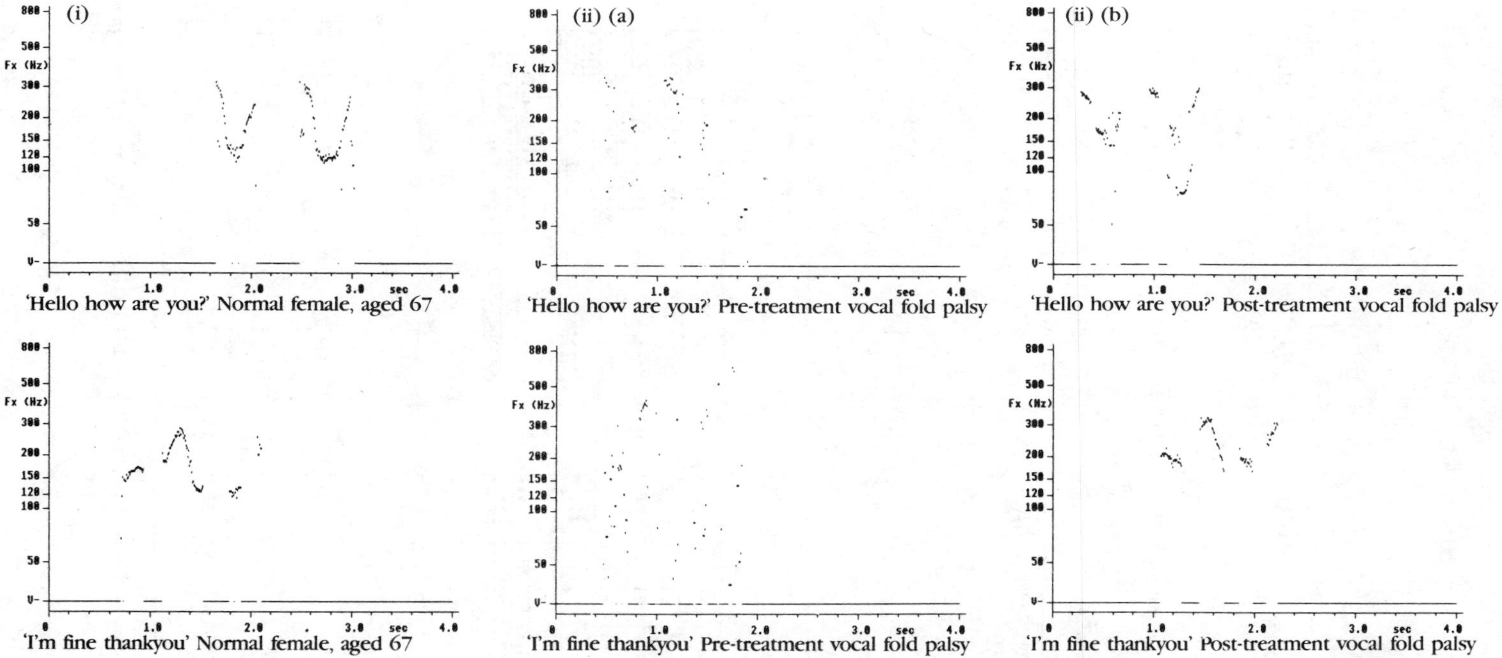

Figure 7.10. *Fx* contours: these printouts with frequency and time scales are obtained by using the recently developed laryngograph program. The contours show cycle-to-cycle variation of fundamental frequency with breaks for voiceless segments. The trace is derived from the input (*Lx*) from the laryngeal electrodes used with the Voiscope. The frequency scale is logarithmic to correspond to our perception of pitch. (i) 'Normal' female, aged 67 years; (ii) 65-year-old woman before and after treatment for left vocal fold palsy. (a) Pre-treatment. The contours show very little evidence of regular vocal fold vibration. The traces show great instability and no control of pitch. The auditory impression was of a high pitched diplophonic voice quality with a great deal of whisper. (b) Post-treatment. After voice therapy the same patient is able to control her pitch better and produce smooth *Fx* intonation contours showing good variation in pitch for the same utterances. 'Hello, how are you?' shows some loss of pitch control, possibly due to difficulty in control of onset of voicing after the voiceless [h]. There is a sudden drop in pitch in the latter part of the utterance to well below anything previously produced.

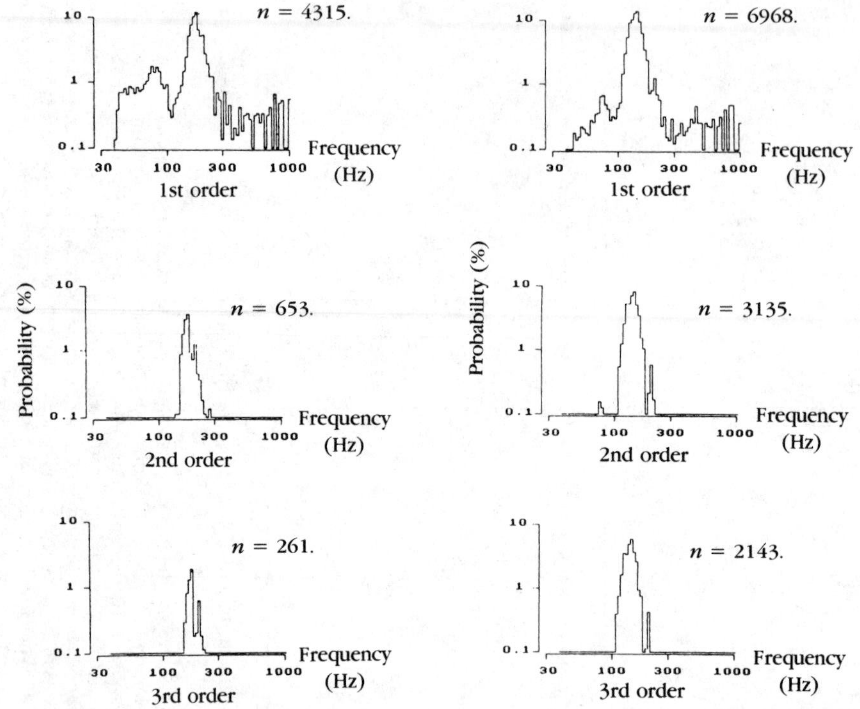

Title: S1	ORDER 1	2	3
Mode (Hz)	177	177	177
Mean (Hz)	158	176	178
Variance	3.07	0.41	9E-2
S.D. (log Hz)	0.248	9.1E-2	4.3E-2
	89/280	143/217	161/197
Median (Hz)	171	175	175
80% (Hz)	70-248	157-208	160-206
	(178)	(51)	(46)
90% (Hz)	54-457	149-224	156-216
	(403)	(75)	(60)
SAMPLE SIZE	4315	653	261

Title: S3	ORDER 1	2	3
Mode (Hz)	147	147	147
Mean (Hz)	151	143	143
Variance	1.62	0.17	0.14
S.D. (log Hz)	0.18	5.9E-2	5.3E-2
	100/229	124/164	126/162
Median (Hz)	144	143	144
80% (Hz)	117-200	124-164	125-164
	(83)	(40)	(39)
90% (Hz)	86-395	119-174	120-173
	(309)	(55)	(53)
SAMPLE SIZE	6968	3135	2143

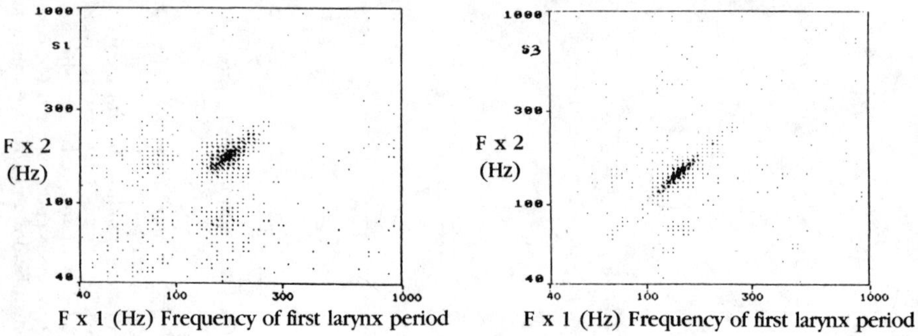

Figure 7.11 (a) (b)

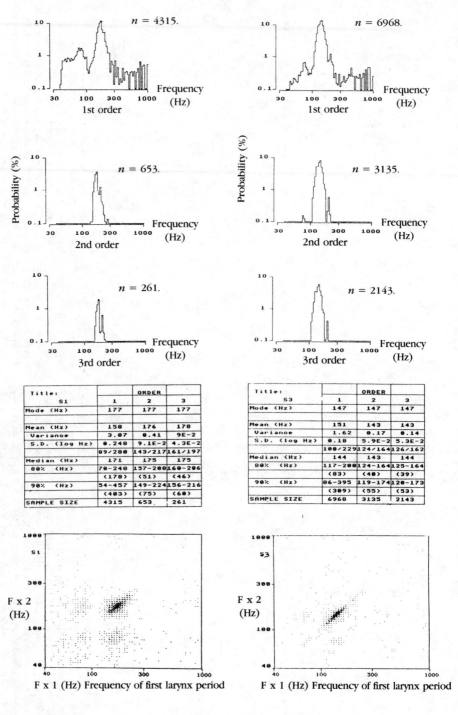

Figure 7.11 (*opposite*). Fundamental frequency distributions, statistics and scatter plots. These illustrate graphically and numerically, pitch parameters in detail. *Dx* plots or histograms, first, second and third order, plot the registered vibrations according to their frequency and probability of occurrence. Second and third order only accept those where two and three adjacent vibrations respectively, fell in the same 'frequency bin'. They offer thereby an illustration of the amount of regularity in the voice. This is also shown by the density and length of the diagonal in the scatter plot or *Cx* distribution. (a) The preoperative pitch range of the young man with vocal fold palsy whose *Lx* was illustrated in Figure 7.9c. The first order speech sample shows bimodality (two 'peaks') and massive irregularity of fold vibrations confirmed by the dramatic reduction in the sample carried into second and third order. The central measurements are extremely high for a man; the mode is best for judging average pitch in this case due to the large amount of both low and high frequency irregularity. The scatter plot shows a very short dense diagonal with a lot of scatter along its full length but particularly at low pitch. (b) Postoperative speech sample showing a reduction in the amount of irregularity of vibrations. A larger proportion of the first order speech sample is carried into second and third order. A longer, thinner *Cx* diagonal shows the pitch range has been generally lowered and increased. This is further confirmed in the statistics, which show lower central measurements, much reduced variance and lower range within 80% and 90% of the distribution. n = number of *Tx* samples in plot.

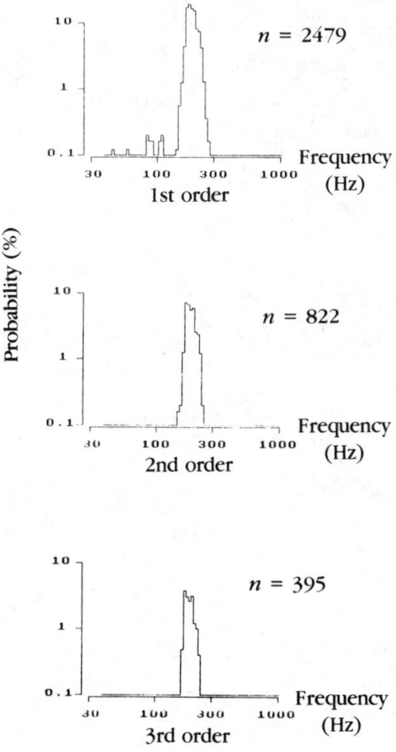

Title:	ORDER		
	1	2	3
Mode (Hz)	186	177	177
Mean (Hz)	193	194	193
Variance	0.3	6E-2	6E-2
S.D. (log Hz)	7.7E-2	3.7E-2	3.4E-2
	161/231	178/211	179/210
Median (Hz)	193	192	192
80% (Hz)	174-224	175-220	176-217
	(50)	(45)	(41)
90% (Hz)	167-233	173-227	174-225
	(66)	(54)	(51)
SAMPLE SIZE	2479	822	395

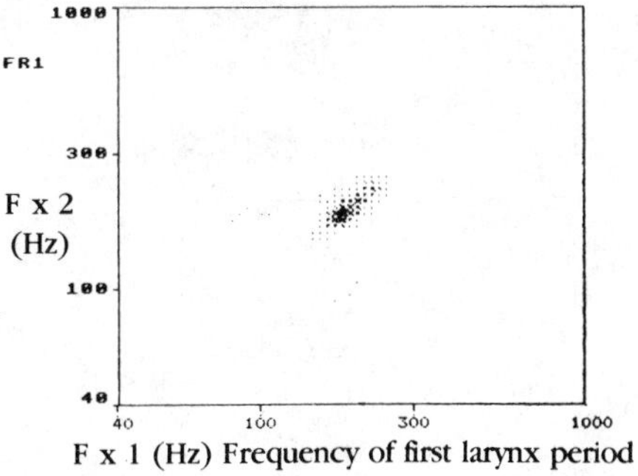

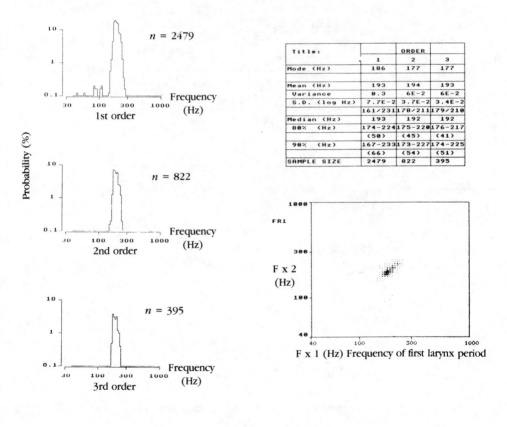

Figure 7.12. The very narrow range of pitch used in reading aloud by the female with oedematous vocal folds, illustrated by *Lx* in Figure 7.9b. n = number of *Tx* samples in plot.

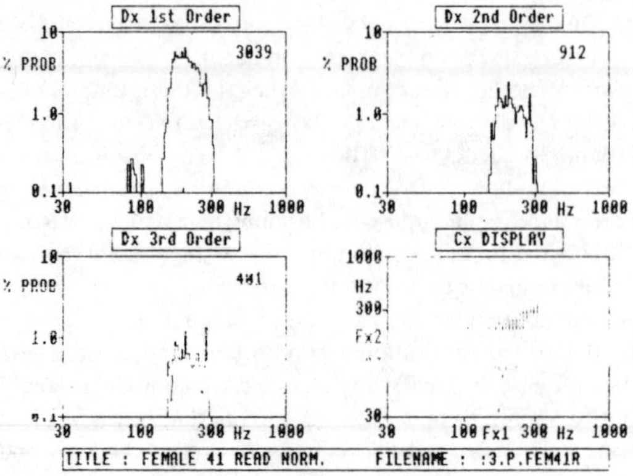

STATISTICS TABLE

TITLE : FEMALE 41 READ NORM. FILENAME ::3.P.FEM41R

DISTRIBUTION TYPE	Dx 1st Order	Dx 2nd Order	Dx 3rd Order
SAMPLE TOTAL	3039	912	401
MEAN	201.3 Hz	212.7 Hz	212.7 Hz
MODE	[illegible] Hz	206.9 Hz	287.5 Hz
MEDIAN	206.9 Hz	206.9 Hz	212.7 Hz
STANDARD DEVIATION	0.11 LOG-Hz	0.07 LOG-Hz	0.08 LOG-Hz
80% RANGE	166.2 272.2 Hz	170.8 279.7 Hz	170.8 287.5 Hz
90% RANGE	157.3 287.5 Hz	161.7 287.5 Hz	161.7 287.5 Hz

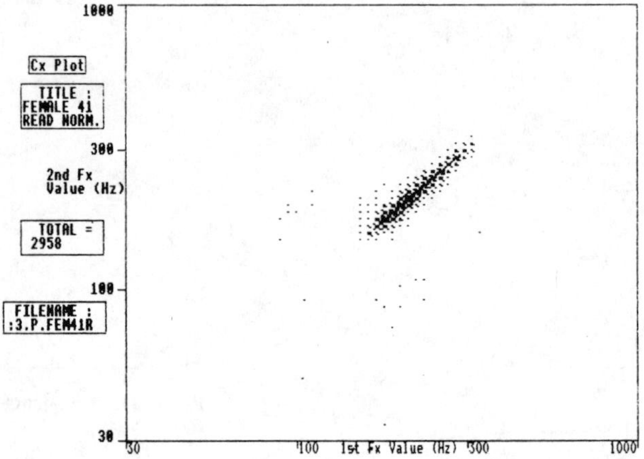

Figure 7.13. A normal female voice reading the same paragraph as in Figure 7.12.

Glottal imaging by processing external signals (GLIMPES)

This is a voice analysis programme which uses acoustic and glottographic signals to assess the configuration of the glottis. Inputs used include combinations of airflow, electroglottograph, photoglottograph, accelerometer and microphone signals (Titze, 1984).

Vocal Tract Imaging

Radiography

Radiography allows the visualisation of internal body structures by projection of roentgen rays through, for example, the pharynx onto a fluoroscopic screen. The image can be observed directly or photographed and recorded on cine film or video tape and synchronised with phonation. An image intensifier can be used to magnify the image. This technique is not suitable for the observation of the vocal fold because it is only possible to obtain lateral or frontal views. It is invaluable for the observation of lateral pharyngeal wall and soft palate movement and tongue positions. Radiography has replaced the lateral X-ray with barium outline used earlier (Calnan, 1955) which provided sagittal stills of the soft palate in emission of vowel sounds. Exposure to radiation must at all times be carefully controlled. Films can be used in treatment but direct fluoroscopy cannot be used routinely in therapy (McWilliams, Morris and Shelton, 1984).

Xeroradiography

This radiological process, originally developed for mammography, is used for imaging the vocal tract. An electrostatic image (still image) is produced on a xerographic plate which registers X-rays on an electrically charged plate instead of the conventional radiographic screen. Lateral life-sized views are photographed showing clearly the edge enhancement of soft tissues in three-dimensional depth as well as the contours of soft tissues, bones and cartilages seen in ordinary X-ray photography. Pharyngeal, lingual, soft palate and laryngeal 'gestures' are shown and are useful in observing undesirable muscular tensions and constriction. After therapy, restoration of relaxed positions can be shown to the patient and compared with previous tense gestures (Berry *et al.*, 1982).

The technique is expensive and, because it subjects the patient to higher dosage of X-rays than conventional procedures, it has strictly limited use. Gordon (1986) draws attention to the fact that there are other procedures which are cheaper and safer to administer, and readily available. These she claims give an equally clear definition.

The combination of xeroradiography and electrolaryngography (XEL) to provide objective analysis of vocal tract function has been developed by Berry *et al.* (1982).

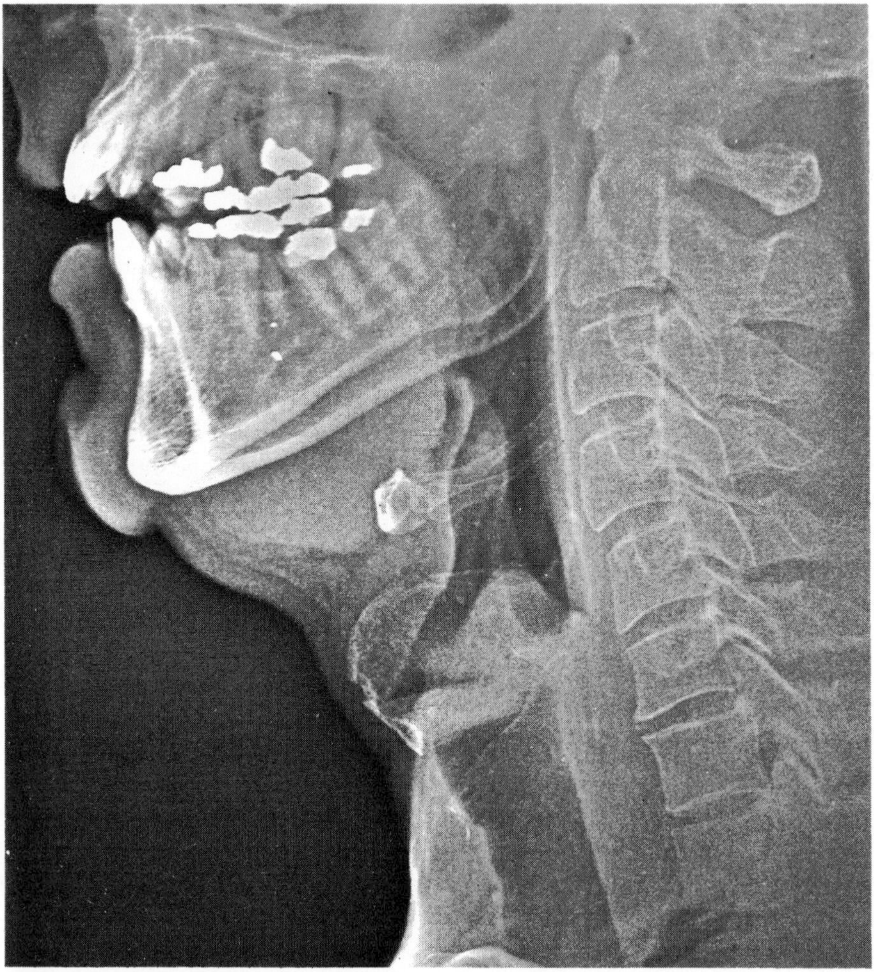

Figure 7.14. Xeroradiograph: normal vocal tract (phonating on /i:/). (By permission of Dr Frances MacCurtain, National Hospitals College of Speech Sciences, London.)

Acoustic Analysis

Oscilloscope

The amplitude and frequency of a sound wave is displayed on an oscilloscope screen. Some displays are temporary but others can be fixed on the screen for analysis. A permanent record of the displayed waveform is made by an attached chart recorder or by photography.

Sound spectrography

The spectrograph analyses sound. The spectrogram produced shows frequency on the vertical axis of the graph and duration of sound on the horizontal axis. The *intensity* is shown by the degree of blackening from the tracing pens. *Fundamental frequency* is shown by temporal separation of

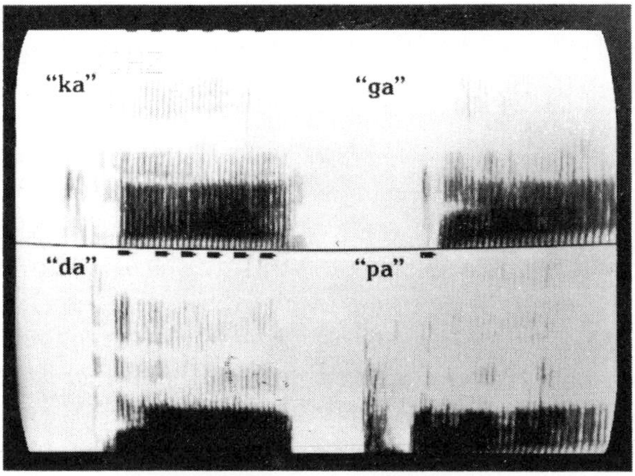

Note consonant differences.

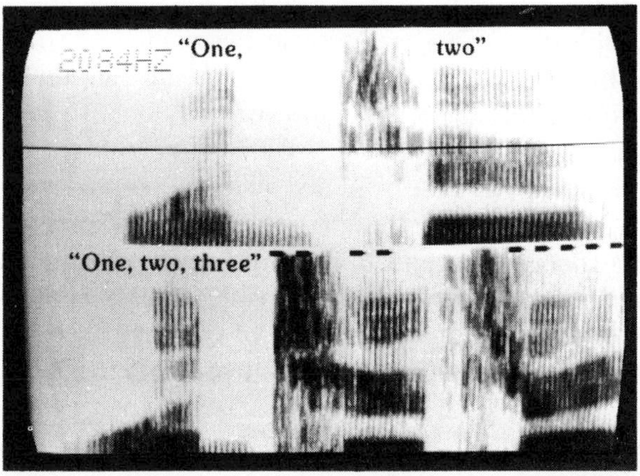

Cursor positioned at 3rd formant and digital display of cursor position.

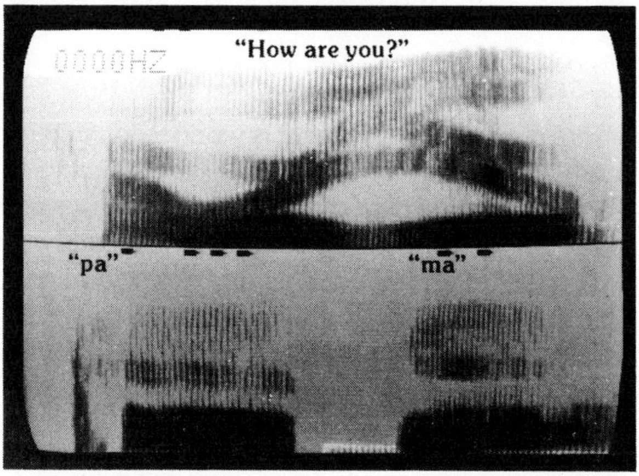

Note difficulty in word segmentation in running speech.

Figure 7.15. Spectrograms. (Courtesy of Kay Elemetrics Corp, NJ, USA.)

successive vertical striations in a wide band-width analysis. A narrow band-analysing filter can be used which shows frequency separation of successive harmonic lines occurring in the vowel formants.

The spectrographic analysis should be able to provide a reliable diagnostic method of describing voice disorder but, although valuable in assessment of individuals, a strong correlation between spectrogram and dysphonia type has not been established in order to render a standard classification possible. Yanagihara (1967a) investigated harmonic changes and noise components spectrographically during utterance of vowels in hoarse voice. Also the physiological mechanism (Yanagihara, 1967b) was examined with high speed cinematography. The harmonics-to-noise ratio can be measured clinically by computer (Yumoto, 1983).

The spectrogram is most useful for the assessment of an individual speaker's pronunciation of vowels. It provides an enormous amount of information, much of which is redundant and creates difficulty in defining which frequencies are responsible for particular vocal effects, especially in dysphonia. Establishing the characteristic harmonics of vowels and diphthongs should be relatively easy but in actual fact a great number of readings is necessary from different speakers in order to establish averages. This is because the spectrograph is so sensitive that it reveals the fact that every time an individual pronounces the same vowel the spectrogram is somewhat different from preceding ones. Added to which, different speakers have rather different modes of articulation of the vowel under acoustic analysis. The 'ear' solves this problem by being capable of classifying speech sounds within bands of frequencies by a system of comparison (contrastivity) between acoustic cues. The 'ear' has the cognitive ability to identify a particular acoustic system - hence the ability to understand the wide variants in the vowel systems encountered in dialects of English and, of course, the harmonic distortions in dysphonia.

Some of the commercial instruments available for acoustic analysis are listed below.

Kay DSP Sona-Graph Speech Analysis Workstation

The Sona-Graph is a complete signal analysis workstation incorporating a real-time spectrograph and a computer-based data acquisition system. It is a dual channel analyser with a split screen capability so that, for example, the lower screen can display a spectrographic analysis simultaneously with a laryngograph waveform on the upper screen. The playback system provides auditory feedback which can be listened to in conjunction with the visual display. Hard copies of the visual display can be obtained. Figure 7.16 shows a Sona-Graph Workstation.

Visispeech

This display system was developed by the RNID (Royal National Institute for the Deaf). It displays frequency, intensity and phonation time and can be used for assessment and to provide feedback during treatment.

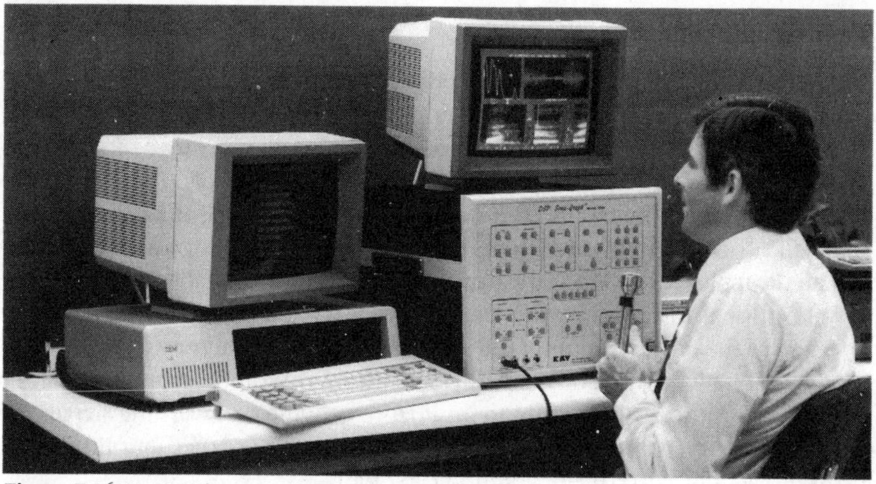

Figure 7.16. Kay DSP Sona-Graph Workstation. (Courtesy of Kay Elemetrics Corp, NJ, USA.)

Kay Visi-Pitch

This electronic instrument extracts fundamental frequency and relative intensity of the in-put signal and can be used for assessment and biofeedback procedures. The vocal parameters are displayed on a screen and visual representation of features such as pitch and intensity levels, glottal attack, voice quality and syllabic stress can be observed. It can be used with the laryngograph and a computer interface is available.

Tunemaster III

This instrument registers fundamental pitch and is strongly recommended by Boone (1987) for pitch assessment and remediation programmes.

Glottal Frequency Analyser

This compact equipment provides information concerning fundamental frequency and has the facility for providing a hard copy. It is manufactured by Entomed AB.

Instrumentation which measures intensity alone is available in various forms. The VU (volume unit) meter on a tape recorder is useful for providing visual feedback of loudness when measurement is not required.

Sound Level Recorder (Brüel and Kjaer model 2307)

A strip-chart record is produced by this complex instrument which is able to record rapid changes in intensity.

Sound Level Meter (Brüel and Kjaer model 2230)

Intensity level is shown on a meter but there is no permanent output record. Baken (1987) suggests that it is best for measuring the intensity of steady-state sounds such as prolonged vowels.

TAM (tactile acoustic monitor)

TAM is a biofeedback device which provides tactile stimulation from a small instrument strapped to the wrist. Incoming sounds are amplified and these signals operate a vibrator which is sensitive to a frequency range of 100 Hz to 10 kHz. In conjunction with the temporal pattern of sounds in the environment it renders sound sources recognisable to the profoundly deaf, the blind and cochlear implant patients for whom the instrument was designed by the medical physics group at the University of Exeter in collaboration with the Royal National Institute for the Deaf. It has a volume control which can be adjusted to the requirements of the wearer against ambient noise. There is also a light which flickers on and off in unison with sound stimuli. A battery charger is provided. Although primarily an invaluable generator of warning signals for the deaf, it may also be used in voice therapy to monitor voice amplitude and prosodic accent patterns in dysphonic patients.

Vocal Loudness Indicator (Jedcom)

This portable, battery-operated, biofeedback device displays relative levels of voice loudness on a display of eight lights. It has an integral microphone and a sensitivity control for adjustment.

Vocal Intensity Controller

A portable instrument used by Holbrook, Rolnick and Bailey (1974) in which a throat microphone activates a tone generator which sends signals to earphones, registering excessive vocal intensity. It can be worn continuously. Eleven patients out of 32 in this experiment experienced complete resolution of vocal abuse.

Airflow and Volume Measurement

Airflow pressure and respiratory volumes are of such direct relevance to normal voice production and dysphonia that aerodynamic studies have been the basis of considerable number of research projects. Respiratory volumes, control of expiration and temporal aspects are an essential feature of assessment. Gordon, Morton and Simpson (1978) reported that in a corpus of 73 cases of 'mechanical dysphonia' (vocal misuse), 47.9% showed disturbed breathing patterns at rest and 79.5% were unable to maintain steady flow rate in phonation.

Spirometry

The first spirometer was built in 1846 by John Hutchinson who wanted to measure the amount of air an individual could exhale after full inspiration. These simple instruments are still used in hospital respiratory function tests (Boone, 1977). Vital capacity, tidal capacity and complemental air are measurable.

Wet spirometer

This simple instrument works on the gasometer principle and is known also as a pulmometer. An inverted glass cylinder is situated inside a cylinder containing water. As air is blown into the inverted receiver through a rubber tube the volume of air expired is measured. The receiver is displaced in cubic centimetres against calibrations on the external frame of the instrument.

A simple, non-invasive, home-made device based on similar principles has been suggested by Hixon, Hawley and Wilson (1982) in order to assess whether an individual has sufficient 'respiratory driving pressure' for speech.

Dry spirometer

A dry spirometer is also used which consists of a small aerometer in a container with a calibrated dial. It is less reliable as it is sensitive to the force with which breath is exhaled (Steer and Hanley, 1959; Boone, 1977).

A simple spirometer measures expiratory volumes and can provide a useful measure of respiratory function but in the light of present electronic technology it is somewhat primitive and limited in the information it provides. However, it is inexpensive and reliable and easily available from hospital chest departments.

Electrospirometer

Electrospirometers have been developed in accordance with the needs of speech therapy departments. These instruments provide an accurate measure of lung capacity and function, e.g. vital capacity, reserve volume. A mask is worn by the subject during this procedure (which children may not tolerate) and airflow measurement in speech is not easy. Airflow studies during vowel production in measurement of maximum phonation time have tended to be the focus of assessment (Isshiki, 1965; Isshiki, Okamura and Morimoto, 1967; Yanagihara, 1967a; Yanagihara and Koike, 1967).

Pneumotachograph

A pneumotachograph is used for calculating airflow rate. The airflow volume over a given time can also be established. A specially designed face mask allows separate measurement of airflow from nose and mouth. When these measurements are being made in relation to phonation a mask is worn in order to leave the mouth as free as possible although even this can constrict mandibular movement and affect the sound. Some investigators then prefer to use a modified plethysmograph in which the subject is completely sealed within a box (Proctor, 1980; Baken, 1987).

A Mercury Electronic pneumotachograph system incorporating a spirometer was used by Gordon (1977) to measure breath flow rates and volumes. The flow-head attached to a rubber face mask was fitted with a microphone. Sound was recorded on a Ferrograph audio-tape recorder. A laryngograph was also used to monitor *Lx* waveform in production of vowels. Over a period of 18 years valuable contributions to the understanding of respiratory function in dysphonias have been published by the team of the dysphonia clinic at the Victoria Infirmary, Glasgow under the direction of Simpson (1971). Their papers are worthy of study (Simpson, 1971; Kelman *et al.*, 1975, 1981; Gordon, 1977, 1986).

Mercury (Scotland) Ltd produce an extensive range of lung function analysers which use screen pneumotachographs. Certain models are microprocessor based and are designed to extract relevant values from the maximal expiratory flow-volume curve. The displays are in numerical form.

Pneumography

Two types of instrumentation are used in registration of respiratory movement of the rib cage and abdominal wall at rest and during speech. These are magnetometry and impedance pneumography. Both methods are non-invasive.

Magnetometry

The magnet coils which are encased in polyethylene are glued to the chest wall. The basic principle is that of sensing with the coil the strength of a magnetic field when measuring body diameter (Baken, 1987). Hixon, Mead and Goldman (1976) measured hemicircumference anteroposterior diameters of rib cage and abdomen in upright and supine postures during conversation, reading and singing. Among many pertinent observations they noted that the abdominal wall occupies an especially important role in running conversation. The abdominal wall mechanically times the rise of the diaphragm to express air for speech.

Impedance pneumography

This procedure can be used in tracking vegetative respiratory movements in infants, a function for which magnetometry is not suitable. Mercury-filled strain gauges (strain gauge pressure transducers) are strapped to the chest wall. They are completely comfortable and can be worn for long periods. Normal changes in the posture of the baby leave them undisturbed. Impedance pneumography monitors movement of chest and abdominal walls but the true relevance of such movements in phonation requires linkage with measurement of lung volumes used in phonation and maintenance of pressure. Unfortunately, electrospirometry or spirometry of any sort is not applicable to infants (Langlois, Baken and Wilder, 1980).

Nasal Resonance

Nasal anemometry

TONAR

Oral and nasal sound intensity are measured as indices of hypernasality by the TONAR (The Oral Nasal Acoustic Ratio) developed by Fletcher (1970). Microphones are placed in the oral and nasal cavities which process frequencies from 50 to 20 kHz. The oral and nasal sound intensity ratio by which 'nasalance' (Fletcher, 1970, 1972) is registered can be adjusted by the clinician to selected levels of performance. Nasalance is the acoustic correlate of perceived nasality. The ratings are displayed digitally and a reinforcement panel lights up and provides biofeedback when the target is achieved. The clinician's judgement of imbalance between oral and nasal resonance and necessary adjustments is crucial.

TONAR II was produced to provide biofeedback but was expensive, bulky and technically demanding according to McWilliams, Morris and Shelton (1984). The Kay Elemetrics Corporation now produces the Nasometer which measures, in real time, the ratio of acoustic energy from the nasal and oral cavities. Calculation of the ratio is immediate and a visual feedback system provides instant graphic and statistical information.

Exeter Nasal Anemometry System

This anemometry system developed by Ellis *et al.* (1978) measures nasal airflow during speech and provides an index of palatal efficiency by means of a digital display. If good quality audio-recordings of the patient are made they can be sent to the university centre for processing. A dual trace chart is subsequently returned with the tape to the speech therapist showing speech on the upper trace and associated airflow on the lower trace (Ellis, 1979). The anemometer can be used to measure improvements in palatal efficiency after using a palatal training device produced by the same team (Curle, 1979). A visual aid is also available (Tudor and Selley, 1974).

The Exeter Bio-Feedback Nasal Anemometer (EBNA) has been designed specifically as a biofeedback device and is less expensive than the previously described piece of equipment which is primarily an assessment instrument.

SeeScape (Winslow)

The SeeScape detects nasal emission of air during speech rather than nasality. The nasal tip is placed in one of the patient's nostrils, and any nasal emission of air causes a float to rise in the rigid plastic tube which is calibrated.

Muscle Function

Electromyography (EMG)

Surface electromyography

The action potential of external laryngeal muscles can be displayed on an oscilloscope by placing electrodes upon the skin of the throat. The amplitude of the electric impulses as the muscles contract is displayed. Surface myography supplies only limited information concerning muscular activity.

Intrinsic laryngeal muscle EMG

In order to measure the potential of individual muscles, for example the cricothyroid, lateral and posterior cricoarytenoids, a needle electrode is inserted into the muscle being investigated. This potentially uncomfortable, invasive technique is only practised by doctors. It is used in cases of vocal fold paralysis and may be helpful in diagnosis, planning surgical intervention and in making a prognosis (Hirano, 1981).

Exeter palatal training device

Selley (orthodontist) in collaboration with Tudor (speech therapist) (Tudor and Selley, 1974) devised a palatal training appliance coupled to a visual display for treatment of hypernasal speech. The palatal appliance consists of a 'U'-shaped loop of orthodontic wire attached to an acrylic base plate and extending backwards to touch the resting soft palate at the level of normal maximum lift for the patient. The patient is soon able to lift the palate off the wire as a voluntary movement. The appliance increases awareness of palatal movement and brings it under voluntary control. This produces good results and can be worn permanently. It can be used with cleft palate patients and in selected cases of dysarthria. When this palatal training device is linked to the visual display, so that a light indicates whether or not the palate is elevated, there is a further marked improvement. Improvement has frequently been achieved by biofeedback where lengthy traditional methods of speech therapy have failed.

The palatal plate has to be carefully fitted and moulded. Fitting of the insulated steel electrodes at the end of the wire loop for link-up with the visual aid presents further work and expense.

Amplification

Amplifiers can be used to ensure that the patient with a quiet voice can be heard and can also provide feedback during therapy. The most commonly used amplifiers can be worn in a shirt or jacket pocket. Larger table top equipment is available for talking to small groups or a larger audience. In addition to hand-held microphones, some amplifiers can be used with either a headset or throat amplifier.

Pocket models

Thackraycare	Cooper-Rand Amplifier
Jedcom	De Luxe Speech Amplifier MkII
	Summit Amplifier
Mediquip	Model Freiburg
	Medici Speech Aid Amplifier
	Mediquip Amplifier

Portable public address systems

Thackraycare	Voicette Amplifier
	Porta-Amp

Information concerning telephone amplifiers is available from the local sales offices of British Telecom in the UK or from the appropriate telephone company in other countries.

Researchers utilise techniques, such as ultrasound, in addition to those described in this chapter. Zagzebski, Bless and Ewanowski (1983) conducted a study of the larynx using pulse echo imaging and rapid ultrasonic scanners. The advantage of this method is that there is no known radiation hazard or interference with sound production, while the equipment is available in most hospital settings. Multidimensional views of the larynx were obtained by Fukada *et al.* (1983) by using X-ray stroboscopy and an ultra-high-speed camera. Investigations of laryngeal adjustment for the initiation of sound have been conducted by Hirose, Sawashima and Yoshioka (1983) using simultaneous EMG and fibrescopic study. A developing area of research related to laryngeal function is the use of computerised mathematical models (Titze, 1981).

The addresses of manufacturers are given in Appendix I at the end of the book.

Chapter 8
Hyperkinetic Dysphonia: Vocal Misuse and Abuse

Before proceeding with details of patient management and remedial therapy, a brief explanation is necessary of the rubric the authors agreed upon in presenting the considerable range of data involved.

Dysphonia due to mechanical misuse is the most common problem the speech pathologist working with dysphonic patients will have referred for treatment. A fundamental consideration in rehabilitation is instruction in the mechanics of phonation and the correction of faults leading to normal function and recovery of vocal health. This is achieved by giving the patient insight into aspects of behaviour which affect phonation such as tension, respiratory patterns, posture and various psychological factors. *The broad base of the rehabilitation programme used in the treatment of hyperkinetic dysphonia is therefore applicable as a foundation to the treatment of all other types of dysphonia. The basic principles pertain whether the voice disorder is the result of a cleft palate, laryngeal palsy or laryngectomy.* Physiological, acoustic and linguistic features of normal voice have to be matched against normal function of every sort. When the damage cannot be cured, as in neurological or anatomical anomalies, compensating strategies have to be devised which are dependent upon knowledge of normal physiological function.

Therefore the rubric in Part II is the presentation of hyperkinetic dysphonia in Chapter 8 followed by remediation procedures. In subsequent sections where the characteristic symptoms in different types of dysphonia need special attention, suggested remedies will be described as addenda to the basic aetiology and symptoms manifest. Appropriate exercises for specific aspects of dysfunction will be provided after presentation of other dysphonias not due to vocal misuse.

Vocal Misuse (Strain)

Hyperkinetic means excessive expenditure of energy in muscular movements. With regard to voice production the term refers to excessive tension in all the muscles involved in phonation, especially the intrinsic laryngeal muscles. Subglottic expiratory pressure builds up below the vocal folds which offer resistance to airflow. Excessive energy goes into phonation and the easy rhythmic vibratory cycle is lost. Gordon, Morton and Simpson (1978) term the dysphonia arising from incorrect voice production as 'mechanical dysphonia'. Another term used is 'habitual dysphonia' (Fawcus, 1986b) because of the habit factor involved in misuse. 'Muscular tension dysphonia' is preferred by Morrison, Nichol and Rammage (1986).

Vocal features

The chief symptom in hyperkinetic dysphonia is hoarseness which varies according to the degree of misuse. This is frequently accompanied by visible excessive tension of the external laryngeal muscles during phonation which can be felt if the neck and suprahyoid muscles are palpated. The larynx may be seen to rise dramatically at the onset of phonation. The predominant voice features are likely to be breathiness and, more variably, harshness with frequent hard glottal attack (Morrison, Nichol and Rammage, 1986). In the early stages of vocal misuse the chief complaint may be that of muscular fatigue – a tired and aching throat which increases during the day but recovers with rest. The voice may be hoarse but not necessarily so, though forcing of the voice to maintain volume will be evident. There may also be increased sensitivity of the laryngeal mucosa so that a particularly rapid intake of air, temperature changes or certain foods will cause coughing. However, there is no stable correlation between damage to the vocal folds and type of hoarseness (Zilstorff, 1968).

Yanagihara (1967b) analysed the formants in hoarse voices spectrographically. He found the acoustic properties of hoarseness in the cardinal vowels analysed were noise components occurring in the main formants, especially the second formant, and loss of energy in high frequency harmonic components. On this basis he postulated that confusions in subjective evaluation might be eradicated and classification of hoarseness on a basis of noise components and loss of harmonics might be arrived at. However, the extreme irregularity of the glottal waves and the fact that the spectrographic tracings showed wide variance from vowel to vowel each time the same vowel is uttered, makes such classification impossible. Subjective judgement by ear remains the most reliable means of evaluation for the practical purposes of voice remediation.

Respiration in vocal strain

While concentrating upon the laryngeal symptoms and state of the vocal folds in cases of chronic misuse, the need to assess lung volumes and airflow must not be overlooked. Cheerleaders whose role is to shout at the tops of their voices provide a useful population for the study of vocal abuse as they commonly suffer from intermittent dysphonia. Reich and McHenry (1987) reported a study of female cheerleaders with histories of dysphonic episodes. Subjects were divided into two groups. Group 1 consisted of cheerleaders who reported acute cheer-related dysphonic episodes. Group 2 reported minimal or no such history. Vital capacity, inspiratory capacity, inspiratory reserve volume and tidal volume were measured. It was found that group 2 exhibited significantly greater vital capacity and inspiratory reserve volume than group 1. This confirms the often stated fact that respiratory efficiency is the basis of healthy phonation and protects the larynx in very demanding performances.

Laryngeal features

Laryngoscopy may show over-adduction of the vocal folds in the anterior section but an open posterior glottic chink between the arytenoid cartilages. Morrison, Nichol and Rammage (1986) report these features to be the main laryngoscopic aspects of increased laryngeal muscle tension. In cases of excessive tension the ventricular folds may be involved in movement medially and downwards, constricting the ventricles. The voice is harsh, with vocal fry evident and is referred to as 'ventricular band voice', although it is the constricted vocal folds which actually produce phonation. There is a strong psychogenic background to this disorder.

The throat may become so tired as a result of the effort used in speech that the vocal folds cease to be over-adducted and exhibit, in contrast, a slackness and insufficient approximation described by the laryngologist as 'bowing' of the vocal folds. The voice is husky and weak, a condition often described as phonasthenia. In these cases it may indicate anxiety and depression and feelings of hopelessness in contrast to the more aggressive personality which employs a laryngeal action indicative of a fighting spirit.

Vocal strain may exist for years, with a history of hoarseness after much talking and loss of voice with colds. Discomfort is increased with exposure to pollutants such as dust, fumes, dry atmosphere, spirits and especially smoking. Shouting and speaking against noise, stress at work or in the domestic situation, fatigue and poor health all aggravate the condition. As time progresses, a habit is established in which the speaker attempts to increase loudness because of the inadequacy of the voice. Vocal quality deteriorates further due to increased effort and as a result the muscular tension is again increased, and a vicious circle is established.

If vocal misuse and strain can be diagnosed early and given appropriate treatment, the sufferer can be cured and patterns of good voice production established with relative ease. If it is not identified and the damaging patterns of voice production and other sources of laryngeal abuse are allowed to continue the situation will deteriorate. It is unlikely to remain static or to improve spontaneously.

Vocal misuse can develop into vocal abuse when continuous over-exertion of the vocal folds produces actual damage to their surfaces and penetrates into the layers of the lamina propria. The acute symptoms of damage are often precipitated by a respiratory infection and persist after the infection has passed. At this stage otolaryngological examination is essential in order to investigate the laryngeal condition and the health of the chest, ears and sinuses.

The necessary medical and, possibly surgical, treatment must be prescribed prior to speech therapy.

Vocal Abuse

Chronic laryngitis

Chronic laryngitis is a long-term condition involving generalised oedema and inflammation of the mucous membrane of the vocal folds. A dry cough, tickle and constant throat clearing often accompany the disorder and aggravate the laryngeal inflammation. Respiration for voice production is uncontrolled, lacking the necessary rhythmic central movement and exhibiting a 'clavicular' pattern of thoracic movement. This condition may follow an acute viral infection and sore throat or may develop insidiously (Ballantyne and Groves, 1982). Faulty voice use appears to be a prime factor and Morrison, Nichol and Rammage (1986) reported that they had usually observed the condition in adult males, particularly those at the beginning of a singing career without the benefit of good singing tuition. Chronic laryngitis is also associated with excessive smoking, spirits, dust and fumes or continual coughing due to infection or allergic rhinitis. It may be a precursor to polypoidal degeneration.

Polypoidal degeneration (Reinke's oedema; polypoid corditis)

Acute laryngitis and vocal abuse can produce an oedematous swelling along the full length of the vocal folds. Sometimes this is described by laryngologists as a 'polypoid fringe'; it tends to be regarded as a separate condition from vocal fold polyps (Bennet, Bishop and Lumpkin, 1987). The space between the mucosal cover of the fold and the superficial layer of the lamina propria, known as Reinke's space, fills with fluid. The mucosal cover of the vocal folds becomes less stiff and increases in mass because of the increased blood and fluid. The oedematous swelling is usually bilateral and symmetrical but it may be unilateral.

The voice deepens due to the bulk of the vocal folds and is severely hoarse. In their study of phonatory characteristics associated with polypoidal degeneration, Bennet, Bishop and Lumpkin (1987) found that the speaking fundamental frequency became much lower than normal and even lower than in conditions such as laryngeal cancer. For this reason they regard it as a diagnostic indicator. Their work also showed that the extremes of the pitch range are affected, with both the upper and lower range significantly lowered.

The fluid can be removed by suction, and the 'fringe' appearance disappears as the membrane is restored to its natural position. In more severe conditions stripping or decortication of the vocal folds may be necessary (Kleinsasser, 1968). A strip of epithelium is removed from the surface of one fold and the undersurface of the opposite fold to prevent the danger of adhesion of raw surfaces in healing. Alternatively, the second vocal fold can be operated upon some weeks later. The voice should be given total rest for at least a week after surgery (Fritzell, Sundberg and Strange-Ebbesen, 1982) and not used before healing has been confirmed by laryngoscopy. The voice improves and rises to normal pitch spontaneously.

Although microendolaryngeal surgery ensures a laryngeal image of extreme clarity, greatly magnified, rendering a slip of the knife unlikely, excellence of surgery nevertheless varies and is dependent upon experience. This may account for the fact that full vocal recovery does not always take place with the complete healing of the epithelium. Prolonged hoarseness and fatigue may continue and may well be due to damage to the mechanoreceptors (Wyke, 1967, 1969, 1983). Fritzell, Sundberg and Strange-Ebbesen (1982) note that the voice may take between 6 and 12 months to recover fully.

It may be necessary to take a biopsy so that the possibility of malignant disease in a persistent inflammatory condition can be excluded. Speech therapy can be started before surgery, if thought necessary. Much can be done in assessment of origins of vocal abuse, and instruction and breathing can be given without using the voice.

In Kleinsasser's (1968) experience polypoid degeneration occurred most commonly among smokers of both sexes over the age of 40 years and this finding was confirmed by Bennett, Bishop and Lumpkin (1987). Morrison, Nichol and Rammage (1986) report that it is most common in older women. However, although prolonged smoking is accepted as a causative factor, opinions regarding the contribution of vocal abuse vary. Kleinsasser is of the opinion that postoperative speech therapy is necessary only when patients have used their false folds in phonation prior to operation. Bennett, Bishop and Lumpkin (1987) regard both smoking and vocal abuse as contributory. Their study indicated that prolonged smoking was the major factor, with only 25% of the subjects exhibiting vocal abuse. In view of the fact that habitual vocal abuse is a possible cause of oedema in some patients, it would appear advisable that assessment by a speech therapist be arranged as a matter of course postoperatively if not preoperatively. Fritzell, Sundberg and Strange-Ebbesen (1982) describe a patient who did not have speech therapy and subsequently developed vocal nodules.

The interested reader is strongly advised to study the beautiful colour photographs in Kleinsasser's (1968) book *Microlaryngoscopy and Endolaryngeal Microsurgery* in which the conditions in this chapter are illustrated and details of surgical and postoperative management are given.

Vocal fold polyps

Kleinsasser (1968) noted that vocal fold polyps are the most common laryngeal disease. They arise as a result of vigorous laryngeal use resulting in a submucosal haemorrhage which with connective tissue forms a polyp (Wilson, 1987). Histologically there are several types of polyp, chiefly the 'gelatinous' polyp which appears as a soft translucent structure and the fibrous polyp which may be a more advanced form. The great majority occur singly. In a series of 100 operated cases Kleinsasser found 79% were simple and 21%

presented with two or more polyps. The typical site is 3 mm behind the anterior commissure and on the subglottic surface of the vocal fold.

It is generally believed that hyperkinetic movement of the vocal folds is the chief cause of vocal polyps (Luchsinger and Arnold, 1965; Morrison, Nichol and Rammage, 1986). Speech therapy is therefore usually recommended following their surgical removal.

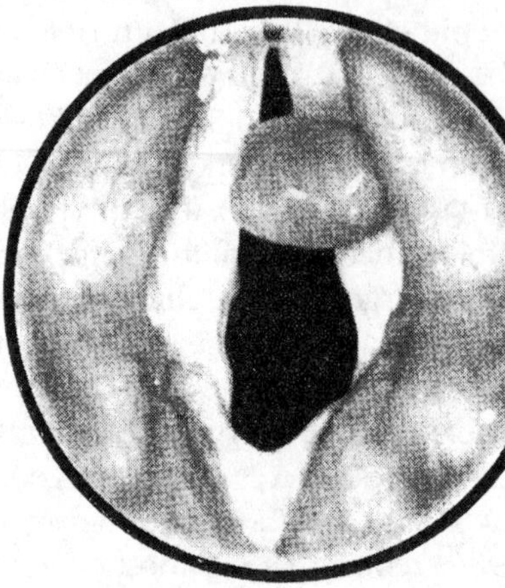

Figure 8.1. Vocal fold polyp.

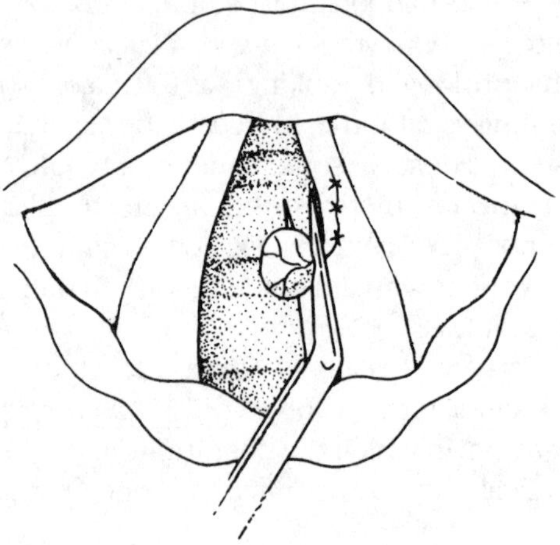

Figure 8.2. Surgical removal of vocal fold polyp.

Vocal nodules

Vocal abuse has to be persistent to produce lasting changes in the epithelium covering the vocal folds. An isolated trauma such as shouting, a scream of fright or an exacting singing performance may produce a tiny submucous haemorrhage in a capillary but this will be absorbed and disappear after a day or two if there is no repeat of the performance. Continuous misuse, however, can perpetuate and aggravate the damage. Initially, laryngoscopy shows the beading of mucus on the folds at the predestined site of nodules which is at the junction of the anterior two-thirds of the vocal folds – their vibratory section. They are comparable to callouses and formed by friction between opposing surfaces of the vocal fold. They are generally bilateral but occasionally unilateral in which case some reddening or slight swelling will be apparent on the opposite side, caused by the abrasive action of the opposing node.

Vocal nodules or nodes, sometimes called singers' or screamers' nodes, are entirely non-malignant minute neoplasms seldom exceeding 1.5 mm in diameter. Starting with local inflammation and oedema they appear as soft red swellings on the edges of the fold where amplitude of excursion is greatest and maximum contact and velocity in the vibratory cycle occurs. In time the swellings gradually fibrose and harden as connective tissue proliferates and chronic nodules, white in colour and conical in shape, become established. The tissue surrounding the nodule may be oedematous.

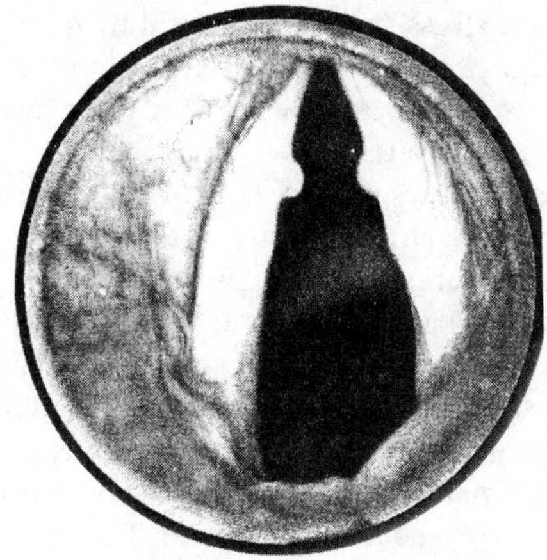

Figure 8.3. Vocal nodules.

Rest and vocal rehabilitation may be sufficient treatment to disperse nodules which have not yet fibrosed, but at the advanced chronic stage surgical removal under general anaesthetic is necessary, followed by speech therapy. After removal of the nodules, the voice should not be used until the mucous membrane is healed. Whispering can also cause damage at this stage. In forced whispering the anterior two-thirds of the vocal folds are tightly adducted and air passes through the triangular posterior aperture. Written messages should be used for a day or two.

Vocal nodules occur most commonly in children and more frequently in boys than girls under the age of 20 years (Heaver, 1958; Kleinsasser, 1968) After adolescence the incidence decreases in males and increases in females when the highest incidence appears to be in young to middle-aged females.

Personality factors

There is a constitutional and personality factor common to individuals who develop vocal nodes and polypoid conditions. They are mostly energetic, active, hard-working and anxious besides being talkative. Arnold (1962) and Luchsinger and Arnold (1965) state that vocal nodules present the reaction of local tissue to mental strain imposed by difficulties in adjusting to the demands made by society in persons of a certain personality structure. Arnold (1962) notes that the disorder is common in pyknic and athletic types and rare in asthenics. Nodes develop in vociferous and aggressive individuals rather than in soft-spoken and gentle-mannered people. However, we have seen patients who do not speak excessively loudly but with such tension and use of hard glottal attack that the folds have been damaged. There is such a strong anxiety component in the personality structure of these individuals who suffer from vocal abuse that one is led to believe that they are akin to psychosomatic disorders. Morrison, Nichol and Rammage (1986) reported that the majority of individuals with muscular tension dysphonia seen in their clinic had problems coping with stress. A fact confirmed by many others.

The individual who produces psychosomatic symptoms as described by Linford Rees (1982) is not necessarily neurotic but may be well adjusted and successful. They are anxious, tense, ambitious and self-driving, always competing with their fellows and trying to excel over them. The business executive, the singer and actor have this tension, ambition and drive besides many housewives and committee women on a smaller stage. They may be perfectionists and find it hard to delegate responsibility and resent offers of help which they regard as interference. It is not surprising that they develop fatigue, even exhaustion. They are of course, productive, responsible and reliable. The old saying 'if you want something done ask your busiest friend' takes advantage of this personality type which cannot refuse to undertake an interesting job and enjoys social commitment. Therapy for vocal abuse must always take into account the anxieties of the individual, and must attempt to bring them out into the open, so that patients can recognise stress and take steps to protect themselves from strain and overwork.

Contact ulcers

These present an extreme form of vocal abuse. The aetiology of ulceration of the folds in the arytenoid region was first related to vocal abuse by Jackson and Jackson (1935). They gave the condition its now accepted name of 'contact ulcer' on account of the trauma of 'hammer and anvil' with which the arytenoids strike each other in the forced type of phonation employed by these individuals. This action causes inflammation and eventually ulceration and granuloma or neoplasm on the mucous membrane covering the arytenoid region of the fold. Kleinsasser (1968) defines contact ulcers as contact pachydermia, the two names being synonymous for the one condition. He states that the lesions are not true ulcers nor granulomata. They consist of crater-like forms with highly thickened squamous epithelium piled up over connective tissue with some oedema.

In the UK where contact ulcers are a rarity there is some confusion over terminology and diagnosis. Thomson, Negus and Bateman (1955) did not recognise the existence of contact ulcers and insisted that the condition was pachydermia. Negus stated 'we have no experience as an entity but only of similar but variable appearance of hypertrophic laryngitis sometimes due to misuse of the voice, especially in foul air with excess of tobacco or alcohol, or syphilis or early and especially senile tuberculosis and what is generally recognised as pachydermia'. Arnold (1962) distinguishes between contact ulcers which consist of granuloma of the cartilaginous portion of the folds and pachydermia of the posterior commissure. This is the area between the arytenoids over the cricoid elevation, where no hammer and anvil or crater appearance is present. This interarytenoid pachydermia is caused by chronic infections and pollutants, especially smoking, and has nothing to do with vocal abuse.

Laryngeal appearance

The classic description of raised granuloma on one side and a crater on the other which fit together on contact like a ball and socket applies only in very advanced cases. In the early stages the arytenoid (cartilaginous) portions of the folds may simply appear oedematous and reddened. The anterior two-thirds of the folds may not appear healthy and exhibit some thickening of the epithelial cover. Bowing of the vocal folds anteriorly is often observable. The ulcer may be confined to one arytenoid region or both may be involved.

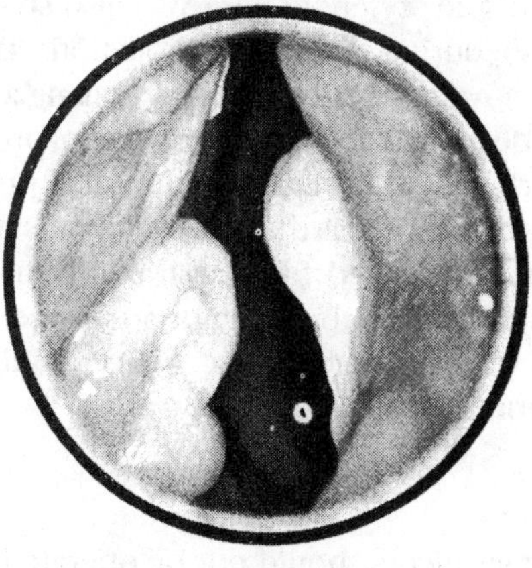

Figure 8.4. Granuloma.

Incidence

Contact ulcers are almost exclusively a male complaint. Vibration of the arytenoids occurs naturally in the pulse register (vocal fry) and contact ulcers develop in persons with deep voices. Women do not employ similar methods of voice production and do not develop contact ulcers. This condition is far more common in the USA, it seems, than in Europe where the condition is very rare (Brodnitz, 1961). Landes (1977) draws attention to the proclivity of American men to cultivate bass voices and comments: 'Somehow our culture seems to dictate that a bass voice is a mark of masculinity.' The high incidence of contact ulcers in the USA would appear to be a social phenomenon with many American men using a lower part of the pitch range than British men (Giles and Powesland, 1975).

In a period of 20 years in the busy ear, nose and throat department of St Bartholomew's Hospital, London, we had only three cases referred, all men. One with advanced lesions was operated upon and another cured by speech therapy alone. In the third case which was diagnosed early there was only oedema over the vocal processes. Interestingly, two of these patients were referred with a diagnosis of 'vocal nodes' by the laryngologist. This indicates that more cases may occur but be given the wrong name. Speech therapists, not having access to the medical notes or indirect laryngoscopy, may not be aware of the true condition, although the dysphonia is highly characteristic.

Vocal features

The voice is characteristically very deep, hoarse and hollow, and diagnostically unmistakable. The attempt to phonate may be very painful with a burning sensation in the larynx or shooting pain in the ear. This is understandable when the action of the arytenoids is seen in the high speed cinematographic film by Von Leden and Moore (1960). The arytenoids are seen to bang together in phonation while the pars respiratus is closed providing a 'posterior air shunt' (Proctor, 1974).

The mechanism of the arytenoid joint was also studied by Von Leden and Moor (1960, 1961) during vocal fry phonation. The arytenoids actually perform a rocking movement in two planes, making a wide excursion in low frequencies. In the deep throaty voice there occurs prolonged approximation of the arytenoid surfaces in the region of the vocal processes which exposes the folds to excessive stress and is the cause of contact ulcer. The equivalent of contact ulcer can be produced by anaesthetic intubation traumatising the vocal folds. In this case vocal abuse is not a consideration and vocal rest to promote healing is the necessary course. This condition is described further under laryngeal trauma (see p. 242).

Management

Newly formed contact ulcers should not be operated upon but treated with voice rest and voice therapy. Myerson (1952) claimed that removal of specific irritants could result in immediate alleviation of symptoms if at a mildly oedematous stage. He claimed that heavy smokers had lost their ulcers within 24 hours of ceasing to smoke. With established contact ulcers surgery is necessary. The hypertrophic epithelium, which develops through the effort to approximate the vocal folds as the separation of the arytenoids increases with development of the ulcers, may be stripped from the anterior sections of the cords. Absolute voice rest is advisable after surgery until healing is complete.

Voice therapy is essential and smoking should be abandoned if posible. Although the adverse effects of smoking are not substantiated by Peacher (1961) or Brodnitz (1961) (see below), it must be remembered that smoking is generally considered to be a prime cause of acute oedema and laryngitis in vocal misuse (Kleinsasser, 1968).

In view of the fact that contact ulcers are a rarity in Europe and there are valuable accounts available concerning quite large groups of patients in the USA, it is necessary to draw upon the experience and research of these speech pathologists. One fact that emerges is that the severe cases of contact pachydermia need surgery, sometimes several times, and that treatment is long and difficult in conjunction with voice remediation.

New and Devine (1949) followed the progress of 53 cases of contact ulcer. Six women in the series had ulceration due to intratracheal intubation, and three men. The contact ulcers of the remaining 44 males were of indeterminate aetiology. In this group 39 received surgery and 32 were eventually cured. A total of 73 operations was performed; some patients had as many as five. The patients were all in vocally demanding jobs such as salemen and all lived on a 'plane of high nervous tension'. Vocal remediation was not given.

Peacher and Holinger (1947) reported the results of research into the value of vocal re-education in the treatment of 16 cases of contact ulcer. An experimental group of six individuals who received weekly speech therapy was given instruction in vocal re-education. A control group of 10 individuals was treated surgically or by voice rest or both, but given no special instruction concerning voice. The results of this experiment showed that the contact ulcers did not heal in either the control or experimental groups unless the patient changed the method of voice production. All those who received vocal re-education showed a cessation of symptoms with total or nearly complete disappearance of the ulcer. Ulcers in the experimental group took from 1 month to 4 months to disappear, and in the control group from 7 months to 3 years. The patients in the experimental group were not made to rest their voices at all, the contention being that if the voice is used correctly talking will do no harm.

Peacher (1961) followed up 70 patients over periods of 1–12 years following voice therapy; five had a single recurrence of the condition and one of these developed malignancy. There was an operated and non-operated group: 34 patients had 80 operations before and during therapy, and 36 patients had no operations. The operated patients had an average healing time of 26.52 weeks and the non-operated group 10.05 weeks. The operated patients were not a control group but had advanced pachydermia and required surgery before therapy. There were 62 men and 2 women and mostly engaged in the speaking professions. Some had concentrated voice therapy and others extended over 2–8 months. The average number of hours of treatment was 5.6–8.0 hours but no correlation was found between healing time or number of hours of treatment. There was no correlation between time of healing and other factors such as smoking, drinking, voice rest and ability to carry a tune or duration of hoarseness prior to treatment. This study confirmed that the two main factors contributing to the condition are vocal abuse and emotional tension. The vocal abuse includes glottal attack, too low pitch, poor breath control and excessive coughing and throat clearing.

Brodnitz (1961) reported on 26 cases and confirms the relation of contact ulcers with stress; four of his patients developed stomach ulcers and a fifth a duodenal ulcer after healing of a contact ulcer. He also found no correlation between incidence and smoking and drinking. A constant urge to clear the throat and also a characteristic pain which radiates to the ear were present. He comments on the difficulty in effecting a cure which is admitted by all therapists.

Cooper and Nahum (1967) reported on 16 patients of whom 13 were cured and the rest were improving. These authors stressed the need for early diagnosis and voice therapy and described three stages or degrees of severity, it being far easier to treat a patient in the first stage, and to obtain a cure, than in later stages when all reports agree that treatment is long and difficult and relapses occur. They describe the first stage as one characterised by vocal fatigue and hoarseness by the end of the day with an oedema developing in the arytenoid region which may improve with rest. The second stage exhibits continual hoarseness and fatigue with occasional pain on swallowing and severe inflammation over the arytenoids. The third stage exhibits constant severe hoarseness, fatigue and pain in swallowing and talking, and ulceration of the cords which may require surgery.

Gastric reflux

Cherry and Margulies (1968) described three patients suffering from contact ulcers which failed to heal when treated by conventional voice rest and voice therapy. These patients were found to suffer from pharyngo-oesophagitis due to peptic acid reflux. Peptic reflux while the patient is asleep can seep into the posterior larynx and cause inflammation and ulceration. Gastric acidity was treated with suitable medication and the patients were advised to sleep on raised pillows. The ulcers were cured after a period of 3–6 months. Cherry and Margulies do not deny that vocal abuse is also a contributory factor and that voice therapy is advisable, but stress the need for peptic reflux to be included as a factor in assessment and diagnosis since this may be a precipitating factor. Cherry and Delahunty (1968) experimentally painted the vocal folds of dogs with gastric juice and found this produced inflammation and then ulceration.

> Case note
> Contact ulcers were diagnosed in a young man of 23 years who, after achieving a good university degree, was employed by a firm of merchant bankers in the City of London. He was extremely ambitious and determined to achieve rapid promotion. In an unconscious attempt to sound as mature and substantial as possible, particularly on the telephone, he had lowered his vocal pitch dramatically; this was accompanied by a posture of tucking his chin in towards his neck which maintained the larynx in an uncomfortably low position in the

vocal tract. A therapeutic programme of establishing awareness of this behaviour and the reasons behind it combined with improved voice production eventually solved the problem.

Vocal Misuse and Abuse in Children

Children can also develop changes in the laryngeal mucosa as a result of vocal abuse. Laryngoscopic examination may reveal chronic laryngitis, nodules or polyps. Polypoidal degeneration is less frequently seen in children than in adults (Wilson, 1987). The resulting dysphonia is not noticed by the child because it is not an inconvenience until the late, severe stages. However, the laryngoscopic examination of any child who remains dysphonic in the absence of upper respiratory tract infection is essential in order to exclude disease and to provide a basis for remediation.

Incidence

In view of the fact that most children shout during play it is perhaps surprising that more do not suffer from chronic hoarseness. Seth and Guthrie (1953) reported that in Germany 40% of school children had hoarse voices. Boys are more commonly afflicted than girls, and the incidence is high below the age of 10 years and diminishes considerably as children grow older (Curry, 1949). Baynes (1966) found 7.1% of children suffering from chronic hoarseness with the highest incidence in children in the first grade at school. Silverman and Zimmer (1975) found 23.4% of children with similar symptoms in their study.

Vocal behaviour

The dysphonic child with symptoms of vocal misuse or abuse probably talks loudly, shouts frequently, uses hard glottal attack and talks incessantly. Talking may continue regardless of the level of background noise and there may be no awareness that effort is increased in an attempt to counteract the competition. The voice is frequently misused in games and when imitating mechanical noises. These phonation patterns can be part of the speech pattern of an exuberant, extravert child who is involved and integrated in the peer group, is a leader of activities and directs with enthusiasm. The same vocal patterns can be heard in the tense, angry, frustrated child who uses the voice as a means of expressing his negative feelings. The habitual level of vocal loudness used in the family will also affect the child's vocal volume. The dynamics of family relationships can contribute significantly to vocal abuse or be its prime cause. For example, a mother with vocal nodules had three children, all of whom had the same condition.

Airflow studies

Observers note the throat tension and poor respiratory patterns for speech in dysphonic children. Sedlackova (1960) studied the pneumographic records of a large sample of children and reported:

1. A rapid drop in thoracic pressure at the end of phonation.
2. Exaggerated contraction of abdominal muscles.
3. Expiratory movement far exceeding the normal.
4. Arrests in expiration when talking.
5. Inverse breathing movements.

Gordon, Morton and Simpson (1978), using a pneumotachograph and a laryngograph, found considerable disturbances of airflow in all their patients (children and adults). There were two predominant breathing types:

1. An exceptionally high flow rate with short phonation time due to poor closure of the glottis.
2. Exceptionally low flow rate with prolonged phonation time but considerable laryngeal tension and glottal resistance.

Medical features

General health can be a primary factor in vocal abuse or make a significant contribution to the problem. Frequent upper respiratory tract infections may give rise to an acute laryngitis from which the child has little time to recover between each episode. These infections also lead to mouth-breathing so that dry air is drawn over the vocal folds and has an irritant effect. In addition, an infected postnasal discharge may aggravate the situation.

A mild laryngitis is often associated with enlarged tonsils and adenoids. There may be an intermittent or long-term hearing loss with this condition and others of the upper respiratory tract which results in children speaking more loudly in an attempt to hear themselves. Seeman (1959) observed that many children with hearing loss develop vocal nodes for this reason. Conductive hearing loss is a common symptom in cleft palate children in whom vocal nodules also occur frequently. McWilliams, Bluestone and Musgrove (1969) found that 27 children with repaired clefts and hoarseness had developed vocal nodules. The follow-up 5 years later showed that 70% of these children still had some abnormality of the vocal folds. It is not clear whether these children had incompetent palatopharyngeal sphincters and therefore used excessive laryngeal effort in compensation (see p. 214), or suffered from emotional disturbance. Renfrew (1988), in a personal communication, confirms the high incidence of vocal nodules in cleft palate children with incompetent palatopharyngeal sphincters. Surgery to improve the sphincter can disperse the nodules.

Allergic reactions in children are common; the allergen may be air-borne or ingested. Wilson (1987) cites a study by Senturia and Wilson who found a family history of allergy present in about 25% of children with laryngeal dysfunction. Dust (the house dust mite), fur, feathers and many other substances can cause a perennial rhinitis which gives rise to well-recognised symptoms. There are dark circles under the eyes and the child constantly performs the 'allergic salute' which consists of rubbing the nose with the finger, hand and even the arm, in one action, in an attempt to deal with the ever present moisture and itching. Pollens and moulds give rise to seasonal rhinitis (hay fever). In both types of rhinitis there will be sneezing, running nose, watery eyes and congested mucous membranes. The voice lacks nasal resonance and is breathy. Asthma may also be linked with vocal abuse because of incessant coughing during attacks and as a result of the respiratory involvement. In any condition of the upper respiratory tract which produces excessive secretions, resultant coughing and throat clearing predispose the child to vocal abuse because of the vigorous approximation of the vocal folds. The throat clearing may also become an habitual element of the vocal abuse pattern (see 'Psychosomatic aspect in anxiety state and disorders of nasal resonance', p. 163).

Wilson (1987) also notes that allergies to certain foods, especially dairy products, may produce mild to severe oedema of the laryngeal structures. Any portion of the larynx which looks pale and glistening may be indicative of an allergic reaction. Whatever the organic basis, there is also a psychogenic aspect in allergic reactions (Linford Rees, 1982). If the mother is obviously anxious and over-protective symptoms are exacerbated.

Management

Family involvement

Parental involvement and, if present, resolution of the child's anxieties are essential factors in successful voice therapy. Resting the voice cannot be imposed on the child in most cases and rigid rules for the avoidance of vocal abuse laid down by the speech therapist may only increase anxiety. If parents understand the underlying aetiology, the problem will resolve with their help and the laryngeal symptoms will disappear. Reassurance for the mother that the condition is not serious or harmful will allay anxiety.

Voice therapy

Even if there are vocal nodules, most laryngologists prefer not to operate but refer the child to the speech therapist. Others prefer to do no more than reassure the parents that the trouble is not serious and that their children will grow out of the symptoms. This is often the case, for as children grow older they shout and scream less. Moreover, as the larynx grows in puberty, especially in males, the pitch drops. The point of maximum excursion of the vocal folds alters position and the original site of mechanical trauma is no longer affected. If nodes are so large that a child becomes aphonic they will need surgical removal. Vocal nodules in children are seldom fibrosed and usually soft and oedematous, which is why they resolve if vocal abuse can be cured.

The speech therapist must identify the actual activities in which vocal abuse occurs by careful questioning of parents, teachers and the child. It may be reported that the child is noisy and excitable in the playground or yells at football matches or the situation requires correction of vocal abuse. Therapy must concentrate on relaxed breathing patterns and phonation, and should be interesting and as much fun as possible. The child's cooperation is essential in order to obtain carry-over of new patterns of voice conservation and production into everyday situations. Wilson (1987) describes suitable treatment procedures in detail.

Other professionals

In certain cases referral to a child guidance clinic or enlisting the help of a social worker or health visitor may be more beneficial than direct voice therapy.

Case histories

1. A 13-year-old boy was referred by his general practitioner to the ENT department following his teacher's concern about his permanently husky voice which occasionally became aphonic. Bilateral vocal nodules were diagnosed and he was referred to the speech therapist. The boy was unconcerned by the 'problem'. When he was interviewed with his mother it gradually became clear that his academic abilities were limited and he had little interest in school work, but he had a wide circle of friends with whom he was popular and who regarded him as the initiator and leader of their games. The boy lived on an open-plan housing development with extensive open spaces and the games involved a great deal of running, chasing and shouting instructions to different groups. He was an out-going, communicative individual at home, school and in the clinic, with a boisterous sense of humour. The family, consisting of mother, father and sister, was happy and supportive. Management of the case without surgical intervention was based on helping the boy to understand the functioning of the larynx and the aetiology of the nodules. It was pointed out to him and his mother that the condition would not remain static but that with his cooperation the nodules would completely recede; the alternative was steady deterioration. Speech therapy chiefly consisted of creating awareness of his damaging vocal behaviours and giving advice on more appropriate phonation. Apart from minor transgressions he maintained the suggested regimen and subsequent laryngoscopy 4 months later revealed normal vocal folds.

2. A 2-year-old girl was referred because of the child's hoarse and breathy voice; it did not worry her but her mother's concern had initiated the referral to the ENT department. Initial discussion revealed that the child had the expected tantrums of this age group which involved shouting and screaming; her vocal behaviour was

apparently not exceptional. However, bearing in mind that some degree of vocal abuse had played a part in her symptoms and that all 2 year olds do not have dysphonia, further information was necessary. It transpired that there were five older children in the family and that the little girl was frequently driven to a fury of frustration when she was ignored or unable to take part in the general conversation. The only ways in which she ensured attention were by shouting more loudly than her brothers and sisters or screaming in uncontrollable rage. Management of this case could only take place with the mother's understanding and cooperation. A year later the voice was within normal limits.

3. A woman of 27 years was receiving treatment for a unilateral vocal nodule. She was a vivacious and assertive individual who always spoke extremely loudly. On one occasion she brought her 3-year-old son to the clinic. He also spoke excessively loudly and his voice was hoarse and breathy and showed vocal behaviours similar to those of his mother.

Vocal Misuse and Abuse in Singers

It is generally accepted that singers who are properly trained and who use the techniques of good voice production do not damage the vocal folds (Zilstorff, 1968; Bunch, 1982). Even so, an excellent singer may have some vocal strain following lengthy rehearsals or a demanding performance. A tiny vocal fold haemorrhage can occur but will gradually disappear when the exertion is over. However, if the voice is poorly produced and excessive effort is being used in an attempt to 'project' it or to achieve notes above or below the natural range, the long-term result will be damage to the laryngeal mucosa and, eventually, vocal nodules.

Vocal nodules are most likely to occur in untrained or poorly trained singers, members of amateur choirs and groups, nightclub, pop, country and western singers, and rock band singers. The classical singer who is badly trained and has an unscrupulously ambitious singing teacher who concentrates on the aria at the expense of technique will inevitably develop symptoms of vocal abuse. The non-classical singer is particularly vulnerable to vocal abuse for a number of reasons. The particular sound of the voice that is produced and which is required by the audience may be the antithesis of well-produced voice. An aggressive, forceful, harsh quality may reflect the anarchic quality of the music. There is also evidence that this group does not use the singer's formant (see Chapter 4; Sundberg, 1974, 1977) which allows optimum resonance. As a result the singer uses increased effort in an attempt to project the voice. In addition, the singer's surroundings are often noisy, dusty and smoky. Some performers admit to drinking alcohol and taking certain drugs before a 'gig' in order to give an uninhibited and confident performance. These substances will exacerbate the effects of vocal abuse. The vocal contortions of many pop singers form the basis of their popularity and voice therapy would ruin their careers, thus they opt for a short life but a profitable one.

Correct voice production in these singers, however, prevents breakdown as is demonstrated by the long and trouble-free career of Cliff Richard. Many aspiring singers fall by the way-side and never last long or, as in the case of Elton John, encounter trouble in the course of time and as they are caught in the ageing process.

Management

Small vocal nodes do not require surgery. Voice therapy, with the singer's cooperation, will return the folds to normal. Nodules which go on increasing in size and cause aphonia are removed surgically. Sometimes there is a sudden flare-up of a polypoid fringe (see 'Polyps', p. 121) along the median edge of the vocal fold following laryngitis or a particularly severe bout of vocal abuse. In this case the vocal fold is 'stripped'. It is advisable to tape-record the singing and speaking voice preoperatively as a precaution in case of litigation, besides being essential to the vocal rehabilitation programme (Kleinsasser, 1968). After stripping of the vocal folds the voice may take as long as 3 months to recover fully. Although the folds appear to heal very quickly, the complex vibratory patterns of the mucous membrane take some time to become re-established. Singers become anxious during this interval and it is necessary to warn them that there will be a delay in full vocal recovery despite learning to produce the voice more satisfactorily.

Voice therapy will follow the programme outlined in the next chapter. When the vocal folds are recovered and healthy in appearance the singer must be referred to a competent singing teacher so that techniques for producing loud voice without strain can be learned. It must be remembered that sheer volume of voice in itself is not damaging. All singers must be particularly aware of the importance of not using a hard glottal attack in place of a clear and controlled initiation of the vocal note. Appropriate diaphragmatic breathing with optimum capacity and control is essential if there is to be sufficient breath support for the vocal note at the end of phrases; without it, the vocal folds will be forced to the mid-line in an attempt to continue to produce some sort of sound.

Singers, even the most successful, are anxious before performances and the emotional volatility and temperament of artists is well known. Their anxiety aggravates the vocal symptoms and they need sympathy and understanding as Punt (1968, 1983) emphasises. A laryngologist is often present in the opera house when major performances are in progress, ready to administer medication and reassurance behind the scenes. Although trained singers can, in emergencies, sing with a cold and infective laryngitis (Zilstorff, 1968), the untrained or poorly trained singer with signs of vocal abuse and chronic laryngitis should never do so. The performance will be disastrous and this will not only aggravate the condition but be psychologically traumatic. All singing should be forbidden until the larynx is reported by the laryngologist to be healthy.

Many singers distinguish between their 'speaking voice' and their 'singing voice' but for the purposes of avoiding vocal abuse it is important for the singer to be aware that everyday habits of vocal abuse when speaking will be reflected in the 'singing voice'.

Case histories

1. A 35-year-old woman had sung without training in amateur choirs for many years. Her choral activities ceased for 2 years during which time she had two children. When she resumed her singing she frequently found that her throat was uncomfortable after choir practice. As time progressed the voice became breathy and the upper singing range was lowered although she reported no problems when speaking. Her vocal folds were mildly inflamed. It transpired that there were two main contributory factors to her vocal abuse. She had always sung as a soprano and had associated feelings of exertion and effort with singing; it was found that she sang the alto part much more comfortably. Although this was an important factor it did not produce difficulties until she had her two boisterous, noisy children with whom she used a loud speaking voice. The laryngeal abuse which she perpetrated during the day was fully realised in the evening when she attempted to sing the soprano part which was not ideal for her particular voice.

2. A quietly spoken solo-singer with a rock band was transformed during concerts into a yelling, frenetic performer whose voice was heard, albeit with a microphone, above the accompanying instruments and the screaming audience. He frequently 'snorted' cocaine before performances and drank spirits afterwards. The vocal folds were hyperaemic and 'thickened'. The voice was hoarse and breathy and was beginning to fail to reflect the excessive effort he used during performance. His dilemma was that the sound he produced was the sound his fans wanted and which made him such a marketable commodity but to continue to produce it in this way would also ensure its complete loss. Following the appropriate explanations he continued to give his usual stage performance but was able to maintain the voice by attention to vocal hygiene and voice conservation when not performing.

Chapter 9
Hyperkinetic Dysphonia: Remediation

The management of the individual who is suffering from the effects of vocal misuse and abuse is described in this chapter and a suitable therapeutic programme is suggested.

Therapeutic Advice

The advice which is given to the patient exhibiting hyperkinetic dysphonia is fundamental to restoration of normal vocal function and is of equal, if not greater, importance than the application of direct remedial strategies. In most cases a regimen which avoids vocal abuse and laryngeal irritants can be formulated. It is helpful if advice can be given to each patient in written form at the end of the first interview. Suggestions can be grouped into three major categories: vocal hygiene, vocal rest and voice conservation.

Vocal hygiene: avoidance of laryngeal irritants

1. Stop smoking or drastically cut down the number of cigarettes smoked. Avoid smoky atmospheres.
2. If working in a very dusty environment at home or at work, wear a mask. Some individuals exhibit a marked adverse reaction to paint fumes; the throat becomes very dry and there is laryngeal irritation.
3. Avoid very dry atmospheres or take steps to improve the situation with humidifiers or regular fluid (non-alcoholic) intake. Air-conditioning affects the voice and respiratory tract in vulnerable individuals (Ferguson, 1988). Steam inhalations are helpful in some cases, e.g. with Friar's Balsam.
4. In some individuals very hot or spicey food appears to have an aggravating effect and should be avoided. Patients who suffer from frequent gastric reflux with its known effect on the laryngeal mucosa may need to see a dietitian to discuss a suitably bland diet which will reduce the symptom as much as possible. Very hot or very cold food may aggravate already sensitive mucous membranes in the upper respiratory tract.
5. Alcohol, particularly spirits, should be avoided in the early stages of remediation.

Vocal rest

The question whether to rest the voice or use gentle voice in cases of laryngitis and vocal abuse arises at the outset of treatment. The decision depends upon the laryngological report, the degree of disability and the personality of the individual. Complete rest while healing of the vocal folds is awaited following stripping of the vocal folds, or other surgical procedures, is of course necessary. In other conditions, such as chronic laryngitis (see p. 233) it is not necessary unless prescribed by the laryngologist. The need to keep joints mobile and muscles exercised is considered to be essential. Immobility is conducive to loss of physiological function and vocal activity in moderation is to be encouraged. In the case of the dysphonic patient, anxiety and exasperation can be greatly exacerbated by being told to write everything down and to stay off work. If the throat is painful the patient will not want to talk much.

Patients on complete vocal rest can be given instruction in a whole range of practical training without using phonation.

Voice conservation

The regimen which is outlined to the patient must stress the lack of effort which is necessary for phonation. It is inadvisable to recommend use of a whisper which may result in a forced sound requiring considerable effort and friction damaging to the folds. The patient is encouraged to speak quietly and to stop talking for a short period if the voice quality deteriorates or if throat discomfort increases. The reasons for each item of this regimen should be carefully explained. The outcome of therapy is the patient's responsibility. The speech therapist can give entirely appropriate advice and treatment but without the patient's motivation and cooperation vocal improvement cannot take place. Certain vocal behaviours should be avoided if maximum improvement is to be achieved quickly:

- Talking against background noise.
- Excessive talking.
- Use of loud voice and shouting whether in the normal routine or in anger.
- Very rapid speech.
- Prolonged conversations.
- Use of the telephone. Many patients admit that the voice deteriorates more rapidly on the telephone. This appears to be due to the fact that an excessively loud voice is frequently used combined with different vocal behaviour which constitutes the 'telephone voice'. The lack of visual feedback and elements of non-verbal communication also appear to put more onus on the voice.
- Hard glottal attack.
- Vigorous throat clearing and habitual cough.
- Singing.

Laryngeal relaxation

Aronson (1980), describing musculoskeletal tension and vocal hyperfunction, also advocates the immediate treatment of the extrinsic and intrinsic laryngeal muscles. Gentle massage is administered to relax the throat muscles and lower the position of the larynx, particularly if discomfort in the throat is a complaint. The therapist places a thumb and forefinger on either side of the hyoid bone and gently massages the muscles. The patient must be comfortably seated and the chin lowered and the shoulders relaxed. Massage relaxes the muscles and relieves pain.

Remedial Strategies

The following plan of rehabilitation incorporates five basic steps:

1. Reassurance and relaxation.
2. Breathing techniques.
3. Phonation.
4. Articulation and resonance.
5. Vocal flexibility, prosody and interpretation.

Naturally the above is an artificial demarcation of function and early in treatment all these aspects begin to be fused. A vocal note involves a balance between relaxation, tension and confidence, besides breath control. Flexibility involves control of expiration and glottal tension, besides self-expression. Treatment depends on the needs of the patient after careful assessment of difficulties and faults in voice production. A sufferer from slight vocal strain will need different treatment from one with vocal nodes or contact ulcers. One patient may need little instruction in breathing technique and concentration upon laryngeal tensions, another may be found to have recovered from laryngeal tension when breathing technique has improved. Treatment must be flexible and imaginative and suited to the patient's needs as these change during the course of treatment.

Every treatment should allow time for a discussion of how the patient is coping. This gives opportunities for making suggestions concerning lifestyle and for counselling as problems in the family or at work are exposed. Some individuals will show excellent adjustment and are simple casualties of their personalities and of driving themselves too hard, trying to get the utmost out of work, sports and social activities. Others will need encouragement, the building of confidence to participate in activities and to live life more fully. A sympathetic and understanding yet impartial confidante found in the therapist may bring about recovery far more successfully than a series of voice training exercises.

Throughout therapy the procedures involved should never be regarded as drills which will bring about improvement purely because they are practised regularly. They have validity only if the patient fully understands the rationale behind them and realises their importance in establishing tactile, kinaesthetic and proprioceptive awareness of appropriate methods of healthy voice production.

Relaxation therapy

Relaxation used to be regarded by speech therapists as the panacea for many speech and voice disorders. They now use relaxation far less than formerly. The custom of laryngologists prescribing tranquillisers for anxious patients dispensed the need for working intensively on physical relaxation. However, diazepam (Valium) and chordiazepoxide (Librium) have been found to be addictive and when they are withdrawn their effect generally ceases and the tension and anxiety remain. For this reason they are less likely to be the treatment of choice for the tense individual.

It is interesting to note that the decline in use of traditional methods of relaxation has occurred while speech therapists have grown increasingly interested in instrumentation. The generation of the 1960s discovered Eastern philosophies and were influenced by gurus, meditation and spiritual healing. John Lennon and Yoko Ono had a great impact on the young. Relaxation instruction became available in evening classes and expectant mothers started to attend routinely relaxation classes as part of their pre-natal care. A swing back of the pendulum in speech rehabilitation is now due 20 years on which is about the length of such a cycle in medicine.

Psychiatrists and psychotherapists have continuously used the couch in analytical situations since Freud. The link between anxiety (angst) and bodily tension is universally recognised. Barlow (1959) in discussing anxiety and muscle tension notes that anxiety has been termed the 'mal du siècle'. He writes as follows:

> We know very little about angst which may even proceed from the birth trauma or be a primitive version of original sin. Freudians consider anxiety to arise from the repression of anger or love. Theologians associate it with the Fall; behaviourists with undigested food in the stomach; Kirkegaard with the vertigo that precedes sin. Buddha and many philosophers regard it as concurrent with desire. Anxiety is inherent in the uncoiling of the ego; it lurks in old loves, in old letters and in our despair at the complexity of modern life.

Barlow also quotes the work of Mitchell (1908) who drew attention to the fact that neurotic patients benefited from rest, relaxation and physical therapy, including a light stroking massage given over the entire body to induce relaxation.

Jacobson's book on progressive relaxation (1929) is the classic source of reference on the subject. Wolpe (1958) used Jacobson's methods of relaxation when employing reciprocal inhibition of neurotic responses as an aspect of behaviour therapy (Eysenck, 1960). Rippon and Fletcher (1940) wrote much earlier of reassurance and relaxation, and based therapy for relief of anxiety and fear on 'induced relaxation'.

It is fashionable among speech pathologists to discard relaxation therapy but it must be remembered that there is a wealth of well-documented evidence that reaction to stress is far less when a patient is relaxed and at ease than when tense and upset. In a scientifically controlled experiment (Linford Rees, 1982) the reaction of patients suffering from allergic asthma and hay fever to artificially introduced pollen was found to be measurably greater when tense than when relaxed. Relaxation does not remove anxiety and conflict but alleviates the bodily somatic accompaniment. Relaxation can be deliberately cultivated and can assist in slowing down the over-active nervous system. It eases panic and allows the intellect to take stock of situations and analyse problems more rationally. Suggestions then are received from the therapist more readily and may be almost unconsciously absorbed and accepted and even acted upon. This is the psychological value of relaxation, but there is also the purely mechanical and physiological aspect which must be appreciated.

Physiology of muscular tension

Bodily movement requires the rhythmic coordination of three groups of muscles: the agonists, the antagonists and the synergists. The agonists (the prime movers known as flexors) initiate the voluntary movement. The antagonists (the extensors) are responsible for the opposing movement and have to relax in order to allow the agonists freedom to act. The synergists are bracing muscles which hold the limb in position. A classic example is the clenching of the fist. The agonists are the flexors of the fingers, the antagonists extend the fingers and the wrist extensors act as the synergists.

When excessive muscular tension overflows into all muscles the delicate coordination of the system is thrown out of balance. The muscles do not give way easily but oppose each other which gives rise to fatigue. Precious physical energy is constantly wasted throughout the day quite unnecessarily. This nervous tension is quite unconscious and can persist when standing, walking and while seated. It often produces harmful postures and strained muscles (Barlow, 1959; Linford Rees, 1982). Aching shoulders, neck and back may be due to rheumatism or arthritis and need medical investigations. When no disease or injury is present it must be concluded that it is of psychogenic origin and chiefly the result of excessive muscular tension and bad posture. Problems are common in sedentary occupations, for instance when individuals sit for long periods in front of computer monitors. Discomfort is easily preventable (Jayson, 1987) when its cause is recognised.

Relaxation strategies

For all relaxation procedures the patient must be comfortable, warm and have eyes shaded from bright light. Once the patient's attention has been drawn to muscle tension and the kinaesthetic difference between relaxation and tension is realised, the habit of relaxation has to be established. The various methods in use are described below. The therapist must select the procedures best suited to the individual. Some people may resent being treated as a 'nut case' and being asked to lie on a couch and may regard the therapist with suspicion, fearing that they are at the mercy of a 'shrink'. Others genuinely enjoy supine relaxation and find it remarkably beneficial. Children and adolescents are often just embarrassed by it and therefore alternative methods should be used if one procedure is to be productive.

Before starting relaxation therapy the therapist should fully explain the reasons for thinking it desirable and thus obtain the cooperation of the patient. Otherwise it is perfectly natural for embarrassment and astonishment, if not suspicion, to be felt at being asked to lie flat on the back when expecting nothing but vocal exercises.

The fundamental principle in teaching relaxation is the development of kinaesthetic and proprioceptive awareness by contrasting muscular tension with muscular relaxation. Feedback and monitoring are as essential in re-education of the neuromuscular training as in hearing training. Although muscular relaxation can be taught separately, the ultimate aim is to link auditory and muscular mechanisms in speech production as previously described.

In order to convey the idea of relaxation, which is very often a totally foreign experience, the therapist should ask the patient to flex the therapist's arm while demonstrating the following three degrees of muscle tension:

1. A considerable degree of tension in which the arm is tensed to resist manipulation.
2. A lesser degree of tension in which manipulation is not resisted but anticipated, which is the degree habitually exhibited by the patient.
3. Full relaxation in which the muscles do not in any way support the arm which falls limply to the side by force of gravity when dropped.

Supine relaxation

The speech therapist explains that it is impossible at first to obtain voluntary relaxation of particular muscles of the larynx, chest and throat but, since the body works as a whole, tension or relaxation of any part tends to overflow into all parts of the body at the same time. If voluntary relaxation of the neck, arms and legs is achieved this will spread to the muscles of speech and voice and the desired result will be automatically achieved. Relaxation of limbs, torso and neck can now be taught. Instructions should be given quietly and slowly, suggesting relaxation through both manner and movement.

1. The patient lies in a supine position with shoulders on the couch and head supported by a low pillow, and is instructed to let one arm relax and become heavy. The therapist supports the patient's arm just above the elbow and subsequently gently manipulates the elbow, shoulder and wrist joints. Tension is felt in the limb at first, like a rod resisting manipulation, as the patient tries to anticipate it. Attention must be drawn to this behaviour and tension brought into the focus of consciousness.
2. Relaxation of the legs is taught in the same way. The therapist supports the

patient's thigh with a hand just above the back of the knee and lifts and drops the leg. The patient's ankle is rotated.

3. Following removal of the pillow, the therapist supports the back of the patient's head with interlocked fingers and gently lifts, lowers and rotates the head which should appear extraordinarily heavy when the neck is properly relaxed. Attention is drawn to any tension in the patient's facial expression. Should such exercises prove ineffective, stretching exercises are often helpful, contrasting tension in forceful, purposive movements with the relaxation and relief which accompanies its abrupt cessation, as recommended by Jacobson (1929).
4. The patient is asked to stretch the arms stiffly downwards, trying to touch the therapist's hands with the finger tips. The feeling of strain in the arms and shoulders, and the contrasting relaxation of the resting period, should be noted by the patient. This exercise is repeated three or four times.
5. The patient stretches the legs and points the toes to touch the therapist's hands, while feeling tension in the back of the legs. After relaxation the exercise is repeated.
6. Following arching the back, so that the small of the back is lifted off the couch, the patient relaxes and repeats the procedure. The therapist encourages the feeling of ease, passivity and helplessness while flexing and testing the patient's arms, legs and head as in exercises 1, 2 and 3.

Relaxation through suggestion

Some individuals respond less well to physical manipulation than to suggestion through mental imagery, while lying with eyes closed, listening to the description of a peaceful scene or to serene music which creates an image of ease and peace. The patient then goes on to imagine or consciously develop peace of mind. This type of individual frequently claims to be perfectly relaxed until tested, when tension occurs involuntarily. The irregular and shallow breathing which accompanies failure in relaxation, however, is generally evident if one watches the rise and fall of the chest which testifies to the persistence of tension in the supposed state of relaxation. Every patient should be able to relax voluntarily and when the limbs are flexed and tested. If this is not achieved it is certain that mastery of the art is quite insufficient to stand up to the far greater demands made upon the individual in everyday life.

Instruction in relaxation should be followed by 5 minutes in which the patient lies undisturbed, resting peacefully with hands folded over the abdomen. If during this interval breathing becomes deep, easy, regular and rhythmic, attention should be drawn to the change in breathing, and to the movement beneath the hands. It is explained that this is the natural way to breathe and approximately the correct way when speaking, and this is what to aim for in everyday life.

The patient who relaxes in the peace of the clinic is very open to suggestion, and this factor can be utilised to good effect when suggesting ways in which the patient may cope better with difficulties at home and at work.

Relaxation when sitting

Some people feel particularly vulnerable if asked to lie down in order to relax and will achieve a relaxed state much more easily if they are sitting in a comfortable chair.

1. The patient's eyes are closed and the therapist, using a suitably gentle voice and slow rate of speech, asks the patient to breathe slowly and deeply as if becoming drowsy before sleep. The head should be dropped forward onto the chest with an increasing sensation of heaviness.
2. The therapist describes each part of the body - feet, legs, trunk, arms, shoulders, face - as becoming increasingly heavy and immobile. The patient should be observed carefully for signs that full relaxation has not been achieved, e.g. rapid breathing rate, flickering eyelids, tense facial expression, movements of the hands and feet, and these areas should be talked through again.
3. When maximum relaxation has been reached the therapist asks the patient to remain in the same position with eyes closed and explains that gentle manipulation of the head and neck is to take place.
4. The therapist places one cupped hand under the patient's chin and the other supports the back of the head. Tension will frequently be felt in the neck. If fully relaxed the head is very heavy to lift and move. The patient remains passive while the therapist gently moves the head from left to right. As the neck relaxes the head may be gently tilted backwards and forwards while fully supported. The therapist must not remove this support without warning the patient. If the patient has arthritis of the cervical spine this procedure must be discussed with the patient's doctor prior to its use.
5. The patient remains in a quiet relaxed state for a short period after head and neck manipulation is complete.

Relaxation when active

Relaxation is not difficult to achieve when supine and concentrating upon nothing else, but when up and about it is far more difficult. The habitual tension of the individual generally returns on rising from the couch, but can be dissipated by further exercises directed at relaxation of head, neck, arms and torso when sitting or standing.

1. Sitting at ease the patient lets the head hang forward and swings it gently from left to right feeling the head as heavy as a cannonball swinging on a rope.
2. The patient stands with feet apart and lifts the arms up from the sides to a horizontal position, imagining the fingers are attached to the floor by strong springs which resist stretching. This resistance is pulled against as the arms lift and uncomfortable tension is felt in the axillary musculature. The arms are then relaxed and dropped heavily to the patient's sides with the force of gravity alone. They should not be brought down to the sides.

3. The therapist flexes the patient's arms as they hang limply. Then the patient swings both arms together from side to side in an easy rhythmic motion.
4. Standing with feet apart, the patient drops the body forward from the waist allowing the arms to swing loose with fingers brushing the floor. When gentle pressure is applied between the shoulders the whole body should swing loose from the waist.
5. Sitting in a comfortable chair the patient's eyes are closed, the breathing rate is slowed and inspiration becomes deeper as if going to sleep.
6. Children may respond to acting the part of a cat or floppy puppet settling down to sleep or in contrast to vigorous activity, will sit down quietly and relax.

Breathing Techniques

Considerable discussion has been generated among those who work with dysphonic patients concerning work on breathing techniques. Many believe (Aronson, 1980; Stemple, 1984; Fawcus, 1986b; Wilson, 1987) that the teaching of breathing techniques is usually unnecessary in cases of hyperkinetic dysphonia where relaxed, natural breathing patterns are all that is required as a basis for vocal recovery. It is argued that the introduction of 'breathing exercises' into the treatment programme will create awareness and a resulting increase in tension which will be counterproductive. However, all these writers agree that there are cases where this approach is insufficient and that if breathing patterns are markedly disturbed by tension and anxiety, a more direct approach is required. There is general agreement that for those patients whose voice disorders are the result of neurological involvement the teaching of improved breathing techniques is valuable. The beneficial effects on phonation of training in breathing techniques is noted by a number of writers (Proctor, 1980; Gould, 1981; Bunch, 1982; Wilder, 1983; Hixon, 1987) and should not be disregarded in voice therapy.

The therapist must adapt explanations and suggestions for changes in breathing technique to each patient's needs. The patient will gradually develop an awareness of respiratory function as appropriate patterns are practised. In addition, many patients discover that to practise improved breathing techniques in a relaxed environment has a calming effect which provides an ideal basis for voice therapy as well as a surprising and revealing contrast to their normal respiratory patterns for speech. The crux of the matter is that patients with habitual patterns of breathing which adversely affect phonation just do not know what normal breathing is and are unlikely to develop it unless instructed.

Objectives of breathing techniques

The chief object of teaching breathing technique is to enable the patient to control the volume and expiratory flow of air thus providing the means of controlling phonation effortlessly and easily. Increase in vital capacity is not the aim, but control of expiration in relation to vocal fold resistance. This requires complex muscular coordination which can be developed through an amalgam of kinaesthetic and tactile sensations.

Preparation for breathing techniques

Posture must be checked since a relaxed upright carriage of the torso, head and neck is essential. Cotes (1979) gives a clear account of changes in lung volume induced by postural changes. Round shoulders and a sagging posture which folds the chest at an angle upon the abdomen in a crease at waist level will not allow good expansion of the lungs or control of expiration, nor provide a good chest resonator. Posture is also allied to personality and confidence.

Bunch (1982), in discussing the 'dynamics of the singing voice', defines posture as alignment. The position of the head establishes the carriage of the long axis of the spine. The balance of muscular forces conserves energy and enhances resonance.

Exercises are best demonstrated while the patient is standing when the therapist can gently manipulate the necessary central movement of ribs and abdominal wall. The therapist can demonstrate the desired movement. Tactile sensation reinforces the kinaesthetic sensation. Patients can practise before a mirror, with one hand on the clavicle and the other on the abdominal wall just above waist level thus reinforcing the tactile, kinaesthetic and visual sensations.

Explanation and demonstration

The therapist first describes to the patient how it is difficult for the pear-shaped lungs to expand the upper thoracic region which is encased in a bony cage, whereas it is easier to expand the lower region where the lungs are larger and the ribs are free in front and separated by a large area of elastic muscle. A demonstration is given of the correct breathing action, showing how when the lungs fill the abdomen wall comes forward and the ribs lift, and as the lungs empty the abdominal wall flattens and the ribs fall. The thoracic and abdominal movements can be imitated with the hands, finger tips touching and palms adducting and abducting on expiration and inspiration.

The patient may now endeavour to take a small easy breath with one hand on the abdominal wall just above the waist level and the other on the rib cage so that the forward and lateral expansion of the thorax can be felt. The instructions 'swell up' with air and then to 'squeeze it out' may be given. The verbal cues are important. The simple instruction to breathe 'in' and breathe 'out' may produce the exact reverse of the desired action with the patient pulling in the abdomen on the instruction to breathe 'in' and pushing it out on breathing 'out'. This pattern is known as 'reverse breathing'. There is a widespread and firmly held but mistaken belief that, for inspiration, the abdominal wall should be well pulled in and the chest thrown out like a sergeant major.

Help for slow learners

It is sometimes extraordinarily difficult in cases of habitual dysphonia to obtain the correct response. In such cases the following procedures are helpful:

1. The patient is instructed to breathe out, then sigh noisily on the remaining air, at the same time the therapist should apply manual pressure to the midriff. This pressure is relaxed as inspiration begins, then applied again during the sigh. Manipulation of the abdominal wall in this way assists in the establishment of the easy rhythmic swing on inspiration and expiration which it is difficult for some to achieve voluntarily.
2. The patient imitates a panting dog by pushing out the abdominal wall and then pulling it in. The breath is not held by a closed glottis and the breathing is not thought about consciously until the sharp oral intake and output of air is heard. Then attention can be drawn to the breathing and voluntary control gradually achieved, and the movement slowed down to a normal respiratory rhythm.
3. The patient is instructed to breathe out and then pretend to blow out a candle with the remaining air; this is followed by the rapid ascent of the diaphragm in the need to replenish the air supply.

Home practice

Once the patient is able to perform correctly the required breathing patterns they should be practised several times each day, preferably in front of a mirror so that any movement in the upper thorax can be monitored and corrected. A week's home practice may be sufficient time for the individual to learn to produce central breathing. Frequently, there is no improvement by the second treatment but the temptation to progress rapidly to the next stage should be resisted if steady progress is to be made with each step having been securely mastered. For this reason in the early stages of treatment frequent short visits to the speech therapist are preferable to once weekly.

Hyperventilation

Deep breathing when first practised by shallow breathers frequently induces giddiness and the patient should be warned of the possibility and reassured. A short rest should be taken after giddiness before continuing with practice which should only be carried out for short periods initially. Any tight clothing should be loosened to allow full expansion at the waist.

Common faults

It is important that the therapist should be aware of the most common faults which may occur during acquisition of improved breathing patterns and correct them as soon as they occur.

1. Tension generally obtrudes itself in every attempt to perform any new exercise demanding concentration and voluntary effort.

2. Nearly all patients lapse into old breathing patterns when initially asked to phonate during exercise.
3. Poor posture may prevent adequate thoracic movement.
4. Inspiration may be noisy as a result of laryngeal tension and approximation of the vocal folds.
5. The patient may mistakenly think that a large volume of air is required and this will result in excessive effort being used during the breathing exercises. The emphasis should be on effortless control of both correct respiratory movements and expiration for phonation.

Oral breathing and phonation

Oral inspiration of air during these exercises should be insisted upon; this is the normal method of inspiration for speech and allows air to be inspired rapidly and imperceptibly between phrases. The coordination of expiration with phonation can now be introduced in treatment by production of a clear sustained vowel of appropriate pitch as soon as a correct breathing pattern is established.

Breathing and voice control – preliminary strategy

1. With the hand flat on the abdominal wall just above waist level, the patient breathes in slowly. On the out-going breath count quietly up to four at the rate of one per second. No breath should escape between each count. This is practised, gradually increasing the count weekly.
2. Rib reserve: as counting above 10 develops, the patient frequently quite unconsciously holds the ribs in an elevated position and only lowers them as he comes near the end of the breath. This can be taught as a voluntary pattern to the professional voice user: the singer, actor or public speaker. A deep breath should be taken, the ribs are elevated while counting aloud up to 15 and then gradually relaxed. For ordinary purposes a count of 20, one per second, should be the target but for singers and actors a count of 30 is appropriate.
3. The patient breathes in and then counts aloud in groups of three while holding the breath for a mental count of three between each group.
4. Following inspiration, breath is emitted on a loud sustained voiceless fricative /ʃ, s, f/. The fricative should be maintained at a steady volume and not fluctuate or fade towards the end. The gradual contraction of the abdominal wall is felt with the hand as the breath is expired.
5. Voiceless fricatives are practised on a crescendo and diminuendo of volume:
   sssssSSSSSSSSsssss
6. Voiceless fricatives are emitted in rhythmic patterns.

Phonation: the soft attack

Many patients have been unaware of their use of the glottal attack. It is such an integral part of phonation that they frequently find these exercises, which are directed at introducing a soft attack, very difficult.

1. The patient takes a breath and breathes out on a sustained whispered vowel. Then voiced vowels preceded by /h/ are attempted. Some patients find it easier to begin by producing a voiced sigh on the vowel /ɑ:/ because the vocal tract has to be relaxed in order to produce the sound.
2. The patient breathes in and then breathes out on strings of six different vowels and diphthongs. At first expiration and phonation is continuous. Later expiration between each vowel can be broken while achieving a soft attack on each. The vocal tract and mandible must be relaxed.
3. Sometimes it is not possible for the patient to produce any of the above exercises without a hard attack. This problem is frequently overcome if the patient is encouraged to phonate with the therapist as a vowel is produced. It appears that the auditory and kinaesthetic patterns have become so entrenched in these patients that they are unable to re-set the laryngeal muscles for the required change in the method of vocalisation. Instant feedback of the therapist's phonation seems to assist correct programming for voice. After producing the vowel in unison with the therapist the patient is asked to produce the vowel unaccompanied.

Respiratory rhythm for speech

1. The patient breathes in and out slowly several times and then imitates the therapist's demonstration of quick intake and slow expiration. The abdominal wall should jump forward on inspiration and subside very gradually on expiration. It is important that oral inspiration is used. The nasal passages are too narrow to allow the adequate and very rapid intake of air necessary for the connected speech. Silent inspiration should take place imperceptibly between phrases or word groups; noisy intake is indicative of tension in the larynx and some approximation of the vocal folds, which should not be present.
2. The patient takes a quick breath in and then breathes out, slowly counting six. The natural tendency to count too fast should be corrected. Repeat six times, until the new rhythmic swing is performed easily. A suggestion of the movement required may be given by the therapist by a quick hand movement to one side and a slow, drawn out movement to the other.
3. Gradually the patient increases the count on expiration until able to count to 20 using quick inspiration.
4. The patient practises sustaining a trilled /r/ at constant pitch and volume - this is a real test of breath control, necessitating a constant breath pressure to maintain vibration of the tip of the tongue and relaxation of the oral musculature.

Voice Therapy

Recording and auditory feedback

Audio-recordings must form an intrinsic part of treatment and hearing training. Hearing the voice played back gives the patient the chance to listen to it objectively and critically in a way that is impossible when actively participating in voice production. Many people have tape recorders of their own which can be used in home practice.

A characteristic symptom of patients with vocal strain is poor ability to distinguish between 'good' and 'bad' voice, changes in pitch, resonance, volume and breathiness. It is often thought that tone deafness, or at least poor musicality, is common to these individuals but research fails to prove this. It is only apparent that they are poor listeners. The speech therapist's ear is so acutely trained that it is often hard to realise how little most individuals listen to their own voices and how little awareness there is of their speech mannerisms. Tapes consisting of different samples of dysphonic and normal speech can be compiled easily in a voice clinic and given to patients to evaluate as exercises in developing listening skills. This may usefully precede introduction of evaluation of the patient's own recordings. Children enjoy this exercise, especially if recordings include funny voices and those of popular television characters.

Maximum phonation time

Once a reasonable degree of respiratory control has been achieved, the aim is to produce a prolonged vowel on a steady note and in the middle of the range of the patient's voice. As the voice strengthens, the phonation can be extended and timed until a comfortable maximum phonation time is achieved. Increasing phonation time is a good indication of progress and a matter of encouragement to the patient. This can be followed by practising inflected vowels and intonation exercises.

Optimum pitch

'Optimum pitch' is a term used to describe the range of notes in the individual's voice which generates the greatest resonance. It depends on the maximum mix of the harmonics or formants of which the vocal instrument is capable. It follows the acoustic principles of resonance described in Chapter 4. The laryngeal note has to be pitched to match the resonators to achieve maximum resonance.

Various devices are suggested for achieving optimum pitch but in the final analysis singing up and down the scale is frequently the best solution. A piano or pitch pipe may be helpful. Yanagihara (1967) tried spectrographic analysis but at the present moment no technique can replace the fidelity of the human ear. Production of optimum pitch is achieved by listening to the notes produced and by sensing the epicentre of vibrations in the resonance cavities.

Sundberg's singing formant is the epitome of optimum pitch. It is obtained intuitively rather than by voluntary control and, once achieved, the voice is produced without effort and with a satisfying sense of rightness and of effortless power.

Instruction in relaxation, in the control of expiration without tension, and in phonation with a soft attack, should ensure that the patient finds the natural pitch range in exercises. The therapist is generally able to assess the natural voice pitch and should give the pitch to be imitated in all phonation exercises. If the pitch the patient is using appears to be too high or low, the pitch of optimal resonance must be discovered by singing scales on a vowel. When optimum pitch is reached the voice leaps into prominence, being so much more rich and resonant that there is no mistaking its rightness. The resonance change is far more striking in strained than in normal voices (Laguaite and Waldrop, 1963) and the discovery of the appropriate speaking pitch is not such a difficult matter, but see Zaliouk's method below. The pitch level agreed upon should be the one used in exercises and later in speech. The therapist, by constantly bringing the patient back to it when it is lost, facilitates auditory perception. Eventually automatic auditory control of the voice is achieved which is the most important factor in maintenance of good phonatory habits.

Tactile method for achieving optimum pitch

Zaliouk (1960, 1963) recommended a tactile approach to voice placement which applied successfully to vocal re-education of children with hearing loss and which applies also to hearing individuals with dysphonic voices.

1. The hands are placed lightly over the face and nose while humming so that vibrations may be felt by the fingers. The vibrations become much stronger when the optimum pitch is reached. The patient can feel the therapist's face for comparison.
2. Another procedure is to place a finger-tip between the lax lips and feel the vibration as a gentle hum is produced. Relaxed lips will tingle during humming. Children can use a comb covered with tissue paper and held to the lips to feel this effect when humming.

Ear cupping

Humming with the palms of the hands cupped over the ears amplifies the resonance of the voice and is also a useful device for determining the best vocal range. As the harmonics buzz in the ears they are felt in the jaws, by the hands, as well as heard.

Chest resonance

Use of tactile cues should be made when treating men using habitually a pitch that is too high and lacking chest resonance. Women with immature voices can also practise feeling chest vibration. The hand should be placed lightly on the throat with thumb and forefinger touching the larynx and the lower edge of the hand resting on the clavicles. Tactile sensations when high and low notes are contrasted should be felt.

Voice exercises

1. The patient works through vowel and diphthong exercises first whispering and then introducing voice after /h/ to ensure a soft attack:
   (a) single vowels are sung on an evenly sustained breath;
   (b) unbroken chains of different vowels are sung on one note;
   (c) interruption of phonation is introduced between each vowel in the chain.

   Throughout these exercises there is emphasis on soft attack, soft volume, a clear vocal note and open, relaxed articulation.
2. If avoidance of hard attack is still found difficult, more time must be spent on whispering vowels and 'gliding' into phonation with an uninterrupted breath. Vowels may be preceded by /h/ or a voiceless fricative lasting three or four seconds. The vowels /i:/ and /ɑ:/ cause most difficulty in strained voices, the voice often cracking on these long after all others have become strong and clear. It is sometimes found helpful to preface a difficult vowel with a vowel which is easy for the patient, and then to isolate the 'difficult' one.
3. Resonance can be developed with exercises based on humming (see above):
   (a) humming is practised concentrating on feeling the vibrations on the lips;
   (b) the sensations achieved in humming are aimed for using /m/ followed by vowels, e.g. /m:, mi:/; these syllables are then used to glide up and down the scale covering a third and then a fifth and in varied rhythms;
   (c) these sounds are sung and said in rapid succession to develop use of resonance.
4. Singing: if the singing voice has to be regained, the exercises given so far will have laid the foundation for this, but graded exercises for increasing the range of pitch will be necessary. The exercises of the kind given below are easier than the singing of plain scales. The therapist, if not a singer, need not be alarmed by the prospect of teaching a singer. Patients will be able to compose their own exercises. The therapist's constructive criticism of pharyngeal and laryngeal tension, breath control and knowledge of the need to change the articulation of vowels by flattening and relaxing the tongue on high notes, for example, is adequate for the immediate purpose. Early referral to a singing teacher is necessary.

Articulation exercises

Specific work on articulation may be necessary for a patient whose articulatory patterns adversely affect phonation, as in the individual with little mouth-opening and a rigid jaw. Relaxed but accurate articulation is the aim of therapy.

Consonants are practised in various combinations and rhythms in order to develop coordination of fine muscle movements, also kinaesthetic and auditory appreciation, e.g.

/p-t-k, p-t-k/	or	/r-l-j, r-l-j-/
/t-tt-t, k-kk-k/	or	/kk-kk-kk-k/

Eventually tongue twisters and alliterative sentences can be used for developing articulatory expertise.

Phonation in connected speech

A strong clear voice is achieved first in exercises and only considerably later will this standard of voice production be maintained during connected speech. At first the old speech patterns rule by force of habit, and the practice in mechanical speech has to be carried over into spontaneous conversation. An important aim in the latter stages of treatment must be the provision of interest and variety so that the patient's interest is held and enthusiasm sustained.

1. With quick inspiration before each line the patient chants a jingle, concentrating on good tone and articulation.
2. Breath intake is adjusted to phrase length. The patient chants and then speaks: 'One is all I need; one, two is all I need; one, two, three is all I need' etc. The count is increased until full capacity is reached but reserve or residual air must not be used. Discomfort and tension are immediately felt. The patient must learn to recognise the danger signals and to replenish the breath supply immediately the necessity arises.
3. The patient composes phrases of increasing length:
   It was a cold day.
   It was a cold and windy day.
   It was a cold, windy and wet day.

These exercises should introduce the particular vowels and consonants in which the individual needs practice. Accurate articulation should be encouraged while the vowels must be slightly prolonged in order to develop their full resonance.

Prosody

The development of vocal flexibility and the prevention of a monotonous and limited pitch range should be an integral part of all vocal exercises.

1. The vowels and humming exercises already described should be practised with rising and falling pitch. This may be reinforced by visual clues such as moving the hand up and down in a wave-like figure to denote rise and fall, and smooth gliding from one pitch to another. The fall–rise or rise–fall glide can be drawn on paper.
2. Phrases can be marked with an intonation pattern. The same phrase can be

spoken with as many different meanings as possible. The patient must learn to be expressive and animated without relying almost exclusively, as formerly, on vocal volume.

3. The lines of a poem, or of prose suitably phrased, are repeated after the therapist with careful attention to tone, intonation, rhythm and rate. The patient's faults should be imitated by the therapist and the patient asked to correct them. When this exercise has been worked through, the patient should read the passage alone attempting to rectify previous faults. Playback of tape-recordings reinforces learning.
4. Practice in reading aloud is a much more difficult exercise and should not be introduced until the new vocal patterns are secure. The patient should be stopped immediately if poor phonation patterns recur. Inability to self-correct necessitates further practice of earlier exercises with recording and playback. Some individuals find that it is easier to read poetry and blank verse than prose.
5. Exercises for the correction of a considerable drop in pitch at the ends of phrases is often necessary. Although this is a characteristic of English intonation it may be carried to excess, the voice dropping into vocal fry register as volume and breath pressure fall. The patient can practise the following:
   (a) speak the last word of a phrase with exaggerated rising intonation;
   (b) speak a phrase on a monotone and then repeat with normal intonation pattern;
   (c) speak a phrase with 'and' tagged onto the end as if it were not the end of the phrase; repeat, merely imagining 'and';
   (d) imitate humming the tunes of phrases hummed by the therapist, then speak the phrase with the same tune.
6. Spontaneous speech practice consists of the patient:
   (a) giving short replies to questions having planned the answers, and applying principles of good voice production in a controlled situation;
   (b) describing objects or events;
   (c) giving prepared talks on any subject. If the patient is a lecturer or teacher, for example, sections from teaching material can be given to an imaginary audience. If possible, this can be carried out in group treatment.
7. If a patient's profession requires speaking against a high level of background noise it is useful for this to be part of the practice in the final stages of treatment. A tape recording of traffic, factory noise, children or whatever is appropriate can be used. Played loudly, it assists the individual to cope with the situation and to increase vocal volume without becoming tense and reverting to forcing the voice.

Re-education of asthenic voice

Air wastage is the most conspicuous feature of this type of voice disorder. Van

Riper and Irwin (1958) stressed the irregular respiratory patterns present in such cases, air being wasted before and after phonation with the patient only using a portion of the air available. This they term 'staircase breathing'. Luchsinger (1962) refers to this as 'wild air'. It is generally accompanied by insufficient approximation of the vocal folds, or bowing of the folds, due to internal tensor weakness. The personality, anxieties and environmental difficulties of the patient must be investigated during treatment. The building of confidence, especially in audience situations where the patient learns to overcome self-consciousness and feelings of diffidence and inferiority, must form an important aspect of treatment.

The general plan of direct speech treatment should follow that for the vocal re-education of the strained voice and include a check on physical health. Voice in most cases will be strengthened by establishing better habits of breathing, increase of lung capacity and control of expiration, and the promotion of increased tonicity of the laryngeal muscles so that the vocal folds provide more adequate resistance to the breath stream. This control is best obtained by auditory training which includes contrasting dysphonic and normal phonation, and the imitation of clear, resonant vowel sounds. Placing the finger tips on the thyroid cartilage and feeling the vibration is helpful. Humming exercises incorporating Zaliouk's tactile method of voice placement, and 'ear-cupping', are beneficial in the early stages of treatment.

If these methods prove inadequate it may be necessary to introduce exercises of greater force, but these must be used with care and discarded as soon as possible to avoid causing laryngeal muscle strain and damage to the vocal folds. The patient should only practise these exercises under the therapist's supervision and not at home.

1. Coughing in order to obtain complete approximation of the folds and to obtain a hard attack can be used to develop kinaesthetic and tactile awareness of laryngeal tonicity.
2. The previous exercise is followed by clear articulation of vowels which are initiated with a glottal stop. Each vowel is sustained clearly for several seconds. The vowels are then repeated without the glottal stop onset.
3. Strings of vowels are intoned on one breath, each preceded by hard attack. These are then repeated without hard attack while there are still clear auditory and kinaesthetic images of strong voice.
4. Consonant–vowel syllables are practised using exaggerated plosives.
5. Singing exercises are useful and build confidence and help to overcome inhibitions.
6. Reading and speaking against ambient noise should be practised as described in the voice exercises (see 'Prosody', point (7)).

In all these methods for obtaining closer approximation of the vocal folds and correction of air wastage in phonation, care must be taken to avoid any increase of generalised tension in the patient and interference with breathing technique. The hard attack should be discarded as soon as possible, especially with patients who have a history of vocal abuse.

Ventricular band voice and reverse phonation

Lehmann (1965) described reverse phonation as a new manoeuvre for examining the larynx during indirect laryngoscopy. In order to produce voice on inspired air, the ventricles are opened up and the false cords drawn aside. Williams, Farquharson and Anthony (1975) describe the excellent view reverse phonation provides in fibreoptic laryngoscopy. The patient is asked to phonate on inspiration and then, after a prolonged reverse phonation, to produce a normal expiratory phonation. Boone (1977) recommends this exercise in the treatment of several types of voice disorder such as conversion aphonia and puberphonia. It is also useful in cases of ventricular band voice.

Contact ulcers: therapeutic goals

This severe condition resulting from vocal abuse requires concentration upon the characteristic symptoms listed by Peacher and Holinger (1947) (p. 127). Unlike vocal nodules which will respond to the general plan of relaxation, breathing technique and prolonged vowel phonation, specific correction of the abnormal action of the arytenoids in phonation has to be tackled. The pitch must be raised so that it is lifted out of the vocal fry register and optimum pitch has to be established (Nahum, 1967). At the same time the effortful quality of phonation should be reduced and removed with therapy being directed particularly at eliminating hard glottal attack. The grating voice gives the impression that the speaker is trying to shout. Overloud voice can be modified by use of amplification and biofeedback techniques should be used. The patient's acceptance of a higher vocal pitch has to be obtained, and fears that it is not sufficiently manly discussed and dispelled.

Pedagogic Procedures

Biofeedback

This term originated with biological engineers to describe the process whereby physiological activity of which a subject is unaware is fed back to him by presentation of visual, auditory or tactile signals. By monitoring the signals the unconscious function can be brought under voluntary control. Biofeedback systems are used in psychiatry to treat anxiety unresponsive to drug therapy. The patient may watch alpha rhythm from the electroencephalogram. Surface electromyography (EMG) without needles is used by physiotherapists to induce relaxation. EMG feedback is also used in an attempt to monitor tension in cases of dysphonia (Boone, 1977).

Amplification of speech by means of a pocket amplifier or a portable voice intensifier (see p. 114) can be used effectively during therapy. A patient who habitually uses excessively loud voice will automatically reduce the volume if he has simultaneous amplification. Carry-over of the quieter voice is the aim when the amplifier is switched off. If the voice is too quiet, amplification results in the patient maintaining the increased volume for some time after the amplifier has been withdrawn. By repeating this procedure the patient will learn how to increase the volume of the voice. The use of amplification is one of the simpler instrumental methods available to speech therapists.

Many of the instruments listed in Chapter 7 provide biofeedback systems. The display of voice features on a screen reinforces auditory control and these systems act as a useful adjunct to traditional therapy. The patient can work alone at times and monitor performance without constant intervention by the therapist. However, the behaviour elicited by biofeedback will not necessarily be carried over into daily life. Pronovost (1967) remarked that despite the proliferation of electronic equipment for use in teaching, there are very few, if any, research projects which can prove the greater efficacy of machines with children or adults in comparison with traditional methods of therapy. Prosek *et al.* (1978) studied EMG biofeedback treatment in six cases of hyper-functional voice disorders suffering from laryngitis, oedema, hoarseness and aphonia. They were given 14 training sessions of 30 minutes. Electrodes placed on the cricoid cartilage were linked to a noise generator which was activated when EMG activity exceeded the value selected from a control of normal speakers. After the 14 sessions three patients had improved and three were unchanged. We would certainly regard this result as abysmal after 14 half-hourly sessions of traditional therapy.

The study undertaken by Andrews, Warner and Stewart (1986) concluded that EMG feedback was certainly useful in detecting global increases in laryngeal tension and demonstrating this clearly to the patient. Unfortunately, it did not detect adductor tension in hard attack and some subjects were so irritated by upward swings of the needle that tension increased. The importance of a competent and caring clinician and the acknowledgement of the patient as an individual was stressed in this study. Guidance and encouragement is vital whichever method or combination of methods are used for the treatment of dysphonia.

Froeschels' chewing method

In the UK the teaching of Froeschels (1948) has never been used extensively and consequently tentative attempts at introducing chewing therapy are discouraged by the marked resistance and even ridicule from patients. This was also the experience of Van Riper and Irwin (1958) who found the method successful in lowering vocal pitch in some cases of boys suffering from pitch breaks and some cases of vocal nodules, when other methods had failed. They commented on the possible psychological value of the method in contrast to its manifest achievement in obtaining relaxation of the vocal and speech mechanism. The technique allows for a reversion to an infantile form of behaviour and some of Van Riper and Irwin's cases improved with practice of vocalised thumb sucking!

The enthusiasm for the method among Froeschels' followers is impressive. The fact that it is so widely practised in the USA and on the Continent with such good results would seem to indicate its value. Practically any technique in teaching, however, will achieve good results in a certain proportion of cases but all cure depends also upon the faith the therapist has in the methods used and the faith that can be inspired in the patient. Froeschels was not only a great therapist but a great teacher judging by the faith with which he inspired his disciples and such medical experts as Weiss (1964) and Brodnitz (1959).

Froeschels' method was described in *Twentieth Century Voice Correction* (1948) and *Practice of Voice and Speech Therapy* (1941). He advocated the method chiefly as a cure for stammering. His method is based on the hypothesis that the movements for chewing and talking are almost identical and that chewing is the origin of human speech. He noted that as primitive peoples chew, the movements of the articulators are accompanied by vocalisation and that babies, during the babbling stage, also move their lips and tongues as if chewing while simultaneously vocalising. Froeschels recommended that after this explanation of the theory has been given, the patient should attempt to use voice while chewing. Nonsense syllables are produced with varied intonation used so that the voiced chewing resembles human speech. The therapist and patient have 'chewing conversations' so that 'the patient becomes aware of the fact that there is no fundamental difference between this kind of language and his natural tongue, as far as the use of muscles is concerned'. The patient is instructed to use voiced chewing for a few moments each day as a reminder (Weiss and Beebe, 1951).

However, Froeschels did recognise that in some cases where there is an important psychogenic contribution to the voice disorder, more fundamental, psychological help is necessary.

Svend Smith – Accent Method

A vocal rehabilitation method invented by Svend Smith is widely used in Holland and Scandinavia and is suitable for use particularly with children besides adults. Smith and Thyme (1976) and Damsté and Lerman (1975) have described this method.

The Accent Method is a dynamic approach involving the respiratory and phonatory muscles, with particular attention to the abdominal muscles, and total body movement in rhythmic sequences. The aim is to increase flexibility and elasticity of the vocal folds and ultimately to produce optimal voice function. The voice training is followed by speech training directed at accentuating prosody.

Breathing exercises are taught initially, and subsequently combined with voice exercises. As breath is expressed a stream of sounds is uttered in varied rhythms and pitch changes, e.g. 'ha-ha-haha-ha' etc. Rhythmic beating of a drum and rhythmic body movements accompany voice exercises. Finally, texts are used to establish various vocal patterns.

Psychologically, this method releases inhibitions and self-consciousness. The patient relaxes when the therapy is undertaken in unison with the therapist. It is essential that the therapist and patient should enjoy the Accent Method and not feel foolish because it is not a dignified performance.

Behaviour therapy

Skinner (1953) first described a method of behaviour modification using general conditioning and following a clearly defined series of shaping techniques until the selected goal or target is achieved. Positive reinforcement is given with the aid of rewards and negative reinforcement by withholding approbation or reward, by 'time-out' or an unpleasant stimulus. Approximations to the target are acceptable at first and the standard of performance raised as the responses improve. Material rewards such as sweets are 'faded out' as marks or praise become adequate reinforcing agents. Behaviour therapy is a modification of Skinner's behaviour modification concept. The principle is that of inhibiting undesirable behaviour and developing desirable patterns by rewards and discouragements (not punishments).

Wilson (1987) advocates the use of behaviour therapy, or operant conditioning, in treatment of voice disorders in children and describes in detail the way in which it may be applied. This seems to be a very involved way of replacing, without necessarily improving, the time-honoured system of reward and approbation. Adults like praise and success; children like stars to be stuck in their books, to win marks in competitive games and to gain a sweet.

There seems little real advantage to be gained from such complicated and graduated steps as those involved in behaviour therapy when treating voice disorders in children. The most important reinforcer in the relationship between parent and child, and teacher and pupil, is mutual liking and respect. Behaviour modification therapy ignores this powerful motivating force in social beings and endeavours to replace it by mechanical rituals which may not succeed. Children like candy but cannot be bribed with it under any circumstances and by anyone.

Negative practice

Negative practice is a method of treatment formulated by Knight Dunlays in 1944 and used in treatment of stammering by Mostafa Fahmy, a psychologist (1950). Van Riper (1947) recommended its use in the treatment of stammering and articulation disorders and Wilson (1987) stresses its importance in the remediation of children's voice disorders.

Negative practice when used in the treatment of dysphonia is based on the hypothesis that if a patient is made aware of a particular fault in vocal behaviour and it is then brought under conscious control, it may be used as a contrast to reinforce desirable vocal behaviour. It cannot be used as a therapeutic strategy until good voice is readily produced under voluntary control. It is a useful method of dealing with hard glottal attack. When the patient is able to produce a vowel with soft onset the production of the same sound with hard attack highlights the kinaesthetic and auditory differences. Obviously care must be taken not to use this practice if there is any danger of exacerbating symptoms of vocal abuse by reinforcement of bad voice production.

Chapter 10
Psychogenic Voice Disorders

The normal voice and vocal tract reflect the changing emotional state of the individual. Psychogenic voice disorders are a reflection of underlying psychological problems and can only be successfully treated with respect for this fact.

This chapter is concerned with the description of anxiety states associated with disturbances of the autonomic system and personality. It is beyond the scope of the speech therapist's work to enter into the psychopathological states which can underlie many voice disorders. Mental illness is the domain of the psychiatrist, and one of the functions of the laryngologist is to direct patients to the appropriate channels for treatment. Sometimes it is not easy to distinguish the severely disturbed and the neurotic at first interview and speech therapy may be inappropriately prescribed. It is important therefore that certain vocal characteristics be recognised: dysprosody, for example, can be a diagnostic sign of psychogenic disturbance.

According to Moses (1954), in his book *The Voice of Neurosis*, uniformity of intonation and narrow pitch range are always pathological symptoms and are characteristic of depression. Excessively wide pitch variation, high pitch and fast tempo are typical of manic states. Schizophrenia may be associated with changes in register when spilt personality adopts male and female roles.

Compulsive neurosis can produce various laryngeal spasms and prolongation of vowels and constantly repeated rhythmic patterns, known to speech therapists in a compulsive form of stammering. Similar symptoms also occur in psychogenic spastic dysphonia (see p. 178).

A carefully compiled case history often clearly points to mental illness. The content of the patient's speech is highly significant. One should not be carried away in pursuit of linguistic and paralinguistic observations to the detriment of noticing what is being said. A schizophrenic when free of episodes of mental disorientation can appear misleadingly normal but an emotional detachment and lack of logic in thought and responsibility of attitude may be detected.

Chronic Anxiety State

Anxiety which can be regarded as within normal limits has been described in connection with vocal abuse and misuse. Every normal individual experiences anxiety when confronted by fear provoking events – illness in a child, visiting the doctor or dentist, addressing a meeting, taking exams or a driving test. Normal anxiety is not crippling and it does not last but disappears when the feared event is over. Anxiety is a necessary emotion, it alerts the individual for 'fight or flight' and releases energy and drive. It is necessary in all competitive activity.

When anxiety persists without alleviation and affects efficiency and health it is identified as an anxiety state (Linford Rees, 1982). The state is not produced by current events but is ingrained in the psyche and originates in childhood as a product of parental attitudes. It is in part genetic and is handed down from generation to generation. Skynner (1976) emphasises that parent behaviour reflects the behaviour of their parents since they treat their children in the same way as they themselves were brought up. The case for a genetic component lies in the fact that babies demonstrate from birth very different temperaments prior to falling prey to the family atmosphere and, later, the psychological structure of the family unit. Some children ride the storms better than others: some are equable and happy, others are the reverse. Neurotic individuals tend to be attracted to each other and fall in love, have children and perpetuate their problem (Skynner and Cleese, 1983).

The voice disorders produced by these individuals are not necessarily very pronounced and the larynx does not usually exhibit vocal abuse. Chiefly there are complaints of vocal inadequacy and weakness accompanied by throat discomfort and, in some individuals, cancer phobia.

Personality Disorder

The case history will reveal difficulties and anxieties at home, at work and in social contacts due to the personality of the individual. There may be a recital of difficulties at school, a succession of jobs or marriages, and general signs of instability. Some people are timid, insufficiently assertive, rather humble and apologetic while suppressing normal feelings of anger and hostility. Others are hypersensitive and take offence when none is intended; they brood over injustices and imagined insults and, as a result, withdraw. Then there is the worrier who anticipates problems and is constantly tense, apprehensive and fearful. Another type is obsessional about order, how things are done and routines. Meticulous attention to detail and over-conscientiousness interferes with accomplishing tasks and drives colleagues and family to desperation. Rigid behaviour cannot be altered and changes are fiercely resented since they threaten the security of the routines in which the individual is entrenched.

Anxiety therefore takes many forms and when a traumatic event or a long build-up of worries explodes into a voice problem it indicates that the patient has reached breaking point and that this is due to a breakdown in personal relationships. These anxious individuals are difficult to get on with and their sensitivity, prejudices, intolerances and criticisms of others create disagreements, ill-feeling and lack of cooperation. The patient becomes wrapped up in his or her own miseries and gets a distorted view of events, unable to see both sides of the question. Unable to cope, the voice disorder is a cry for help which cannot be admitted overtly since this would be an admission of failure and inadequacy, and recognition of suppressed fear.

Psychosomatic Symptoms

Chronic anxiety state upsets the homoeostasis of the whole organism; it upsets the regulatory mechanisms of the body which are controlled by the autonomic and sympathetic nervous system thus influencing the endocrine mechanism and release of hormones (Linford Rees, 1982). In this way, psychogenic disorder produces physical disorders known as psychosomatic since mental and physical state are interdependent. When in harmony or homoeostasis, health endures. When out of tune, illnesses of every sort can appear. Psychosomatic symptoms assume many forms and only careful medical examination can determine whether or not such symptoms are organically based. The following conditions generally have a psychosomatic component:

- Respiratory: vasomotor rhinitis, hay fever, asthma, hyperventilation.
- Skin disorders: eczema, urticaria, psoriasis.
- Endocrine disorders: hyperthyroidism, diabetes mellitus.
- Cardiovascular: hypertension, cardiac symptoms, palpitations, headache.
- Hormonal disorders: premenstrual tension, menopausal disturbances.
- Gastrointestinal: ulcer, indigestion, anorexia nervosa, dryness of mouth, urgency.
- Excessive sweating: particularly on forehead, upper lip, palms of hands.
- Sleep disturbance: insomnia and fatigue.
- Thought disturbances: forgetfulness, confusion, disorganisation, phobias.
- Musculoskeletal tension: joint pains and muscle pains (myalgia).

Health Check

A thorough medical examination is necessary to ascertain the validity of the patient's complaints and to prescribe appropriate treatment. Such symptoms as peptic ulcer and high blood pressure are not difficult to diagnose. It is in less well-defined areas such as asthma, migraine and rheumatic pains that the degree of psychological involvement is difficult to ascertain.

Menstrual pains

There are a number of organically based symptoms of ill health which can be mistaken for emotional disturbance. If the patient is not incapacitated by the symptoms it is frequently expected by the doctor that they must be endured although, in fact, they may be helped by medication. For example, hormonal disturbance in females, associated with menstrual and reproductive functions, affect mood and energy. Premenstrual syndrome, postnatal depression and the menopause can produce excessive fatigue, irritability and anxiety. Suitable hormonal treatment is available in many instances; progesterone may be prescribed for premenstrual syndrome. Hormone replacement therapy, although still viewed with caution by many doctors in the UK, is being used increasingly in the USA to relieve the unpleasant symptoms of the menopause. Such treatments can restore the patient's spirits and energy.

Viral infections

Postviral fatigue syndrome may follow an acute attack of influenza and the patient feels tired and depressed for many months without understanding why. These patients may be regarded unsympathetically as neurotic and hyperchondriacal. On the other hand a persisting depression can be purely psychological as in the case of John Cleese (Skynner and Cleese, 1983) who appeared to suffer from 'low grade 'flu symptoms' for 2 years before embarking on a successful course of family therapy (Skynner, 1976).

Myalgias

Myalgic encephalomyelitis (ME) syndrome was not a recognised registered illness until recently. It is a form of postviral fatigue during which the patient is exhausted by minimal exertion and from which it may take years to recover. It appears to be caused by a number of viruses and there is no known drug therapy. The round the world yachtswoman, Clare Francis, suffered from ME syndrome and her problems were regarded as psychogenic for a prolonged period until a correct diagnosis was made. In such cases even the recognition that symptoms are physically based is reassuring. Syndromes such as ME continue to be the subject of debate between doctors regarding the contributions of organic and psychogenic factors. Illnesses have a certain vogue value. Rheumatic pains were 'fibrositis' in the 1950s, now myalgia has taken its place. Polymyalgia is another currently popular term.

Allergy and hypersensitivity

Reactions to specific substances can produce results which resemble psychogenic symptoms. An interesting case is described by Freeman *et al.* (1987). The episodic dysphonia of a young professional woman was initially diagnosed as 'hysterical and/or spasmodic dysphonia'. Although there was no evidence of earlier allergic reactions, careful stroboscopic investigation by the research team revealed a hypersensitive reaction to a particular loft insulation material. This reaction occurred only in the larynx and consisted of oedema and stiffness of the vocal folds. There was complete absence of the closed phase of vocal fold vibration. Freeman *et al.* (1987) concluded that reaction to specific environmental agents should always be considered in cases of psychogenic dysphonia.

Neuropathology

The early stages of neurological disease can mimic psychogenic dysphonia, particularly if the disorder is subject to remissions and relapses. Aronson (1971) describes a case of early motor neurone disease masquerading as psychogenic breathy dysphonia.

Case histories

1. **Mrs E. (47 years)** The laryngologist referred this patient with a normal larynx for speech therapy because her voice grew tired during long conversations. Mrs E. spoke rapidly with few pauses in a light, girlish voice and used frequent hard glottal attack. Sentences were frequently incomplete and she changed subjects rapidly and bewilderingly. She asked questions and either answered them herself or apparently did not listen to the answers because she would ask the same question again a few minutes later. Her first appointment with the speech therapist was delayed because she confused the date for the first visit and as she lost her way on the next visit it began late. She reported that although her voice was troublesome her chief concern was the discomfort in her throat and she admitted that she was terrified that this was cancer which the laryngologist had overlooked. Her father had died of laryngeal cancer and so had a much-loved uncle.

   This patient needed reassurance and sympathetic understanding combined with a matter-of-fact pragmatic approach to establish more relaxed and effective phonation. Throughout her visits over several months she was experiencing stomach pains in addition to her throat symptoms. Gradually she was able to acknowledge when her anxiety was peaking and that it was unfounded. She was the long-awaited only child of over-protective parents upon whom she had been dependent. She married a man much older than herself and retained her dependent role. Much of her anxiety seemed to arise from the fact that she did not feel that she could competently control and organise her own life. These feelings were discussed during treatment. When her throat symptoms were marked she was seen by the laryngologist for indirect laryngoscopy to provide additional reassurance and to confirm that there was no organic basis for her symptoms.

   As time progressed it was possible to discontinue clinical appointments and the patient was able to deal with her anxiety by telephoning the therapist from time to time, and the throat symptoms abated. The voice remained 'girlish' but improved breath support, reduction of hard glottal attack and tempo ensured that it was no longer a problem.

2. Mr D., a lawyer aged 37 years, was referred for treatment of his weak, breathy voice which was also raised in pitch. The laryngologist reported that vocal fold movement was normal.

The dysphonia became apparent within days of a vasectomy under general anaesthetic. Mr D. was a married man with four children and he and his wife had mutually agreed that their family was complete. He reported that he had been reassured by his doctor's explanation that vasectomy was a relatively minor procedure without unwanted side effects although his office colleagues had joked about the possibility of him having a high voice after the operation. However, the post-operative recovery period was traumatic because of marked swelling and discomfort in the genital area which Mr D. felt his doctors had not dealt with effectively or sympathetically.

In the light of the laryngologist's report a psychogenic basis for the dysphonia, precipitated by the operation and its attendant anxiety, seemed probable. At the beginning of therapy Mr D. presented as pleasant but tense, and revealed considerable well-controlled anger concerning the surgeon who had undertaken his operation. During subsequent treatment sessions Mr D. was highly motivated to improve his voice and cooperated fully with voice therapy and with discussion directed at identifying underlying psychogenic aetiology. Apart from being able to achieve stronger voice on single vowels initiated with firm glottal attack, there was no change in phonation over several weeks. It was not possible to establish any primary or secondary gains resulting from the dysphonia.

Further indirect laryngoscopy by the laryngologist confirmed an apparently normal larynx. Mr D. continued with voice therapy and his wife attended sessions occasionally so that the patient's home background and relationships could be explored in more detail. No significant information was revealed but at this point Mr D. willingly agreed to being referred to a psychiatrist in the hope of solving the problem. The psychiatrist reported that he could not identify any underlying psychogenic aetiolgy.

Within the following months Mr D. was examined by three experienced laryngologists while continuing with voice therapy. The vocal fold movement was pronounced normal on each examination. During 18 months of therapy there had been some improvement in vocal quality by ensuring maximum efficiency of all aspects of phonation. The voice remained weak and breathy. It was finally agreed that therapy should be discontinued although Mr D. would be kept under review.

Eventually the advice of another laryngologist was sought and a unilateral vocal fold palsy was diagnosed. Following injection of Teflon into the paralysed vocal fold there was marked improvement in vocal quality.

The history of this case suggested a psychogenic basis to the dysphonia, particularly when the initial laryngoscopic examinations apparently indicated normality. However, it appears that a vocal fold palsy was somehow sustained during the period of this patient's hospitalisation and was not diagnosed.

Hyperventilation Syndrome

This is a serious disturbance of breathing in people suffering from anxiety state. Breathing irregularity is well known to be associated with anxiety and emotional disturbances. Increased heart rate, sweating and muscular tension accompany a breathing crisis. Over-breathing occurs in persons suffering from anxiety state when they are undergoing a panic attack. A frightening situation triggers an attack which will subside gradually, but individuals may become conditioned and react in this way in similar circumstances or even at the memory of an attack (Lum, 1976). Breathing is not only rapid but irregular and may be accompanied by sighing (Innocenti, 1983).

Ventilation of the lungs in excess of metabolic needs produces arterial hypocapnia which is a persistent drop in carbon dioxide level in arterial blood and expired alveolar air. A sudden acute panic attack is accompanied by excessive panting and high clavicular breathing with heaving shoulders. It may be seen in aircraft passengers when going through a period of turbulence or landing in thick fog. Although an acute attack is very alarming to witness it is not fatal. However, it is necessary to be aware that hyperventilation may be provoked, for example, when the patient is given a breathing exercise or if a sensitive topic is touched upon in taking a case history. The therapist should remain calm and assume a reassuring and quietly authoritative manner, exhorting the patient to breathe slowly and from the 'stomach' (Greene, 1984). Tranquillisers may be prescribed by the physician but these are addictive, have side effects and do not solve the patient's emotional problems. Patients treated by Greene (1984) said that the tranquillisers did not help to allay the panic.

Situational anxiety, stage fright, examination nerves, and the fear of flying can best be alleviated by ß-blocking drugs, i.e. ß-adrenergic receptor blocking drugs such as oxprenolol (Gates and Montalbo, 1987). This is also used as a prophylactic treatment for migraine. Administered half an hour before a dreaded ordeal, concomitant anxiety is dispersed without affecting concentration, clarity of thought or reaction time.

Marked over-breathing can exist in anxiety states without any dramatic episodes of hyperventilation. These patients suffer from a wide spectrum of psychosomatic disorders simulating diseases and listed on the previous pages and described by Lewis (1959) and by Magarian (1983) who gives an excellent account of hyperventilation syndrome in discussing 'infrequently recognised expressions of anxiety and stress'.

There is a wide range in the severity of symptoms in hyperventilation. Borderline cases of hypocapnia and chronic anxiety may have only occasional stressful situations. Relaxation is helpful to such patients as it is in many cases of psychogenic aphonia.

Psychosomatic symptoms may be so severe and the patient's complaints so persistent that they frequently result in extensive medical examinations in one hospital department after another. The patient's case notes will provide evidence of many investigations of heart, lung, gastric and endocrine function all proving negative (Greene, Timmons and Glover, 1983, 1984).

Measurement of hypocapnia

Precise measurement of carbon dioxide levels in each expiration can be obtained by passing expired air through a capnograph machine which also indicates the number of respirations per minute. Normal breathing rate is approximately 12 per minute and rates in excess of this indicate the presence of hyperventilation. The capnograph is difficult to operate and testing requires an experienced technician and medical assistant. A 'provocation' test of panting rapidly for 3 minutes is required, after which the carbon dioxide readings are monitored for a recovery period of 3 minutes. The level should return to that of the testing level and, if it fails to do so, hyperventilation is diagnosed (Greene, 1984).

A speech therapist can very easily time respiratory rate with a watch, and note irregularities and sighing especially during relaxation therapy. Confirmation of diagnosis is reinforced by the case history and indicates the need for emphasis in treatment on respiratory training.

Greene, Timmons and Glover (1983, 1984) subjected a number of dysphonic patients attending a speech clinic to capnographic assessment. Two patients who were failing to progress proved to be hyperventilators with positive hypocapnia. They had typical case histories and suffered from anxiety state and a series of unconfirmed physical disorders. Two cases with spasmodic adductor dysphonia were not hyperventilators. Two newly referred patients were tested before being given speech therapy and diagnosed as hyperventilators and then given a course of breathing therapy and counselling. They responded well to treatment.

Breathing therapy

Re-education of breathing is the first requirement. Difficulty in speaking and phonasthenia is the least of the problems. Lum (1976) reported excellent results with a programme followed by physiotherapists (Innocenti, 1983). Diaphragmatic central breathing must be established and slowed down to a normal regular rate of 12 cycles per minute approximately. Brief breath holding pauses can be introduced either at the peak or trough of the respiratory cycle. When normal breathing is established, breathing rhythm for speech can be introduced and vowel prolongations practised, i.e. maximum phonation time (MPT). Poetry and prose reading can help establish respiratory control in speech. Relaxation therapy and breathing rehabilitation is insufficient and supportive therapy is essential. Discussion of problems and fears is necessary and suggestions should be made in an endeavour to guide the patient to meet and manage them.

Case history

Mr W. (32 years) was referred by the laryngologist chiefly for relaxation therapy. He complained of a painful throat which grew worse with talking and made communication difficult. His larynx was normal but the laryngologist reported that the patient was 'terribly tensed-up and quite unable to cooperate in the clinical examination'. He had had treatment for neurosis in the past.

He presented as a self-possessed individual with no worries, just a sore throat. He was happily married with a son of 4 years and a baby of 6 months. He had a job as a clerk in the County Council Office and had been employed there for 5 years. Prior to changing from his previous job he had suffered from severe stomach pains which were, after full investigation, diagnosed as neurotic. He confessed to being 'rather a worrier' over his responsibilities.

His thick file of medical notes covered many extensive investigations over the last 10 years concerning pains in his torso. A pain in the left side was found to have no organic basis and no cardiac signs. He later had a pain in the left iliac fossa but no cause could be identified. Physiotherapy was prescribed by the orthopaedic surgeon for a slight scoliosis.

He was slightly round shouldered and certainly had poor posture. His voice occasionally 'grated', his breathing was shallow and rapid. The sore throat was not there all the time he said, but came and went. A course of relaxation and breathing therapy, and reassurance concerning the worries over his responsibilities, provided at least temporary relief. The sore throat gradually disappeared and he was discharged.

Individuals suffering from chronic anxiety cannot be so easily cured but their condition can be alleviated and sympathetic support helps them to carry on without breakdown or resort to drug therapy.

The Globus Symptom

The globus symptom refers to the sensation of a lump in the throat in the absence of true dysphagia. It may accompany aphonia or dysphonia. It was previously known as 'globus hystericus' but this terminology is now regarded as out-dated as evidence regarding a multiplicity of factors which give rise to the symptom has been amassed.

Many individuals experience the sensation of a lump in the throat at times of strong emotion when they are either unable to express the emotion or when it would be considered inappropriate to give vent to these feelings. This sensation differs from the globus symptom in that it is relatively transitory. The globus symptom is persistent and may recur constantly; the patient may attempt to clear the throat by frequent swallowing and throat-clearing. The condition is distinguishable from true dysphagia by the fact that it is either relieved or not affected by swallowing, while in true dysphagia swallowing is difficult and pain or a sensation of obstruction develops within 15 seconds of the pharyngeal movements of swallowing (Bradley and Narula, 1987). These authors found that approximately 1–4% of new patients seen in an ENT clinic were referred for treatment of globus symptoms and that in women of 50 years or younger the incidence is three times more frequent than in men. After 50 years the incidence is comparable to men (Moloy and Charter, 1982).

Physical aetiology

As the globus symptom may have both psychogenic and physical origins all patients with this complaint undergo careful examination which includes thorough visualisation of the oropharynx and supraglottic region in order to exclude the presence of disease and especially malignant tumour. Malcolmson (1968) found that in a series of 307 patients complaining of lump in the throat 38% had miscellaneous local lesions and 62 distal lesions, of which the most common was hiatus hernia which comprised 69% of distal lesions. It is interesting and significant that there were only 90 males but 217 females in this series. Delahunty and Ardran (1970) discovered that 22 out of 25 patients with diagnosis of 'globus hystericus' suffered from reflux oesophagitis resulting in acid-induced motility disturbance. The feeling of a lump in the throat was eradicated when these patients were placed on an acid-free regimen. On the other hand Moloy and Charter (1982) question the relationship between globus symptom and oesophageal reflux. In their study, of 103 patients the incidence of gastric reflux symptoms was 38% compared to 36% in the general adult population. They found that even when the reflux symptoms were treated successfully the globus symptom did not improve. Gastrointestinal tract roentgenography for all patients with globus symptom is recommended by Nishijima, Takoda and Hasegawa (1984) as a result of their study of 290 patients with globus symptom, 76% of whom had gastrointestinal tract lesions. Other possible physical causes of globus symptom include cervical osteophytes, upper respiratory tract infection, enlarged lingual tonsil and disordered mobility of the oesophagus (Nishijima, Takoda and Hasegawa, 1984). Osteoarthritis of the cervical spine is a common cause of referred pain. Pressure symptoms can be caused by a slightly enlarged thyroid gland. A feeling of a lump in the throat can arise from very tense laryngeal muscles.

Psychogenic aetiology

In those patients where physical causes have been excluded it appears that true conversion syndrome (see p. 172) is uncommon. Studies suggest that depression is the most common psychological feature in the globus symptom. The dysphonic patients we have treated with globus symptoms usually appear to have their emotions under careful control and are reluctant to express their feelings. In many instances their approach to life is stoic and they continue to carry out their family and work commitments in spite of real emotional and practical difficulties. They regard the need for support from family and friends as a sign of weakness and yet there is pride in providing support for others even if, at times, it is accompanied by resentment and feelings of being 'put upon'.

Discussion and support which give the individual insight into the condition will often produce weeping which heralds the initial stage of recovery and appears to be related to the opportunity to be 'weak' in a situation of complete confidentiality. Studies confirm that giving the patient reassurance concerning the aetiology of the globus symptom, particularly confirming that it is not cancer, produces a cure in the majority of cases. Patients suffering from, dysphonia and globus symptom are routinely referred by laryngologists for speech therapy and respond very well to therapy.

> Case history
> Mrs A. (48 years) was referred for speech therapy because of intermittent dysphonia. The laryngoscopic examination was normal although the laryngologist noted that she was 'rather tense'. Mrs A. was extremely thin and her posture was upright and rigid. She had minimal facial expression; this lack of affect was disconcerting for the listener because of the limited feedback from the patient during conversation. Phonation required visible effort and yet the voice was only just loud enough to be heard in normal conversation. As the case history was taken she complained that her throat felt constricted almost continually to the extent that she felt unable to eat at times and swallowing was uncomfortable.
>
> A story gradually emerged of divorce proceedings 5 years previously which had been followed by a very happy relationship with a married man. Unfortunately, without warning, he ended the relationship by letter. The patient was devastated when this happened 3 months before her referral to the ENT department. She was quite unaware of the link between these events and her present problems. During a lengthy interview she revealed that she had felt unable to show her feelings at the break-up of this relationship because her teenage children would have been upset by their mother's distress. She had not been able to express her grief and anger at the termination of the relationship and the way it was ended. As she gave this account she began to sob uncontrollably and she expressed the fear that she would not be able to stop crying. When she did stop weeping she put her hand to her neck as she realised that the 'feeling of a lump in the throat' had gone.
>
> This interview was followed by weekly speech therapy sessions which provided emotional support and traditional voice therapy. As her self-respect increased and as she talked about her feelings of loss, the globus symptom reduced in intensity and eventually disappeared. Her voice returned to normal and her facial expression, which had indicated depression, became increasingly animated and responsive.

Conversion Syndrome (Conversion/Hysterical Aphonia)

The conversion syndrome has a strong anxiety component but it is essentially a psychogenic illness with a characteristic motive of gain of which the individual is unaware. In the case of anxiety state the symptoms from which the person suffers are produced by the reaction of the autonomic nervous system to stress and are not under conscious control. In the individual suffering from conversion syndrome the physical symptoms produced concern the voluntary nervous system although they appear to be involuntary and are outside the patient's control. Aronson (1973) lists the criteria for diagnosis of a conversion aphonia as:

1. The existence of normal structure and function of the affected part of the body.
2. Existence of anxiety, stress, depression or interpersonal conflict and symbolic significance for that conflict.
3. It serves a purpose and extricates the patient from a difficult situation.

The conversion symptom conforms to the patient's concept of the disability and will therefore exhibit various anomalies. A sufferer from writer's cramp with hand and arm going into a painful spastic spasm has the symptom in writing only and in no other movement. An hysterical paraesthesia is found to involve the lower part of a limb and follows a 'glove and stocking' distribution and is therefore not neurologically viable. The vocal folds fail to adduct and produce voice but move normally at other times.

Disassociation

Under intolerable stress the individual evades it by disassociating thoughts from it and directs them into imagined disability which effectively provides a means of escape. For example, loss of voice in a teacher solves the horror of trying to control an unruly class. The primary gain is that the individual is no longer able to carry on in an intolerable situation. The attention and sympathy which the symptom subsequently elicits is the secondary gain which is extremely satisfying to the patient.

Personality of the 'hysteric'

The conversion syndrome is not evidence of malingering which is the conscious assumption of an ailment for gain and known to be false by the subject. Backache or headache can provide an excuse to avoid going to school or work but this is an excuse just as conscious as that of having to attend the fictional 'grandmother's funeral'. The conversion syndrome personality differs from that of the sufferer from anxiety state. The former craves attention and seeks the lime-light, with a proclivity for histrionics and a tendency to exaggerate and dramatise. The craving for love and attention is so acute and the individual can be so demanding that people are driven away. At the same time there may be considerable manipulation of family members, friends, colleagues and even strangers. The hysterical trouble-maker can be detected in all organisations, hospitals, schools and offices. When things are going well a conversion symptom is not necessary.

In dealing with the conversion syndrome, the therapist must remain alert to the possibility of also being manipulated by the patient and caught in the net. To do the 'hysteric' justice, it must be understood that the actual conversion symptom is assumed without conscious awareness of any connection between its appearance and the reason for it and the advantage it represents. The exact nature of the mental process which happens 'when the mysterious leap from the mental to the physical' is made (Freud, 1943) is not fully understood. Freud thought that the imaginary symptom symbolised conflict and reflected the conversion of mental torture into acceptable physical discomfort.

'La belle indifference'

A pronounced feature of the disorder is the detached attitude sufferers exhibit towards their afflictions described by Janet (1920) as 'la belle indifference'. Paralysis of the leg or hand normally produces acute concern about the cause and the future economic consequences of the inability to work. However, the hysteric exhibits indifference and real lack of concern, conveyed positively in the paralinguistic behaviour, although the inconveniences may be expressed verbally. A long-suffering attitude is attenuated by a certain stoicism and the patient obtains sympathy and commendation for being so courageous in the face of such adversity.

Precipitating factors

The onset of a conversion symptom may be precipitated by an emotional shock such as a disaster in the family or at work. In many instances, however, it appears that the gradual accumulation of stress eventually results in the conversion symptom when the individual can no longer cope and suffers the proverbial straw which breaks the camel's back. In such cases it may be precipitated by illness, particularly an upper respiratory tract infection and a viral laryngitis.

The conversion symptom may be an isolated incident or unexplained afflictions may be traced throughout adult life. The reaction is virtually unknown in childhood although we have seen such cases. Nerve wracking, terrifying protracted experience, as during months of combat, can demoralise previously stable and well-integrated individuals who finally reach breaking point. Smurthwaite (1919) and Sokolowsky and Junkermann (1944) reported hysterical voice disorders in soldiers returning from the front in World War I.

Laryngeal symptoms

Smurthwaite (1919) described four distinct positions assumed by the vocal folds in attempted phonation which are significant in the diagnosis of 'functional dysphonia' so familiar to laryngologists. Similar vocal fold positions were noted by Sokolowsky and Junkermann (1944). The types of pseudo-paralysis include:

1. Folds elliptical - paresis of the thyroarytenoideus.
2. Folds in cadaveric position; the folds can be freely abducted but there is no attempt at adduction.
3. Both true and false folds tightly adducted in a spasm of both adductor and constrictor laryngeal muscles.
4. Folds approximate in the anterior two-thirds, but there is a triangular aperture in the posterior third due to paralysis of the transverse arytenoid muscle.

Morrison, Nichol and Rammage (1986) also note that conversion aphonia may present as hyperadducted ventricular band aphonia as well as the more classic bowing of the vocal folds. Their studies reveal no direct correlation in psychogenic dysphonias between laryngoscopic appearance and the various psychiatric diagnoses.

The indirect laryngological examination may be easily accomplished due to a paraesthesia of throat and palate. This is a distinguishing difference from anxiety state.

Incidence

Conversion symptom aphonia is more common in women than men, occurring in a ratio of 7 : 1. Its greatest incidence is between the ages of 18 and 34 years and it is virtually unknown in children. It was thought to be a largely female complaint (Thompson, Negus and Bateman, 1955), hence the term 'hysteria' derived from Greek for the womb.

It is our belief that aphonia as a conversion symptom is on the decrease due to a better informed and more sophisticated public. During the last 25 years we have observed that the conversion aphonias seen in our clinics have become less naive in type and pattern. We no longer see cases where the voice disappears on Monday morning as the unpleasant working week starts, only to return on Friday evening and then continue the pattern as the week begins again. We have the impression that increased knowledge does not allow the individual to produce a symptom of such transparency.

Rehabilitation

Eliciting voice

It is generally agreed that in cases of conversion aphonia the voice should be recovered as quickly as possible, preferably at the first interview. The manner in which the therapist handles this important session is crucial to the eventual outcome. The longer patients perceive that their 'difficult' problem is confounding all treatment, the more entrenched the symptom will become. As these patients are highly suggestible it is important that particular care is taken when giving the usual explanations of normal voice production and the reasons for their symptoms. Many patients, although not unduly distressed by their conversion aphonia, are very distressed to learn at indirect laryngoscopy that the larynx is normal and that the symptom is therefore psychological. They may be appalled by this evidence of their mental disturbance. We have seen patients who have declared that they would have preferred that an organic abnormality had been found.

Most patients find it acceptable to be told, quite truthfully, that the vocal tract and vocal fold movement is particularly responsive to emotional changes. In some individuals this is more marked than in others who may succumb to headaches or abdominal pain. It can be pointed out that although under stress it is usually necessary for individuals to continue with the routine of daily life. In order to do so true feelings are repressed and as a result, in this instance, the vocal folds have become so tense that they will not fully adduct.

Further discussion concerning the psychodynamics of the problem are usually less important at this time than voice recovery. The patient is reassured that there is no physical reason why voice cannot be produced, apart from an element of habit, and the therapist introduces strategies for eliciting voice.

Vocal strategies

A survey of the literature describing the various methods recommended for the recovery of voice in conversion aphonia patients demonstrates forcibly that practically any tactics will succeed if put into effect with sufficient aplomb during the first session with the patient. Smurthwaite (1919) recommended groaning or coughing after deep inspiration, or the application of a laryngeal probe to produce a paroxysm of coughing. Pulling the tongue out with the instruction to say 'ah' was also found to be efficacious. Lell (1941) advocated provoking the gag reflex by probing with the laryngoscopic mirror. This use of the 'surprise attack' was supported by Sokolowsky and Junkermann (1944) who found that strong verbal suggestion and a confident authoritative manner led to a cure in the great majority of their cases at the first session. The administration of systematic voice training techniques which they tried at the outset took time and produced only 60% recovery of voice. Jackson (1940) recommended getting the patient to bring the elbows down to the sides with a thump coincident with a phonatory cough or grunt.

Some patients are helped by the use of white noise through headphones. The patient is asked to sing or talk against the noise. With auditory control of the voice removed, the voice returns and convinces the patient that it is not irrevocably lost (Labarrque, 1952). This procedure will not be successful with those patients who do not vocalise while wearing the headphones. Although the patient often does produce voice while 'deafened' in this way, many do not.

In the past, application of a strong faradic current to the larynx has been used. This method generally produces a scream which is convincing to the patient. If there is an associated anaesthesia - and this is possible - the patient remains impervious to the electric shock.

The majority of conversion aphonia patients respond well to a confident and relaxed approach which involves the speech therapist firmly but gently depressing the larynx. The patient is then asked to cough or clear the throat. Immediately phonation is heard, however brief or 'croaky', the patient is encouraged to extend the sound on a vowel, two vowels, serial speech, automatic speech and so on. The recovered voice frequently sounds strange to the patient but reassurances are given that it will return to normal with use.

It is to be deplored that some laryngologists having restored a patient's voice with the 'surprise attack' send the patient away cured. Instead, referral should be made to the speech therapist. Recovery of the voice is not the sole aim in these cases; a patient needs to gain insight into the reason for the voice loss and be helped to cope with the difficulties from which it originated. There is always a possibility of recurrence of the aphonia or development of another conversion symptom if the mental conflict is not resolved.

Case history

Mrs C. (36 years) was referred for speech therapy with aphonia which started with an upper respiratory tract infection. On direct laryngoscopy there was no laryngeal abnormality. She had been aphonic for 16 months during which time she had visited her general practitioner repeatedly for advice and medication without improvement. Eventually she was referred to a laryngologist.

During the interview with the speech therapist she was vivacious and verbose, all conversation being conducted in a forced whisper. She was not unduly concerned by her lack of voice. Having reassured her that there was no reason why the voice should not recover completely, the therapist gently manipulated the larynx and encouraged relaxation of the neck muscles. She was encouraged to cough and then to give a cough immediately followed by various vowels. Within 5 minutes she was counting, saying the days of the week etc. and after 10 minutes was phonating throughout conversation. The patient was tearful and amazed that her voice had returned so quickly after its long absence. As a result of the explanations given to her concerning the reasons for such symptoms she was soon able to identify the precipitating factor. She had two children, a girl of 14 years and a boy of 10 years. She felt that there had been constant conflict with her daughter over everything from homework, to the time she should come home and the suitability of her clothes. The arguments between mother and daughter were disrupting the whole family with her husband blaming her for not being able to control their daughter. It was significant that the family had been more cooperative since the mother had been voiceless, and that the father fulfilled a more positive role in relation to his daughter since his wife had been unable to shout. Two further appointments directed at establishing a secure voice through traditional voice therapy in combination with counselling ensured the stable return of the voice.

Conversion dysphonia

The acquisition of an unexplained but severe dysphonia is not uncommon and corresponds to the type of pseudoparalysis assumed by the vocal folds. Adduction of both true and false folds can produce a double vocal note (diplophonia), the false folds producing a deeper pitch than the true folds.

Tight compression of both true and false folds produces a high-pitched and raucous voice described as 'ventricular band' voice. The false folds press down and obliterate the sinus and prevent folds vibrating normally. A falsetto or puberphonic-type voice may be produced by male patients and immature high pitch by women. Patients may produce different vocal effects on different occasions.

Remediation philosophy

It is important that normal voice should be established early so that the patient does not manipulate the tender-hearted therapist indefinitely. Damsté (1983) cautions against being drawn into 'playing the patient's game' and advocates firm handling. Linford Rees (1982) advises ignoring the affliction and concentrating upon improvement. If given sympathy, this is just the attention the patient craves and it encourages indulgence in a successful gambit.

Speech therapy is successful with patients in whom conversion is not too deeply entrenched. Prognosis for early recovery are an acute onset, short duration, stable relationships and permanence of occupation. In favourable circumstances the speech therapist may be more successful than a psychiatrist. Psychotherapy may be required in some cases but Freudian psychoanalysis continues over a long period and is not always successful. Skynner (1976) is critical of this approach and in his Family Therapy the psychiatrist plays an active role in helping the family or group to solve their problems.

Linford Rees (1982) presenting the analytical approach cautions against the therapist taking a positive attitude, of taking sides and, above all, giving advice on how to act. It is sensible for the therapist to avoid becoming involved in the patient's personal relationships especially when this is the scenario the hysteric is so skilled at manipulating. On the other hand, the patient needs guidance desperately and friendly support can be given and counselling which gives a positive structure to life. First, the hysteric has to gain insight into why the vocal disability has arisen and to take responsibility for it. Subsequently, the patient is guided through suggestion in other ways of handling the situational circumstances which provoked the conversion symptom.

However, when the patient's voice does not recover after a few sessions the speech therapist is well advised to recommend to the laryngologist that the patient should be referred for psychotherapy.

Voice therapy

It can be argued that voice therapy is superfluous in treatment of conversion aphonia and dysphonia. However, the regimen advocated in Chapter 9 has considerable efficacy, in long-standing cases, in establishing normal phonation after a vocal note has been elicited. Although the aetiology is psychogenic, phonation patterns and their associated kinaesthetic feedback have been abnormal and patients frequently feel that they have 'forgotten' how to produce normal voice. A programme of voice therapy stabilises the regained voice and provides a focus for the interaction between speech therapist and patient as support is gradually withdrawn.

This patient group is generally highly suggestible and will benefit from relaxation techniques as previously described. Tension can be reduced further by slowing and regulating the breathing rate while concentrating on diaphragmatic intercostal breathing patterns. Attention to central breathing also diverts preoccupation with the throat and sensations of pressure or a lump.

The fact that the patient has unconsciously selected a vocal symptom may be due entirely to a failure to communicate in a traumatic social encounter, but it may also be due to the fact that phonation is poorly produced habitually and that there is an element of vocal strain which engenders laryngeal and pharyngeal discomfort. Therefore direct therapy for improving phonation will establish confidence in the voice and reduce the factors which predispose the patient to dysphonia.

Psychogenic Spastic Dysphonia

A particular and immediately recognisable type of dysphonia is that characterised by a spasmodic adduction of the vocal folds. This interrupts phonation, producing the so-called 'strangulated' voice. There is extreme laryngeal and pharyngeal tension, and phonation is interrupted by uncontrolled sphincteric closure of the laryngeal mechanism. The aetiolgy of 'spastic dysphonia' is not fully understood and there is evidence that though this condition has both psychogenic and neurological origins it may be attributed exclusively to one or other cause: either psychological or neurological. The neurological form of spasmodic adductor dysphonia is described in Chapter 14. In this section we confine the discussion to the hysterical syndrome.

The symptoms known as 'spastic dysphonia' have been recognised by laryngologists since 1854 after Manuel Garcia designed the laryngeal mirror and indirect laryngoscopy became available. It was considered to be a conversion symptom because vegetative functions, such as coughing and laughing, are frequently normal. The condition excited no particular interest among speech pathologists until Arnold and Heaver (1959) published a report of a female patient suffering from 'spastic dysphonia' whom they treated as a psychiatric case for years without effecting a cure. Greene saw the patient herself in New York who made an indelible impression of acute distress. The exaggerated attempts at forcing the voice when speaking certainly appeared to be indicative of an hysterical state.

In 1960 Robe, Moore and Brumlik described 10 patients suffering from 'spastic dysphonia' who exhibited frank neurological signs. Since then evidence attributing the disorder to a defect of the central nervous system has accumulated (Dedo and Shipp, 1980). Research and brainstem audiometry now confirms that persistent cases of spasmodic dysphonia are of neurological aetiology (see Chapter 14).

Evidence in the case history and remissions in the symptoms will point to a psychogenic spastic dysphonia. Aronson (1980) established that 45% of the patients he examined had experienced emotional trauma prior to onset of the condition. We have seen male and female patients whose symptoms were cured by therapy and where the aetiology was obviously psychogenic. There are various reports in the literature of spastic dysphonia being cured by speech therapy, and these cases must have been conversion disorder (Damsté, 1983).

Voice therapy in all cases is concentrated upon relaxation, soft attack and quiet voice in an attempt to reduce or prevent the laryngospasm. Considerable reassurance and support must be provided by the speech therapist and combined with diagnostic therapy aimed at identifying the emotional factors related to the conversion sysmptom.

Case histories

1. Mr F. (38 years) a married man with two young children was referred for speech therapy with the diagnosis 'hoarse voice - vocal cords normal'. As he spoke there was frequent laryngospasm and speech involved great effort. The symptoms were those of spastic dysphonia. His manner was incongruously cheerful in the light of his obvious difficulty in phonating; laughter was normal.

   The case history revealed that a 'catch' in his voice had become noticeable shortly after he had been told that he was to be made redundant from his job as an acountant. Phonation had become increasingly effortful in the 5 weeks prior to seeing the laryngologist. He was now in the process of applying for another job. Although he found it difficult to believe that there was any connection between losing his job and his dysphonia, he was highly motivated to comply with therapy because of forthcoming interviews. Relaxation and breathing therapy followed by work on voiced sighs and the elimination of hard glottal attack in order to avoid inducing laryngospasm proved to be the most effective method of remediation. Cheerfully and politely he rejected all attempts at discussion of the underlying aspects of his problem. As he became able to produce vowel-strings with normal voice and his confidence increased in applying these principles to normal speech, carry-over was apparent. Although the voice was not completely normal he dealt with job interviews successfully, started his new job and eventually telephoned the therapist to report that he was too busy to have further treatment and that his voice was fine, which it did indeed seem to be. There was no evidence of the psychogenic spastic dysphonia.

2. Mrs L., a middle-age woman who worked in the hospital, was referred suffering from aphonia. She was devoted to her husband who was retired. (They had no children.) He had not been well recently and had 'passed out' several times and was admitted to hospital for tests. Talking over her anxiety concerning her husband, and having to leave him at home alone when she was at work, her voice returned. It was found that her husband had diabetes and he soon returned home with a strict diet to observe. Some weeks later the wife came to the speech clinic again. She had not lost her voice this time but 'it sounded terrible' and she had difficulty speaking. The dysphonia was of typical spastic adductor type. Was her husband worse, was that the worry? The problem was that her husband's diet was very costly because it was high protein and she was having difficulty 'making ends meet'. Once she had exposed her anxiety and fears, a few exercises restored the voice to normal. She was then referred to the dietitian for advice and the medical social worker for help with financial problems.

   This case, suffering from conversion aphonia earlier and spastic dysphonia later which was curable, was unquestionably a psychogenic disorder.

(We are indebted to Mrs Mary Kirk, LCST for the following interesting case history of Mrs A. who at first had periods of vocal recovery, presented no neurological symptoms and suffered, it seems, from a psychogenic spasm dysphonia.)

3. Mrs A. (50 years) was first examined by a local laryngologist near her home before being referred for speech therapy at a city hospital clinic. This consultant told Mrs A. that her voice problem was psychological but she refused to accept this and was very upset by his remarks. She came to the city hospital complaining of dysphonia and recurrent loss of voice lasting several days. She was examined by a sympathetic consultant who referred her for speech therapy. There was no progress and the speech therapist asked for a neurological assessment but no disorder was discovered. The patient was then referred to the psychiatric department but did not keep the appointment.

   Mrs A. was periodically reviewed by the laryngologist and speech therapist for a year, during which time the larynx looked normal with no signs of inflammation. She was now referred to the department of psychological medicine where she attended as a day patient and received suggestion therapy under pentathol and hypnosis. There was good recovery at first and the voice became normal. Then it deteriorated again. Mrs A. continued to attend this clinic every week.

Mrs. A. had worked as a cleaner most of her life. Her husband was an alcoholic who physically attacked her and treated her appallingly. She had left him 18 years previously. She had three children and was sterilised after the third. She lost all her hair after this operation and said that she kept feeling a choking sensation in her throat, as though she could not breathe, at this time. She became dysphonic after the death of her father, to whom she was very attached. He died of cancer of the lung and larynx and she nursed him through this. She said that she never had any fear of developing cancer herself but immediately after his death the choking feeling returned and then she lost her voice. She said she wanted to cry but could not. Mrs A.'s daughter developed conversion blindness after her grandmother's death. Mrs A. was described in her medical notes as suffering from various psychogenic symptoms for many years.

She presented in the speech clinic with a typical spastic dysphonia. She coughed, sighed and sang normally and her speaking voice was often normal for some seconds and then deteriorated. Her breathing was very tense and clavicular. Despite constant work on this, her breathing pattern remained jerky and shallow. She breathed rapidly when not phonating and often a glottal stop could be heard on expiration. She was unable to breathe in, hold the breath and breathe out, even to a count of three. Therapy consisted of direct voice work and discussion of the factors underlying her dysphonia. She told the therapist very little of her personal history, not because she had anything to hide, but because she thought it had little to do with her case. Her sister gave the therapist most of the information. Mrs A. attended regularly but only, it seemed, to please the therapist. She showed no reaction when a tape-recording of her voice was played to her saying that 'it didn't sound too bad' and that she had become used to it. This lack of involvement was a barrier to progress and more than anything else indicated that a cure could not be achieved by traditional methods.

Chapter 11 Psychogenic and Endocrine Disorders of Pitch

Puberphonia (Mutational Dysphonia)

During adolescence the boy's larynx achieves adult dimensions, the vocal folds double in length and the voice 'breaks' and drops an octave into the male register. Occasionally, despite normal growth and the development of secondary sexual characteristics the adolescent retains his pre-pubertal voice. This is known as puberphonia among British speech therapists but is referred to as failure in voice mutation or mutational falsetto in USA and parts of Europe. There are a number of physical conditions which may render normal voice mutation impossible and these are detailed in Chapter 13. When maturation of the boy and growth of the larynx is normal and the movement of the vocal folds is unimpaired, failure in voice mutation is always psychogenic.

Aetiology

Various explanations for the retention of the child's voice have been suggested. According to Freudian psychology puberphonia is explained by the Oedipus complex. The boy's love for his mother reaches full strength and fantasies of incest which are unacceptable terrify him. Denial of sexual maturity and adulthood requires rejection of masculinity and use of the mature male voice. It seems evident that whatever the fundamental origin and the relationships with his parents, there is in most cases a strong bond between mother and son. Over-protection in childhood leads to over-dependence and fear of assuming adult responsibilities. Frequently the father is seen by the boy as threatening or, at least, as a peripheral member of the family.

Homosexual tendencies may be at the root of the failure to obtain vocal maturity if there is a rejection of those qualities which are associated with masculinity. Many adolescent boys pass through a pseudo-homosexual phase which is regarded as a normal phase of development and is apparent in the 'hero-worship' of an older boy or a teacher. The majority outgrow this phase and form heterosexual relationships in which male voice is an attribute.

Speech therapy

Despite the possible psychogenic, pathological reasons for puberphonia, the results of speech therapy are excellent. The majority of patients will be highly motivated to achieve an appropriate post-pubertal voice because they have been made painfully aware of the social and career disadvantages of the 'unbroken' voice. Treatment is unlikely to be successful if the individual has no real desire to change the voice but has responded to the pressure of others who think that treatment should be sought. Normal laryngeal growth and length of vocal folds ensures that male voice can be produced as long as the patient is cooperative.

Frequently the patient, still with 'unbroken' voice long past the normal maturation period, appears to have adjusted satisfactorily to his own problems in the process of growing up and obtaining economic independence after leaving school. Van Riper and Irwin (1958) stress the force of vocal habits in dysphonia; even if the voice problems start as a psychogenic symptom and the expression of emotional conflicts, they may become purely reflex and habitual.

Shyness at switching over to a new and more appropriate voice may ensure the perpetuation of an undesirable vocal habit. Sometimes a deeper pitch can be produced quite easily but the patient just lacks the confidence to use this in public knowing that it will cause comment and possible ridicule.

Predisposing factors

1. Unusually early 'breaking' of the voice which renders the boy self-conscious among his contemporaries leading him to favour the boy's voice. It becomes so habitual that it is impossible to achieve normal voice (West, Ansberry and Carr, 1957). Late development of sexual maturity may cause similar problems.
2. A desire to retain a 'star' treble voice which has brought distinction when it is known that loss of this singing voice will mean loss of attention.
3. Fear of assuming a full share of adult responsibility or of losing material protection. There is unconscious assertion of immaturity by prolongation of a childish voice, especially when the boy is an only child and there is a strong bond with the mother, while the father is unsympathetic because excluded. The majority of our patients have been only children or, where there are more children, the only male child. We prefer this explanation of mutational dysphonia to the complicated tale of the Oedipus complex.
4. Hero worship of an older boy or man by a boy with a strong feminine inclination, if encouraged, may also result in rejection of the masculine voice.
5. The possession of a natural tenor voiçe or small larynx with short vocal folds would appear to be a predisposing factor in puberphonia, while any of the above factors may help to crystallise the condition. A tenor register seems to occur more frequently than a baritone or bass in the adjusted voices of puberphonic patients, but in this Greene's (1961) observations conflict with those of Weiss (1950) whose experience with many more cases was the exact opposite of her own.

6. Severe deafness and the ability to hear his own voice and appreciate adult male voices, may result in retention of the pre-pubertal voice (Greene, 1961, 1962; Wirz, 1986).

Vocal features

Although the predominant characteristic of the puberphonic voice is its unnaturally high pitch, there are many variations in the voices of these patients. Sometimes, the voice is a true falsetto, high and thin and exhibiting no abrupt vacillation in pitch. It would be logical to assume that individuals consistently using a pitch so foreign to their natural registers would produce vocal nodules. This, however, proves to be the exception rather than the rule, and we have encountered only two patients with vocal nodules: one was aged 26 years and the other 69 years. Some patients experience supralaryngeal pain as a result of the larynx being maintained abnormally high in the vocal tract (Hartman and Aronson, 1983). However, excessive tension does not always exist in association with falsetto voices and, when an individual produces this voice quite easily, vocal strain does not necessarily occur.

Most commonly the pitch of the voice is inconsistent and breaks occur inadvertently. The voice reverts to falsetto as the deep pitch is rejected. Individuals who can produce mature male voice momentarily are much easier to treat successfully than those who can only produce falsetto. Also the younger the better. If treatment is given during the mutational period before years of habit have established the abnormal voice, acquisition of male voice should not be difficult.

Remediation

A laryngologist's report confirming normality of laryngeal growth and structure (see Chapter 6) is essential.

A careful case history is necessary so that comprehensive information regarding the patient's childhood, home background and personality is obtained. It is also necessary to gain the patient's full cooperation at the initial interview to ensure that he has a sincere desire to improve his voice. Frequently vocal 'weakness' is the patient's complaint and he seems quite unaware of the unsuitable pitch of the voice.

An audio-recording should be played back to the young man and his reaction to it discussed. It is unusual for the teenager not to know what his voice sounds like since the majority own tape-recorders. Dislike of the pre-pubertal voice should be apparent. If there is resentment towards parents or teacher who have persuaded him to attend the voice clinic against his will, the conflict has to be sorted out. Willing cooperation on the part of the boy must be gained and there must be no resistance to therapy (Weiss, 1955). Various clinicians are of the opinion that a male therapist is more suitable than a female and will achieve the necessary voice mutation more easily (Hildernesse, 1956). The attendance of a parent who is sympathetic and not critical of the boy, but encouraging, can be a great inducement and relieve the domestic situation of embarrassment when the boy uses his mature male voice at home. The father's involvement in treatment is a great advantage.

When the failure in voice mutation is largely a question of habit and the patient has adjusted psychologically, and especially when voice 'breaks' are present, the mature male voice is established at first interview. The longer the high-pitched voice has persisted past adolescence and into maturity the more difficult it may be to induce the required change of pitch.

Pitch lowering strategies

The authoritative manner and strong suggestion on the part of the therapist are potent influences in therapy. Even though the therapist may be female, she can still demonstrate that she can produce a much lower voice than the adolescent boy and that therefore this is possible for him.

The patient is asked to cough, clear his throat, laugh or sing down the scale in order to produce low notes. The prime aim is to discover a vowel an octave lower than the habitual pitch. This provides the starting point from which normal voice can be developed through exercises in humming and vowel prolongation.

Laryngeal tension may require specific therapy. In order to obtain falsetto voice the larynx is elevated by the suprahyoid musculature while the cricothyroid muscles approximate the cartilages anteriorly and the arytenoids are pulled back by the cricoarytenoids. The vocal folds are thinned and stretched and the voice is raised in pitch (see Chapter 3). Luchsinger and Arnold (1965) describe the Gutzman pressure test. If pressure can be exerted on the thyroid cartilage by pressing on the wings with finger and thumb, while the patient hums and drops the chin over the therapist's hand, the necessary relaxation of the intrinsic laryngeal muscles may be obtained.

Another strategy may produce results. If a laryngectomee's laryngeal vibrator is placed against the thyroid cartilage as the patient is asked to phonate, the sensation and the low pitch can produce a change in phonation. This approach appears to be successful because there is an element of the 'surprise attack' in using equipment apparently designed to change the voice.

Recordings of tenor, baritone and bass voices humming, played loudly and asking the patient to imitate or join in these vocal notes may produce results. If sound can be relayed through earphones as a masking device, the self-conscious individual may succeed in lowering pitch (Van Riper and Irwin, 1958).

The following strategies may also be employed:

1. Using a tongue depressor, the therapist depresses the posterior part of the patient's tongue as the patient emits a groan. This results in descent of the hyoid bone and therefore of the larynx; the resonance pitch of the pharyngeal resonator and the pitch of the vocal note are lowered. For this exercise to be effective the patient must be thoroughly relaxed. The back of the tongue should not be rigid and thus resist the tongue depressor.

2. With head tipped slightly forward and neck and shoulders relaxed, the patient phonates on 'hm' while placing thumb and forefinger on either side of the thyroid alae so that any tendency to elevate the larynx on phonation can be monitored and corrected.
3. The patient holds the arms up horizontally and drops them heavily to his sides while saying 'ah'. The arms must drop through force of gravity and not be brought down to the sides by the patient.
4. Following a period of relaxed diaphragmatic breathing the patient vocalises on a deep sigh on the expiratory airstream.
5. Some patients are able to produce a different, and mature male voice, if they are impersonating another man when they have the protection of assuming another identity (Greene, 1955).
6. Froeschels (1948) advocated chewing therapy and voluntary jaw and chin wagging when vocalising.

It is important that the therapist should present any method used with calm confidence and persist with it for a reasonable time before giving up. Any suggestion from the therapist, either explicitly or in attitude, that there is a desperate search for an approach which works will only confirm to the patient that he is attempting a difficult or impossible task. If speech therapy does prove to be unsuccessful referral to a psychiatrist is advisable if the patient consents.

Establishment of mature male voice

Immediately normal vocal pitch is achieved and seized upon with enthusiasm by the therapist, it can be developed in the usual ways. The deep voice should be practised assiduously in meaningless mechanical exercises which will establish the auditory and kinaesthetic patterns desired and enable their effortless recall. Intoning meaningless vowels and nonsense syllables when using the good voice will be found easier at first than connected speech. In most cases the voice is strong and resonant immediately a pitch appropriate to the adult resonators is used. The contrast in the vocal expression of personality is startling and dramatic for the therapist, and highly rewarding. The first recording should be played and the contrast with the new voice evaluated and praised.

Very great difficulty is often encountered in persuading the patient to use the mature male voice outside the clinic, since he is frequently convinced that it is more conspicuous than the habitual mutational falsetto. This is indeed the fact at first and the 'new' voice does provoke comment. If parent, sibling, friend or work colleague can be taken into the patient's confidence, perhaps accompanying him to the clinic, confidence may be increased. Assignments with hospital staff who understand the problem and give appropriate encouragement and praise extend the situations in which the patient feels sufficiently confident to speak normally.

Case histories

1. Case A., aged 18 years, was apprenticed to a jeweller. He presented with a voice which cracked from falsetto to baritone with great ease and he was able to speak in a mature male voice at the first interview when merely asked to do so. His larynx was normal but his posture was stooping and breathing was clavicular. He had learning difficulties and when asked if he was 'tied to his mother's apron strings' he was astonished and replied, 'That's what my father is always saying'. He had a clever younger brother who was the father's favourite child and who 'picked on' the patient. His mother was kind and protected him from his father. However, he resented the fact that at times she was over-protective and prevented him from doing things he wanted to, such as going abroad with his friends. Both his father and mother came to the clinic separately because trouble had arisen when the patient reported to his parents that the speech therapist said he must develop independence. Father was delighted, saying 'At last I have an expert agreeing with me'. Mother was upset. It transpired that mother would never accept that her elder son was a poor scholar and had insisted that he should stay at school until he was 18 years in order to pass 'O' level GCE examinations with special tuition. He had failed to do so and, with great difficulty, his father had been allowed to find him a job which was acceptable to the mother. Father was a successful self-made man and denied that he favoured the younger son and 'picked on' the patient. He only wanted the boy to be tough.

   Although A. switched to a mature male voice when asked to use it in the clinic, he continued to use the creaky falsetto outside. As pressure increased to use the normal voice he ceased to attend, his mother telephoning on his behalf with a succession of excuses. She refused to let her son be referred to a psychiatrist, which was necessary, and speech therapy was terminated.

2. Case B aged 16 years: the patient sought treatment because his application to become a member of a dramatic society had recently been rejected on the grounds that his voice was unsuitable, and he felt that it was not 'strong' enough for dramatic work. He was the youngest of a not very prosperous family. His speech was fast and accompanied by fidgeting movements of the head, arms and legs. His manner and dress were effeminate. He had a friend some 10 years older whom he admired greatly and with whom he spent most of his spare time. The friend had suffered from a similar disorder and had been cured by a speech therapist, and had advised speech therapy for B.

   The patient was able to laugh on a normal pitch and to sing falsetto, tenor or baritone with facility and had been able to do so since the age of 13 years. He said he could not speak in a deeper voice because it made him feel silly. When a recording of his speaking voice was played, he could hardly bear to listen to it, however, because it sounded to him 'so girlish' - a healthy admission.

A tenor voice was established in exercises but great difficulty was encountered with speech. The matter was decided when the good and bad voices were recorded and contrasted, but even then prolonged discussion and argument was necessary before he could be persuaded to speak normally outside the clinic. He first practised at work by talking to a female typist who was fortunately profoundly and favourably impressed. Eventually he was able to use his deep voice with the men with whom he worked who had previously ridiculed his voice.

The youth had exhibited overt signs of adolescent homosexuality which were apparently arrested when normal voice was established.

Immature Voice in Women

Vocal immaturity in women is less conspicuous than in males as during adolescence the female voice drops only 3 or 4 semitones compared to an octave in young men. However, if the woman's voice does not mature and remains that of a girl, it is an indication of an immature personality. Women who shun acceptance of adult responsibility and desire to cling to the shelter and security of childhood may cling unconsciously to the vocal pitch of childhood as a symbolic expression of their unconscious desires (Moses, 1958, 1959). The immature voice may be accompanied by immature articulation, a lisped /s/ or defective /r/. Father's or mother's little girl never grows up and this, of course, may be very appealing to the protective male in which case it has its advantages, especially in marriage. We have treated several women with conversion symptom aphonia and dysphonia whose habitual voices were inappropriately girlish and immature. In some cases referred with vocal strain and laryngitis, the pitch disorder was obviously psychogenic. In working to produce a lower pitch and improve quality it was also necessary to explore the immature emotional attitudes to people and problems at work and in the home. A common feature was the feeling expressed by these patients of being 'put upon' and being asked to do too much, whereas in reality they were often avoiding full responsibility. They capitalised on the kindness and helpfulness of long suffering colleagues or indulgent relations, using voice to gain protection by emphasising their helplessness.

The Trans-sexual Voice

During the last 20 years, since surgical sex change procedures have been more readily available, an increasing number of trans-sexuals have been referred to speech therapists. A trans-sexual is an individual who is convinced that he or she is of the opposite sex to that of his or her body; this conviction frequently establishes itself early in childhood and usually before puberty. The majority of trans-sexuals seeking medical help are male (Gelder, Gath and Mayou, 1983). Female trans-sexuals can take androgens which have the effect of increasing the mass of the vocal folds with a resulting drop in vocal pitch. For this reason the female trans-sexual is less likely to be referred for speech therapy than the male whose vocal folds are not significantly affected by the oestrogen which is administered. This section therefore deals with male trans-sexuals.

The male trans-sexual

There is a feeling of estrangement from the body and a desire to alter the body to resemble that of the opposite sex. Throughout childhood and into the teens, the trans-sexual is increasingly motivated to live as a member of the opposite sex although social pressures frequently prevent the realisation of this goal. Initially, dressing as a female enables the individual to feel like a woman although this may only be possible when alone. The condition is different from that of the transvestite where the man enjoys dressing as a woman for the purpose of sexual arousal but continues to perceive himself as a man and does not wish to cross-dress permanently or to lose his male characteristics. It is probable that there is an overlap area in relation to trans-sexualism and transvestism. In this respect trans-sexuals are also unlike homosexuals who may dress as women in order to attract other homosexuals. The trans-sexual's sex drive is typically low (Gelder, Gath and Mayou, 1983).

The aetiology of trans-sexualism is not fully understood. Although there does not appear to be a well-defined organic basis for the condition some researchers have suggested that little understood hormonal abnormalities during intrauterine development may be a contributory factor (Gelder, Gath and Mayou, 1983). Others propose psychological and environmental causes although the precise mechanisms involved are unclear (Oates and Dacakis, 1983). A combination of physical and psychological factors may be the reality.

Treatment of male trans-sexuality

The male trans-sexual frequently decides to seek medical help during the late teens or early twenties. The most logical treatment would appear to be directed at changing the individual's conviction that he is a man in a woman's body. However, psychotherapy is unsuccessful and the professional approach is increasingly to approach the problem with a multidisciplinary team (Bralley *et al.*, 1978; Oates and Dacakis, 1983). The team is composed of psychiatrists, surgeons, medical social workers, speech therapists and others because of the complexity of the medical, psychological and surgical issues which must be considered in each case. Treatment is conducted on the basis of attempting to satisfy the individual's aims of taking on a woman's appearance, living as a woman and changing the body to resemble that of a woman.

Presurgical phase

The individual's involvement with the team will be long term. Surgical sex change will only be undertaken when it has been established that the man is able to adjust to living daily as a member of the opposite sex. It is also essential that the man fully appreciates the problems which accompany such surgery. Sim (1981) stresses the importance of thorough psychiatric examination because of the mutilating nature of the operation which leaves the individual sterile and incapable of orgasm. In England, even after surgery, the male transsexual is still legally regarded as male. This presurgical period usually lasts for about 2 years and during this time hormones of the desired gender are prescribed.

For medical, psychological and social reasons it is important that the change should be gradual. In response to the female hormones, breasts and female distribution of body fat develop. Hormones may produce unpleasant side effects such as nausea and dizziness or more serious risks including thrombosis and malignant breast tumours (Gelder, Gath and Mayou, 1983). The lengthy process of electrolysis for the removal of facial hair is started and breast enlargement may be further enhanced by mammoplasty. It is during this transition period that the speech therapist is called upon to give therapy.

Adjustment difficulties

Although there is a compelling desire to become a woman, the onset of femininity brings enormous problems. There is fear that family, friends and strangers will discover the situation if attempts are made to conceal what is happening, but complete honesty may result in rejection and isolation. In some instances the unwanted attention of curious males has to be dealt with. The individual needs encouragement for a considerable time and depression is a common feature. When sex change surgery, which involves castration, penectomy and the creation of an artificial vagina (Oates and Dacakis, 1983), is eventually performed the postoperative period may produce severe depression (Sim, 1981). Linford Rees (1982) questions the legality of such surgery. Moreover, it is extremely expensive and time consuming for the professionals involved, and the person, after much suffering, is never normal nor satisfied.

Having undergone this prolonged pursuit of feminity and assuming female dress, hair-style and make-up the visual result is frequently convincingly female, but the mature masculine voice is a major factor in not being accepted as a woman.

Elimination of male voice

Treatment procedures have as their basis a vocal tract which is anatomically and physiologically normal for a male, not a female. In addition, established patterns of verbal and non-verbal communication remain unchanged and are therefore inappropriate for the female appearance. Possible treatment for these communication problems may be divided into surgery and speech therapy.

Surgery

Cosmetic surgery

Surgical reduction of the thyroid cartilage (Adam's apple), also known as laryngeal shaving, is performed in order to give the much flatter appearance of the female larynx. This is a cosmetic operation which allows the neck to resemble the female neck more closely. It does not affect the quality of the voice (Isshiki, 1980).

Phonosurgery

Phonosurgery (surgery involving the vocal folds) for trans-sexuals is still relatively experimental and does not always produce satisfactory results. Various procedures are advocated to raise vocal pitch by changing the mass, length and tension (or stiffness) of the vocal folds. Isshiki (1980) notes that stiffness is the most important factor. Bralley *et al.* (1978) describe restriction of the anterior third of the vibrating segment of the vocal folds. These authors also note the work of Donald (1982) who describes a procedure in which a laryngeal web is created in order to obtain raised vocal pitch. A procedure which involves removing the anterior third of the vocal folds and then stretching them and reattaching them to the thyroid cartilage is described by Oates and Dacakis (1983). This has the effect of increasing vocal fold tension and decreasing vocal fold mass so that higher fundamental frequency is produced.

Isshiki (1980) regards three types of intervention as possible in these cases:

1. Increasing vocal fold tension by cricothyroid approximation.
2. A longitudinal incision of the vocal folds.
3. Steroid injection into the vocal folds in order to reduce mass. The rationale of the steroid injection is that steroids cause local atrophy but the author reports that the results are unsatisfactory.

Surgical intervention in these cases is still experimental and maintaining an unobstructed airway and avoiding marked deterioration in voice quality are major considerations.

Speech therapy

Voice therapy is only one aspect of a speech therapy programme concerned with many aspects of verbal and non-verbal communication, including a careful analysis of the individual's communicative behaviour. The programme is based on the following factors.

Male/female speech and language features

Voice pitch is generally regarded as the most important factor in identifying the gender of a speaker (Bralley *et al.*, 1978; Oates and Dacakis, 1983). There are several studies which indicate that females may use a greater variety of intonational patterns than males while males tend to speak more loudly than females (Yanagihara, Koike and Von Leden, 1966). The differing dimensions of male and female resonators result in identifiable differences in the quality of resonance. These suprasegmental aspects give some of the most important clues concerning the sex of the speaker (Smith, 1979). Various studies cited by Oates and Dacakis describe female speech as generally having more accurate articulation than males who tend to articulate with less mouth opening and greater degrees of lip rounding than females.

Sex markers in speech also extend to conversational topics and type of vocabulary used. Speech therapy should therefore include discussion of topics with a feminine bias so that the trans-sexual develops this aspect of communication.

Treatment goals

The patient and the speech therapist should be agreed on the goals of treatment. Unrealistic expectations of treatment will eventually cause distress; the therapist must make every effort to understand the trans-sexual's expectations and to clarify the limitations that are placed on the possibility of acquiring a female voice by the size of the larynx and vocal tract.

Discussion concerning well-known trans-sexuals and the patient's view of the degree of their success in presenting as a female may give further insight into the individual's perception of a 'successful' voice. A male trans-sexual was most impressed by the television appearance of a well-known trans-sexual and indicated that it would be a considerable achievement to acquire such a voice. This response was surprising as the voice was definitely male; it was significant that the non-verbal communication and dress were convincingly female.

Most trans-sexuals embarking on speech therapy are highly motivated to cooperate, but this may be the first time that such active involvement in the achievement of goals has been required. Hormonal treatment and surgery require a more passive role. The therapist may need to make it clear that therapy will not consist of a programme of speech exercises alone which will subsequently result in a suitable voice. Reassurance should be given that the therapist is fully aware that both voice and non-verbal communication should avoid creating a caricature of a female.

Increasing the individual's awareness of paralinguistic behaviours

Postures adopted may remain essentially masculine in some individual's although the regular wearing of female clothes tends to encourage more feminine movements. It will be necessary for the therapist to give guidance concerning appropriate postures and gestures as part of a programme in which the trans-sexual learns to communicate femininity. Video-recordings are essential for monitoring all aspects of appearance including hair-style, make-up and clothes.

More subtle aspects of posture which directly affect voice may also have to be considered. For example, if the habitual head posture is for the head to be tipped forward and the chin tucked in, the larynx will be depressed in the vocal tract and the pitch of the voice lowered.

Habitual articulation may enhance an impression of masculinity but hearing training, in conjunction with analysis of video recordings, can be successful in eradicating this problem. The tense jaw with little mouth opening, and flexing of the masseter muscles and clenched teeth when at rest, may result in an aggressive appearance which is perceived as masculine. Similarly, emphatic and explosive articulation is less likely to indicate a female speaker than softer and more gentle contacts.

The individual must be aware of the habitual voice quality. The tendency to use hard glottal attack, harshness, roughness and creak will have to be guarded against if the more female voice quality is to be convincing. It is not that females do not produce these voice features but that distinctively male voice pitch is used when these features are produced by the mature male larynx.

A similar, and difficult, problem is the use of vegetative behaviours such as laughing and coughing. These can be dealt with satisfactorily if performed gently under voluntary control, but the natural male voice remains apparent if voluntary control is lost.

All aspects of speech, language and content of conversation must be considered.

Psychological support from the therapist

The trans-sexual's difficulties in acquiring and maintaining the new behaviours related to voice and communication should not be underestimated. Although highly motivated, translating these new skills into daily life and dealing with responses which are not always favourable may be discouraging and consequently depressing. The speech therapist may be the only member of the team who sees the patient regularly and frequently, and realistic encouragement and support is an intrinsic element of the treatment programme.

Speech therapy programme

The speech therapy programme will incorporate the points outlined above and may proceed according to the following outline:

1. Traditional voice therapy which will encourage voluntary control over the various elements of voice production with increased kinaesthetic and auditory awareness as a basis for changing habitual patterns.
2. Exercises directed at comfortably raising pitch and subsequently increasing the vocal range within the pitch range. It is essential that any voice therapy does not allow vocal abuse and that the therapist notices any signs of voice fatigue or strain.
3. Translation of newly acquired vocal skills into hierarchical tasks in which intonation patterns and prosody are developed.

Studies indicate that although the vocal pitch is raised by therapy it is likely to be distinguishable from the female voice on account of the presence of male resonators and resonance. Bralley *et al.* (1978) found that both the trans-sexual and therapist overestimated the extent to which pitch had been raised and they suggest that objective assessment is probably required. However, if the general appearance of the male trans-sexual is feminine the voice tends to be perceived as female. This was highlighted by a patient in the early stages of therapy who was engaged in conversation by a male who commented on the 'lovely deep voice'; there was no recognition of a male voice. Responses will vary according to the listener and the situational context of the conversation. When the voice is the only indication of gender, for example on the telephone, it is particularly important to give the name immediately so that the listener will be encouraged to accept that the caller is female. Signalling femininity affects the listener's set of expectancy so that the voice is more likely to be perceived as that of a woman.

Endocrine Dysphonia in Males

The endocrine glands secrete hormones which regulate bodily growth, development of sexual and reproductive functions and the emotional stability of the individual. The chief endocrine glands controlling normal development and relating to normal voice are the thyroid, ovaries and testicles. The mutual interdependence of the various endocrine glands is extremely complex and here we intend only to describe the voice disorders which are predominantly related to particular hormonal systems.

Gonadal disorders

Development of male characteristics is dependent upon the release of male hormones during puberty. The growth of facial and pubic hair and the larynx may be delayed by several years in the 'late developers'. The youth then retains a boy's voice while growing in normal bodily dimensions. In many cases normal development of masculine maturity without recourse to hormone treatment takes place (Luchsinger and Arnold, 1965).

Gonadal failure results in maintenance of the high pitched voice of puberphonia. Chaucer's Pardoner in *The Canterbury Tales* is a classic example of the eunuch although we have no information regarding aetiology except that he had strong connections with Rome.

> A voys he hadde as small as hath a goot
> No berd hadde he, ne never sholde have
> As smothe it was as it were late y-shave.

Damage to the testicles before puberty can cause atrophy and prevent development of male sexual features altogether. Tuberculosis, now that it has been almost eradicated in the Western World, is a rare cause. Tumours of the testes are less rare and represent the second most common form of malignancy in young males. Accidents involving the testes are rare.

The connection between the testes and male sexuality has been recognised throughout the ages. Castration of male children was practised in the Orient in order to provide impotent domestic staff for harems. In the seventeenth and eighteenth centuries the barbarous practice of castration was an accepted social and cultural procedure in order to satisfy the demand for the admired castrati singers. The Vatican choir, not allowing female singers, engaged castrati singers as late as the nineteenth century until Pope Leo XIII (1878–1903) banned castrated singers (Luchsinger and Arnold, 1965).

Moses (1960) draws attention to the fact that early castration resulted in abnormal growth of the long bones as a characteristic. The individual grows tall and willow-like. This is clearly displayed in the paintings of Farinelli (1705–1782), a famous castrati singer who was renowned throughout Europe for his marvellous voice and brilliant technique. He settled in Spain for 25 years, gaining great political power at court through his employment by the Queen to sing every night to Philip V to cure him of melancholy madness. He utilised his ascendancy over Philip VI to establish Italian opera in Madrid.

Moses (1960) in an analysis of the psychotherapy of castrati singers explains the popularity of these singers on the basis of the need of the Baroque period for wish-fulfilment of hermaphrodite dreams and desires in the subconscious. The mystical desire for purity, the unity of the male and female in a deity was symbolised in the high voice of those purified by castration and who, therefore, were chaste. Natural tenor singers are occasionally found to have a freak vocal range, able to sing with facility in the falsetto register. The thin and silvery voice of the counter-tenor always has a certain vogue. The fluty, rather haunting quality of the voice is due to reinforcement of a limited range of overtones in contrast to the deep baritone or bass voice which is enriched by a wide range of harmonics. Alfred Deller popularised counter-tenor singing in the 1930s. The voice of the male falsetto singer is rather richer in harmonics than that of the boy by reason of the larger adult resonators and especially the chest resonator. The falsetto voice has a range of 130–784 Hz and uses head and a little pectoral resonance. Counter-tenors still have a certain vogue today and this singing voice is produced by normal males with normal speaking voices. These singers' voices have a range of two octaves (164–698 Hz) and do not use the falsetto (falsettisto) (Jackson, 1987).

Vocal treatment

It is doubtful whether endeavours to lower the pitch of the voice by voice therapy can produce a marked change in cases where insufficient androgens are being secreted. Isshiki (1980) in describing recent advances in phonosurgery suggests a thyroplasty under local anaesthetic suitable for female to male sex change (p. 191). This should be equally suitable for physically irreversible puberphonia. The anterior posterior distance of the thyroid ala is reduced by excision of a vertical rectangular slice of cartilage. Excision on one side may be sufficient. The vocal fold is shortened by this procedure and relaxation and bunching of muscle (an increase in mass) takes place as the thyroid angle (Adam's apple) is moved back. This sounds a feasible procedure but we have no experience of cases treated in this way.

Female Endocrine Dysphonia

In women the endocrine system is active throughout life controlling the reproductive system, initiating puberty and the menstrual cycle and withdrawing at the climacteric. Endocrine changes during menstruation and pregnancy may produce oedematous vocal folds as a result of fluid retention. Muscular hypertophy may be apparent in cases of virilisation (Van Gelder, 1974).

Menses

A slight huskiness due to congestion of the vocal folds during puberty may appear. The oedema may produce hoarseness when aggravated by vocal strain; there is a reduction in muscular tonicity and limitation in pitch range. It is not a great inconvenience for the average teenager but the voice should have no demands made upon it by singing, acting or cheering. A deterioration in the voice and huskiness may recur every month with the vocal folds exhibiting hyperaemia, oedema and, in some cases, haemorrhage (Van Gelder, 1974). Normal tension of the vocal folds is reduced.

During pregnancy the voice can also be affected by hormonal ingestion of the larynx. Tarneaud (1961) observed that these symptoms during menstruation and pregnancy cease after childbirth. Flach, Schwickardi and Simon (1969) reported assessment of 136 professional singers among whom 80 were engaged to sing large operatic parts. Their voices all showed change for the worse in the premenstrual and menstrual period. Two-thirds of the singers becoming pregnant experienced vocal deterioration and in a quarter of these cases the voice change persisted after delivery. Professional singers frequently have a clause in their contracts excluding performance during the menstrual period (menses).

Sexual excitement can evoke vocal change and the 'sexy voice'. Réthi (1963) explains that the recurrent laryngeal nerves contain both sympathetic and parasympathetic fibres. A vasomotor rhinitis, hoarseness and cough may develop soon after marriage and, with attendant difficulties in establishing the new interpersonal relationship, the slight dysphonia may become a focus of anxiety.

> Case history
>
> A young woman, an only child who had lived at home and never had to cook, shop, wash and clean the house, experienced great difficulty in managing her home and full-time job when she married and the honeymoon was over. Her voice, which was of markedly immature pitch and underwent menstrual changes, became permanently weak and husky with a chronic mild laryngitis. Sympathetic discussions of her difficulties and help in planning her daily programme, including her domestic arrangements, reduced her troubles. Voice therapy formed only a minor part of treatment as the vasomotor symptoms were physically and psychologically based.

Climacteric

The menopause is another time in a woman's life when vocal difficulties can occur. There is a reduction in the secretion of ovarian hormones and a relative increase in adrenal cortex androgens which results in the vocal folds becoming oedematous. This is often accompanied by vasomotor rhinitis and the voice may become husky and noticeably deeper. It is, besides, a time of life when the middle-aged woman often feels ill, irritable and excessively tired with a tendency to nervousness and depression. The most troublesome symptom is the 'hot flush' and, at night, sweating which disturbs sleep. Short courses of hormonal treatment can greatly relieve the symptoms but if administered for a long time can damage the voice.

Women also put on weight at this time and may need to diet strictly if they are to remain slim. This is another cause of anxiety and also fatigue. Women complaining of dysphonia at this time need sympathy and support, and help from their families must be enlisted. Adolescent children and husbands frequently have little insight into the difficulties of the mother of the household until these are explained. The family should be patient and tolerant in order to tide her over these difficult years.

Menopausal voice changes are aggravated by excessive smoking which produces a chronic laryngitis, cough and considerable drop in vocal pitch. If the woman has to use her voice much at work it may become a real inconvenience and the laryngeal condition may be aggravated by vocal strain. No improvement will be achieved without drastically cutting down the number of cigarettes per day.

Thyroid Disorders

Thyrotoxicosis

The thyroid gland, which is controlled by the anterior pituitary gland, is concerned with the maintenance of the metabolism of the body by discharging thyroxine into the blood. The regulation of all life functions, as Arnold (1962) points out, is dependent upon the hypothalamic-pituitary-thyroid-adrenal system. Disturbance of the thyroid will upset the whole chemical and emotional balance of the body. When the normal secretion of thyroxine is diminished (hypothyroidism) in children cretinism is the result. Hypothyroidism in adults results in myxoedema. When the secretion of thyroxine is increased (hyperthyroidism) the individual suffers from thyrotoxicosis; if this is associated with protrusion of the eyes it is called exophthalmic goitre or Graves' disease. The gland may be visibly and palpably enlarged, but not necessarily so.

Graves' disease is characterised by well-recognised symptoms: tachycardia (abnormally rapid pulse), a warm moist skin, increased sweating and diarrhoea. Appetite is increased but there is loss of weight as a result of increased body metabolism. There is also a pronounced nervousness and excitability associated with the physical condition (Wittkower and Mandelbrote, 1955). Women are prone to fits of weeping. There are menstrual changes in both hyper- and hypothyroidism.

Pseudo-hyperthyroidism

it is not easy to distinguish between hyperthyroidism due to over-secretion of thyroxine, and pseudo-hyperthyroidism which is largely psychogenic but with psychosomatic symptoms. Enlargement of the gland may be minimal and toxicosis not prove positive in the blood analysis yet vocal changes may present themselves (Sonninen, 1960) and warrant thyroidectomy. These problems are discussed further under laryngeal palsy (see p. 304).

Many dysphonic middle-aged women diagnosed as suffering from 'functional dysphonia' may be suffering from endocrine imbalance during the climacteric with its well-known association with emotional lability, depression and anxiety. Incipient thyrotoxicosis is a possibility, however, and with it compression symptoms from the thyroid gland. These encompass muscular weakness due to compression of the recurrent laryngeal nerve and sensations of a lump in the throat (globus symptom – see p. 169).

Psychosomatic problems

Wittkower and Mandelbrote (1955) say:

> The thyroid hormone is primarily a stimulator of cell metabolism and as such it promotes intellectual activity and performance and increases sensitivity and alertness.

It is especially active in adolescence and accounts for the heightened emotional reactions, vitality and growth of intellectual interests at this time. Over-secretion has profound psychological effects upon the individual. The clinical picture of thyrotoxicosis so often closely resembles an anxiety state that diagnosis is extremely difficult. Here we see the psychosomatic 'servo-system' of the body at its most complex. Thyrotoxicosis can be precipitated by shock and it is to be remembered that conversion aphonia and dysphonia frequently develop after shock or periods of ill health, overwork and mental strain. Thyrotoxicosis can in some cases be cured by rest and the relaxation of a holiday. The families of thyrotoxic patients tend to show nervous traits and over-reaction to the trials and tribulations of life. Disturbed interpersonal relationships between all thyrotoxic patients and their mothers are apparently a phenomenon.

Speech therapy should follow the remedial strategies recommended for anxiety and conversion aphonia (see Chapter 10).

Hypothyroidism

Myxoedema is the disorder of metabolism which results from under-secretion of the thyroid gland. The congenital form of thyroid deficiency causes mental and physical handicap known as cretinism. If recognised and treated early in childhood with thyroxine the condition can be arrested. The cry of the baby with this condition is recognisably abnormal at birth with a fundamental pitch conspicuously lower than normal and with constricted pitch range (Michelsson and Sirvio, 1976).

Juvenile myxoedema may arise from failure of thyroid function in childhood but this is not as serious as cretinism because normal development will have taken place in the fetus and in early childhood. The vocal folds appear odematous and the voice becomes gruff and hoarse. The gradual onset of the disease may at first go unrecognised but early diagnosis and treatment are essential. A lifelong regimen of thyroxine therapy has satisfactory results.

> Case history
> A girl aged 6 years 6 months was referred for speech therapy with a diagnosis of oedematous vocal folds and hoarseness. She was not noisy at home or school and did not get on well with other children and was quarrelsome and aggressive at times. Her laryngeal condition did not appear to be due to vocal strain. She was short and thick set and overweight, slow in her movements and suffered from nasal catarrh. Her cheeks were noticeably rough and chapped. She was having reading difficulties and her IQ was estimated to be in the region of 80. She presented, in fact, the typical symptoms of hypothyroidism and was referred for investigation.

Myxoedema in senescence

Myxoedema can occur in normal individuals in old age. The skin becomes rough and dry and the hair thin; the individual may gain weight and become slow in movements and thought. An early sign is a slowly progressive deepening of the voice and a slight huskiness which is less conspicuous in men than in women. The vocal fold movements remain intact but the folds increase in bulk due to deposits of mucopolysaccharides in the submucosa. Ritter (1967) advocates stripping the vocal folds along their edges with the aim of reducing bulk or inducing scarring which increases tension. Isshiki (1980) also suggests various surgical procedures to improve voice, but in the elderly drastic steps are uncalled for and thyroxine medication is all that is required.

Heinemann (1969) investigated 42 cases of myxoedema and noted the fact that if the voice has been allowed to deteriorate substantially, administering thyroxine does not result in improved voice quality. The elderly, particularly if living alone, may not realise nor care that their health is slowly deteriorating. If there are no acute symptoms to alert them any changes may be attributed to natural ageing. One elderly lady who was hard of hearing was not in the least concerned by her gruff voice. She had not really noticed it herself and as her only companion was her cat, vocal improvement was unnecessary.

Androphonia (virilisation of the female voice)

Gynaecological carcinoma is frequently treated by male hormones (androgens) and it is to be anticipated that the female patient may develop male characteristics with growth of the clitoris, and hair on the face, legs and arms and development of a male voice. It is a different matter when testosterone is administered in order to alleviate climacteric complaints.

Damsté (1964) described six patients who presented with dysphonia due to administration of testosterone-containing drugs by their doctors with no conception of the connection between the drugs and the voice. He describes voices as becoming unsteady with fluctuation between chest and falsetto and this may continue for some time before the voice settles into the male register.

Damsté (1967) noted a striking difference in the length of the vocal folds on high and low notes, with an increase in extensibility of the connective tissue. The folds also appeared greyish. The changes in the larynx were irreversible and treatment with oestrogens (female hormones) did not lead to any improvement. Some patients can be helped, especially the younger ones, by speech therapy during which it is possible to learn to obtain a new balance between glottic tension and respiratory pressure and to use the upper vocal range.

Shepperd (1966) reported five cases of women who had also been treated for climacteric complaints for periods varying from 6 months to 2 years with commercial preparations incorporating methyltestosterone and oestradiol, the presence of which was not suspected by their doctors. All women developed hoarseness and increased growth of hair. Withdrawal of the drugs resulted in disappearance of excess hair but the voice remained unchanged. Shepperd comments on the fact that the voice is not hoarse but strong and deep. This agrees with our experience, the voice being smooth and agreeable if it were not so inappropriate. It is quite different from the rough and broken contour of the heavy smoker's female voice due to oedema.

The development of male characteristics is naturally very distressing to the female patient. The phonosurgery recommended by Isshiki (1980) in connection with the myxoedematous voice may provide a solution.

> Case history
>
> A 62-year-old woman had been operated upon 2 years previously for mamillary cancer and had then retired from teaching and removed to the coast to live with her sister which had not proved a happy arrangement. She was referred for speech therapy with a diagnosis of functional dysphonia, the larynx appearing normal. The masculine character of the voice led to the enquiry by the speech therapist whether she could be on testosterone. This proved to be the case and she was switched to oestrogens, but no improvement in pitch was achieved. Vocal exercises and hearing training did, however, help her to speak in the upper limits of her chest register.

Anabolic steroids contain androgenic components and are prescribed in some cases of back pain and polymyalgia. The voice changes, which consist of lowering of pitch and subsequent narrowing of register, are generally regarded as irreversible (Van Gelder, 1974; Tanabe *et al.*, 1985). Phonatory abnormalities have also been reported in chronic asthmatics following prolonged use of aerosol corticosteroids which cause oedema (Watkin and Ewanowski, 1985). However, voice quality may be considerably improved by voice therapy and by eliminating features of abuse which may have evolved.

Chapter 12
Disorders of Nasal Resonance

Before embarking upon discussion of nasal resonance dysphonia, it is advisable to pay attention to the sociolinguistic aspects of nasality in normal speech. A degree of nasal tone to the voice is acceptable in some cultural settings. Native English speakers cannot believe that their speech sounds nasal to the Dutch, but apparently it does. To the English, some American accents have a marked nasal twang. Nasalised vowels are phonetically correct in French but not in English. The nasal consonants /m, n, ŋ/ are common to European languages, and adjacent vowels (as in man, name etc.) assimilate slight nasality which is far more marked in American English. Increase in nasality can be achieved by constriction of the oropharynx and elevation of the back of the tongue which creates a nasal resonance chamber. When nasal consonants are substituted by their oral counterparts /b, d, g /, as in 'by dose is ruddig', it indicates a nasal obstruction such as a cold in the head and a type of nasal dysphonia not acceptable in a healthy speaker.

Disorders of nasal resonance can be considered under two distinctive categories: excessive nasality and insufficient nasality. There are a number of terms used to describe these types of dysphonia: hypernasality and hyponasality; hyper- and hyporhinolalia or rhinophonia; rhinolalia aperta or clausa. Nasalised and denasalised are simpler terms in use. Nasal escape is associated with excessive nasality and describes the audible emission of turbulent air via the nose during articulation of consonants.

Causes of excessive nasality (hypernasality)

- Cleft palate.
- Submucous cleft.
- Congenital short palate.
- Deep and wide pharynx.
- Palatal paralysis - congenital/acquired.

These conditions can prevent the necessary closure of the nasopharyngeal valve in speech. This is referred to as palatopharyngeal or velopharyngeal incompetence.

Causes of insufficient nasality (hyponasality)

- Enlarged adenoids.
- Nasal congestion.
- Polyps associated with allergic rhinitis.
- Deflected septum - commonly associated with trauma and cleft of the hard palate.

Hyponasality is due to obstruction of the nasal resonator and the exclusion of the nasal resonator system.

Hypernasality (Palatopharyngeal Incompetence)

Cleft palate

The two halves of the lip, hard and soft palate normally fuse during the first 3 months of fetal life. Fusion can fail entirely or in part. Unilateral or bilateral cleft of the lip can occur in isolation or involve the alveolus and part of the hard palate. The uvula can be bifid and the cleft of the soft palate be isolated or extend into the whole or part of the soft palate. A complete cleft runs right through from lip to uvula. It is the posterior cleft of the palate which engages us in the study of hypernasality.

Submucous cleft

Rarely, the mucosal cover of the soft palate is entire, concealing a cleft of the muscular segments of the palate beneath. This is known as a submucous cleft. Because the cleft is invisible and suckling and swallowing can function adequately, the submucous cleft may be unsuspected until hypernasal speech develops in the child. A translucent line may be detected running down the centre of the palate and a notch may be felt in the posterior edge of the hard palate. These are easily performed clinical tests carried out by a speech therapist in assessing nasal dysphonia. The incidence of submucous cleft palate is about 1 : 1200 but only 5–10% have palatopharyngeal incompetence. Those children who have submucous cleft frequently have other associated abnormalities according to Bumsted (1982), deafness and mental handicap being the most frequent.

Congenital palatal paralysis

This condition also occurs rarely and may be confused with submucous cleft until thorough investigations eradicate this possibility. Surgical treatment is not successful but a palatal prosthesis can help.

Acquired palatal paralysis

Hypernasality occurs in motor disorders of the nervous system, described in detail in Chapter 14, and involves palatal and pharyngeal paralysis.

Diphtheric neuritis

The palate is sometimes paralysed temporarily after diphtheria on account of a peripheral neuritis which prevents the conveyance of nervous impulses to the palatal muscles. Movement of the palate is soon recovered and speech therapy should not be necessary. Anxiety with regard to impaired speech and a superimposed neurotic disorder and prolongation of hypernasal speech is possible. In this event speech therapy will be necessary.

Patients suffering from diphtheric peripheral neuritis are now exceedingly rare since infant immunisation is generally practised. However, following an outbreak of diphtheria among unimmunised children in Buckinghamshire, England, in 1963 speech assessment was carried out. Two children had gross nasal escape which was far more conspicuous than in any case of cleft palate or postadenoidal hypernasal speech we had encountered. Speech therapy was not given in these cases and speech recovered with the movement of the palate and the subsidence of the illness.

Congenital short palate, deep pharynx

Incompetent palatopharyngeal closure and hypernasal speech may also be caused by a congenital short palate with the associated deformity of an unusually deep and wide nasopharynx. This may only become evident after removal of adenoids which have hitherto reduced the dimensions of the nasopharyngeal cavity, and made closure by the palate possible. Damsté (1962) states that the condition though rare is twice as common as submucous cleft. Pharyngoplasty as for cleft palate is the usual curative surgical procedure.

Postadenoidectomy hypernasality

Removal of grossly enlarged tonsils may result in a temporary palatopharyngeal incompetence and hypernasality. There has to be a mechanical compensation for lack of the adenoidal pad against which the soft palate made contact. Nasal escape may only last a few days and then a satisfactory adjustment is made (Greene, 1957).

Psychogenic hypernasality

Hypernasality may be due exclusively to emotional disturbance in the presence of a competent speech mechanism. Speech in these cases is generally variable and characterised by hypernasality rather than audible nasal emission. It can be an hysterical manifestation or it may persist for psychological reasons after adenoidectomy as a means of attaining attention and enjoying the spoiling received from an anxious mother in hospital.

The full nasopharyngeal assessment will need to be carried out if hypernasal speech persists for months. A congenital short palate is a possibility but functional use of the palate can be misleading. The differential diagnosis between congenital short palate and psychogenic hypernasality should never be made hastily. Diagnostic speech therapy in doubtful cases should be given while the child's emotional stability is explored and the possible need for such a symptom is investigated. A period of 9 months to a year should elapse before pharyngoplasty is seriously considered.

Case histories

The following case histories illustrate the complexities of differential diagnosis in cases of hypernasality where the aetiology is not immediately apparent.

1. A girl of 14 years had a pleasant singing voice and was in demand at local charity concerts. She had developed excessive nasal escape after a recent adenoidectomy and after 6 months' duration of the symptom, clinical and lateral X-ray assessment showed without doubt that this girl suffered from a short palate in relation to a deep pharynx. The surgeon in charge fortunately decided to postpone carrying out a Hynes pharyngoplasty. Three months later speech and singing reverted to normal suddenly. In this patient one can only conclude that there was some psychogenic reason for long-lasting nasal escape.

2. Tonsils and adenoids were removed from this little girl (B.I.) at the age of 7 years 9 months. Her parents declared that speech was entirely normal before the operation but that when she arrived home from hospital, suffering from a severe cold and high temperature, her speech was almost unintelligible.

   When examined in the speech therapy clinic 3 months later there was gross nasal escape and grimace throughout speech and she failed to displace even one cubic centimetre in the Windsor measure. There had been no nasal regurgitation at any time and the ear, nose and throat surgeon described this as 'phoney'. Nevertheless, the palate appeared paralysed and did not rise when touched or in articulation of the vowel /ɑ:/.

   Speech therapy was commenced and after a few weeks the palate showed a flicker of elevation on vowels. In the meantime, a plastic surgeon had examined the girl and suggested that she had contracted a focal attack of poliomyelitis following tonsillectomy, with paralysis of the palate as a result. She was accordingly examined by a neurologist who found no grounds at all for confirming this diagnosis and stated that since the palate was beginning to move the prognosis for eventual recovery was good.

   Speech therapy continued and it was noticeable that hypernasality and nasal grimace, although always present, varied greatly in degree from week to week. The child, once shyness wore off, was discovered to be seriously maladjusted. She was uncooperative and wilful in clinic and drove her parents to distraction at home by her disobedience. She was the only child of elderly parents whose relationship was far from harmonious and whose business commitments provided constant anxiety and overwork. Nerves were frayed and little time or patience were left for a troublesome though much loved and spoiled daughter.

Seven months after the commencement of speech therapy it was possible to take later X-rays of the palate. Previously the little girl's nervousness had debarred this procedure; the sight of a new tape-recorder, for instance, had at one time thrown her into a state of terror. The X-rays were instructive. Although the palate failed to elevate in blowing and articulating vowels, the camera had by chance caught a photograph when crying, and this showed excellent elevation of the palate and complete occlusion of the palato-pharyngeal isthmus.

These X-rays confirmed the suspicion which had been steadily growing that hypernasality, though originally due to postadenoidectomy palatal weakness, was now a psychogenic symptom. Her parents, when this was explained to them, were most resentful at the suggestion that their daughter was 'playing them up' and alternately demanded surgery and hypnotism which were not provided.

Speech exercises were discarded early on because they were resented, and play therapy alone was given, through which B.I. developed a strong affection for the therapist. As confidence and cooperation increased, she would sometimes speak without a vestige of hypernasality especially if she were 'top dog' in a game and issuing orders. Hypernasality and grimace returned dramatically as soon as she was returned to one or other parent in the waiting room.

A change of school at 8 years 5 months and a new uniform and friends produced normal speech, even at home, for a week. Then something upset her and she developed a non-inflammatory earache, followed by mysterious tummy-aches which the doctor pronounced 'psychological'. Speech, of course deteriorated. After 3 weeks she returned to school and gradually settled down happily. Speech 6 months later was normal.

The resemblance of these nasal symptoms to conversion symptoms is an interesting feature of the case (see Chapter 10). When we had news of this child some years later, she was attending the child guidance clinic on account of 'night terrors'.

3. A.C.: this boy of 9 years who had always stammered had been diagnosed by various doctors and surgeons as having 'breathing difficulty' on account of clonic expiratory spasms. He also exhibited variable degrees of hypernasality 'according to how he felt', as his mother accurately described it. His mother had twice been admitted for in-patient psychiatric care for treatment of depression. Her emotions found an outlet in alternately abusing and beating the boy for his naughtiness, or insisting that something should be done about his speech.

He was eventually referred to the plastic surgeon. Lateral X-rays revealed incomplete nasopharyngeal closure and pharyngoplasty was performed. We were not in agreement in this case that the palatopharyngeal mechanism was incapable of competent closure. We agreed that its function was incompetent but we believed that this was a psychogenic symptom. The boy was very upset by his hospital stay and his speech was even more hypernasal postoperatively. The palate appeared to be paralysed but this proved to be a conversion symptom and it recovered normal function during his first visit to the speech therapist as an out-patient. After 6 months, following speech therapy, his speech was no longer hypernasal on the whole and his stammer improved. Hypernasality and stammer both returned whenever he was upset at home or school.

4. Miss B., 22 years: the mother of this young woman first wrote to Greene on the advice of the speech therapist who had given her daughter speech therapy for 6 months while at boarding school when aged 8 years. Therapist and mother had met quite by chance this many years later. Miss B. had spoken normally until 17 years old when her tonsils and adenoids had been removed on account of infection and deafness. After this her speech was unintelligible and hypernasal. She had various ear, nose and throat check-ups and it was reported that nothing was wrong and that the trouble would clear up in time. At age 15 years she had more speech therapy and after lateral X-ray investigation, her mother was told that she had 'a lazy palate' and that probably when she got a boyfriend she would take more trouble and speak normally. Her mother said that she had not only no boyfriend but her speech was interfering with her career and social life and asked if the problem could be habit or nervousness. Greene agreed to see Miss B. and then learned from Mrs B. that she would have some trouble persuading her daughter to attend for speech therapy. Eventually, after a year, Miss B. telephoned quite late one evening, obviously in the hope that nobody would be in the speech clinic – her speech was so hypernasal that there was no need to ask her name. It transpired that she was telephoning from outside the hospital and she was invited into the clinic. A drab, nervous person arrived. At first she was defensive and rather aggressive, making it plain that she had only come to pacify her mother, to whom she was devoted, and that she resented any further attempts to improve her speech. She did not mind it herself and her friends never noticed it. She had become a committed Christian recently and was planning to become a missionary. Gradually she relaxed and spoke of how hard she had tried despite being told she was lazy, especially by her father, who blamed her for not speaking well. It was then not difficult to persuade her to agree to an assessment by a really expert plastic surgery team. It was obvious that pharyngoplasty operation would improve her palatopharyngeal

closure; on saying /ɑː/ the palate elevated well but just did not reach the posterior pharyngeal wall. Her facial bones were rather broad with eyes set wide apart, which may be associated with a wide pharynx. Articulation was good and when pronouncing single words with open articulation resonance was normal.

Miss B. was referred to the Plastic Surgery Unit at Oxford. Dr Adran reported as follows on cine-radiographic data:

> The line of this patient's hard palate is level with the arch of the atlas or even slightly below it. The first three vertebrae of the cervical spine show some congenital abnormalities, vertebrae 2 and 3 being fused. Adenoidal mass small. Pharynx large. Superior dental plate *in situ*.
>
> On saying 'ee' the palate elevates well enough though it is rather thin, but fails to make contact with the posterior pharyngeal wall by about ¾ cm.
>
> Counting 4, 5, 6, 7 the palate remains elevated and the gap is considerably reduced and momentary contact may be made with the posterior pharyngeal wall, though this is not complete.
>
> Blowing was effective with no evidence of nasal escape, partly with the aid of a diffuse Passavant's ridge.
>
> Swallowing: no significant abnormality. The palate does not, however, make closure with the posterior pharyngeal wall until finally pushed up by the tongue at the end of swallowing.
>
> Conclusion: I would have thought that a pharyngoplasty would have produced a good result.

A Hynes pharyngoplasty was performed and immediately afterwards, as is usually the case, speech was hyponasal and there was some nasal obstruction. After 3 months speech became entirely normal. This transformed the patient's personality; she left the secretarial work which she had been undertaking intermittently and took a job in the accounts department of a large clothing store for women, in London. Here the girls persuaded her to have her hair restyled, use make-up and dress fashionably. When last seen she was scarcely recognisable, looking happy, smart and beautiful and on her way to a party.

This patient's problem was not hard to solve; it is only sad that help was provided so late owing to the ignorance or sheer lack of experience of those who had tried to treat her.

Cleft Palate

Incidence

Cleft lip and palate are the most common of all congenital deformities and have been reported throughout history world wide and discovered in Egyptian mummies. There is some difficulty in ascertaining the incidence due to incomplete records but a central system of registration has pertained in Denmark for the last 45 years. Incidence was estimated at 1.3 per 1000 live births during the first five years but there has been a steady increase, rising to about 2 cases per 1000 (Fogh-Andersen, 1980).

A genetic influence is recognised. Cleft lip and cleft lip and palate are more common in males. Cleft palate alone is more frequent in females and is not generally hereditary, which indicates that the aetiology in these cases is exogenous. Drugs taken in pregnancy are the most suspect factor; cleft palate occurred among thalidomide casualties.

Postnatal management

Postnatal management involves primarily counselling the mother and reassurance immediately by all members of the medical team: the obstetrician and nurses, general practitioner and health visitor, and later the plastic surgeon and supporting hospital team. It is a disaster and shock to be presented with a baby with cleft lip and so visible a deformity. Anxiety and guilt haunt the parents. The way in which parents, particularly the mother, are handled at this time will affect the mother–child relationship. Sympathy and explanation of surgical procedures and presentation of photographs before and after surgery are mandatory. Assurance must be given that the baby will look normal and develop normal speech and that normality will be achieved ultimately (Bernstein, 1979).

Feeding difficulties cause anxiety as the necessary intraoral pressure for sucking is reduced and also swallowing action expresses milk down the nose (nasal regurgitation). Breast feeding is attempted by some mothers of cleft palate babies and may be successfully achieved if a nipple shield and teat are used. If breast feeding is difficult the milk can be expressed and given by bottle spoon.

Many cleft palate babies thrive on feeding from a spoon although there are various types of specially designed teats for bottle feeding. There is also a feeding bottle with a spoon attachment available. The nurse will show the mother how to position the child. The feeding situation should be a relaxed and satisfying one for both infant and mother which establishes a close bond and must not be disturbed by anxiety and failure (McWilliams, Morris and Shelton, 1984).

Some speech therapists think that they should be called in at this early stage to talk to the mother about swallow patterns and speech and language. In most cases the mother has enough to cope with adjusting to her child's difficulties and speech development is not one that needs to be added to them at this time. However, parents are reassured to know that a speech therapist is available for advice and discussion. In most cases follow-up after surgical repair of the palate is completed is early enough and then regular periodic monitoring of speech development is very necessary.

If properly handled, the negative feelings the parents may experience at first sight of the child need not become embedded in their attitudes towards the disability. Cleft palate children are not in fact found to be more maladjusted than non-cleft palate children. Clifford (1979) in reviewing an extensive literature found that pronounced signs of maladjustment, personality disorder, mental handicap, social adjustment and domestic stability were no different from the rest of the population. The happy lack of psychogenic disturbances in cleft palate children is due to the enlightened handling of the situation by the cleft palate team.

Primary Surgery

The lip is repaired first as early as possible for aesthetic reasons. The child needs to be gaining weight steadily. The popular age for operation under general anaesthetic is 10 weeks. The cleft in the alveolus may be closed at the same time. When the plastic surgery centre favours orthodontic treatment to move the free alveolar segments into alignment, surgery may be later but this should be possible at 3 or 4 months of age (Foster, 1980a, b). There are a bewildering number of possible techniques for repair of the lip and also the palate and these are well reviewed by Bernstein (1979) and Watson (1980).

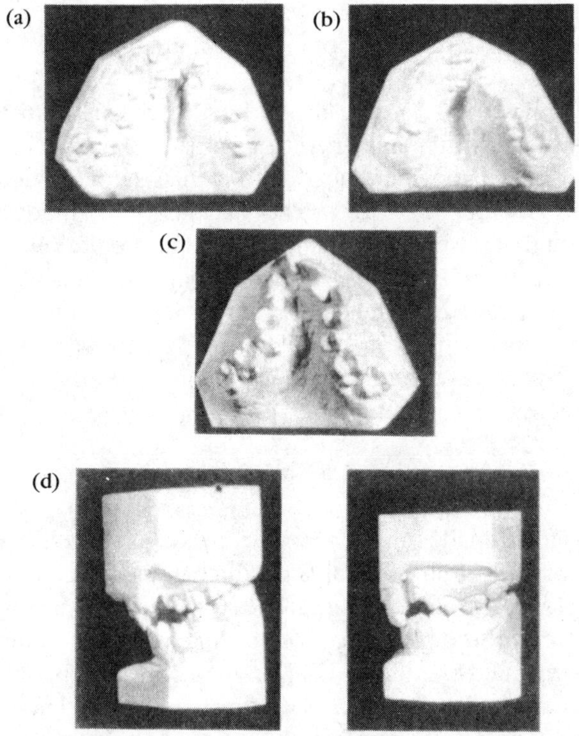

Figure 12.1. Orthodontic moulds of cleft palate patients. Models of upper jaw of patients with cleft of lip, alveolus and palate (a) showing collapse of the alveolar arch; (b) showing medial collapse of the left maxillary segment; (c) showing bilateral collapse of the maxillary alveolar arch. (d) Upper and lower models of two patients showing the lateral open bite produced.

Success as in all plastic surgery depends upon the skill, care and experience of the surgeon but also the severity of the cleft (Greene, 1960). The width of gap between the confronting segments of lip and palate and the amount of tissue available is variable and in some cases lack of fetal growth may militate against a good result. In this event secondary surgery will be necessary at a later stage when the competence of the velopharyngeal mechanism can be judged from the quality of the child's speech.

Closure of the hard and soft palate should be completed before 2 years of age – at 18 months is better. This offers an excellent prospect of normal speech and before compensatory muscular movements and abnormal articulatory patterns have become established (Barimo *et al.*, 1987). However, some American experts believe strongly that repair of the palate and transposition of the palatal flaps after freeing them from the bony palate, irrevocably damages the bone growth centres subsequently. Maxillary and facial deformity may occur with collapse of the alveolar arch and dental irregularities (Foster, 1980a). Orthodontic treatment is required until growth is complete in late adolescence. It has not been conclusively proved that early closure of the hard palate is related to abnormal maxillary development. Those who disagree maintain that failure in growth is due to the original fetal failure. Two schools of thought exist. In England surgeons have always put early surgery and speech first. In the USA both regimens are followed, it seems with equal conviction (Foster, 1980).

The oral deformities such as the inside bite of prognathism and dental irregularities associated with maxillary retrognathism do not necessarily affect the voice, but the articulation, and need not be enlarged upon here (Greene and Canning, 1959; Greene, 1961). The excellence of modern surgical techniques is such that normal speech and resonance are the rule rather than the exception. Speech and language retardation may occur as a result of other handicaps, low intelligence, deafness and poor social environment. Once the programme of primary surgery is complete one has to wait for speech to develop. Normal speech is the rule in England demonstrating the efficacy of early repair (Greene, 1960; McWilliams, 1960).

Speech Assessment

A distinction has to be made between normal delays in speech development and the articulatory substitutions infants produce in the process of acquiring mature pronunciation of adult speech. These phonemic substitutions and omissions will reveal the presence of an incompetent velopharyngeal sphincter if accompanied by audible nasal escape and hypernasality and if they have the compensatory characteristics of 'cleft palate speech'. These are glottal stops for plosives, especially velar plosives, and nasal pharyngeal fricatives for fricatives and affricates. Such features are not characteristic of normal speech development but are compensatory adjustments to nasal escape and lack of pressure.

Speech and language development

Late speech development can be expected if the child has spent some time in hospital or been given rather less attention than was needed from a busy mother with a family to look after. In some instances the mother may react negatively to the child and not provide the necessary language stimulation. Primary surgery occurs during a vital linguistic stage in the toddler. Details of hospitalisation and family reactions and support are important to complete the psychosocial and sociolinguistic background.

Hearing

Testing of every cleft palate child's hearing is essential and it should be monitored throughout childhood. There is a prevalence of otitis media in cleft palate infants which persists in 50% of older children and often into adulthood. Lencione (1980) reviews the research reports regarding conductive deafness in cleft palate patients.

The eustachian tube drains the middle ear and ventilates it, maintaining equilibrium between atmospheric air pressure and pressure behind the tympanic membrane. The exit of the tube into the pharynx is closed except when opening in swallowing and yawning. Opening of the eustachian tube is executed by the tensor palati and its efficiency is impaired in cleft palate surgery (Honjo, Okazaki and Kumazawa, 1979). Help from the otologist is necessary with medication to reduce infection and if necessary the insertion of grommets to provide artificial drainage of middle ear secretions (glue ear). This procedure is known as myringotomy. Tonsils and adenoids also become enlarged and infected and cause further problems.

The child who is not conspicuously deaf and only hard of hearing intermittently can be severely handicapped in noisy surroundings and can become educationally retarded. This must be recognised and adequate help given in school. Too often the problem is undetected or thought not serious. A teacher of the deaf should be enlisted to advise teachers and the mother. Parents should have problems explained to them so that the child is given encouragement and does not suffer the stigma of being dull, lazy or not heeding instructions. A speech therapist may replace the teacher of the deaf if the hearing problem is not severe.

Adenoidectomy

The removal of adenoids in children with repaired cleft palate and normal speech may produce hypernasality if the palate is short and nasopharyngeal closure has hitherto been obtained by contact of the palate with the projecting adenoidal pad. Removal of adenoids is recommended for patients with cleft palate only if the ears and hearing are affected. Pigott (1977) states that 20% of cleft palate cases suffer from a 30 dB hearing loss.

In the normal course of events the adenoidal pad atrophies during adolescence. Children with short cleft palate and enlarged adenoids appear not to lose their good speech as they grow up, even though slight incompetent closure may develop as the adenoids atrophy. This appears to be because this process takes place by imperceptible degrees and the child automatically regulates speech production to conform to the already established auditory patterns.

Assessment of nasality

The perceptual judgement of hypernasality and audible nasal escape is a valuable aspect of the speech therapist's contribution to the plastic surgeon's remedial programme (Morley, 1980). The speech therapist's report must embrace a description of deviant resonance, nasal escape and articulation. Deviant resonance is due to abnormal coupling of oral and nasal resonators which produces an imbalance of harmonic structure. Most cleft palate speakers with inadequate velopharyngeal closure develop abnormal tongue posture to compensate. By elevating the back of the tongue and tensing the jaw and pharynx an attempt is made to reduce nasal escape. The pharyngeal constriction can increase nasal tone. Sometimes the muscular effort is such that a nasal grimace is present and constriction of the nares is visible. The Vocal Profile Analysis (see p. 88 and Appendix II) can be used in this assessment. Consonant substitution must be carefully noted. The fricatives, especially /s/ may be laterally articulated due to the collapse of the alveolar arch. The lateral sigmatism only occurs in cleft palate cases with palato-pharyngeal competence (Greene and Canning, 1959).

The voice may be perceived as having an indeterminate hollow tone with nasal emission, sometimes described as 'mixed nasality' (Morley, 1970), rather than being obviously hypernasal. This may be due to deviation of the nasal septum associated with deformity of the palatal bones which contributes a blocked, 'cul-de-sac', resonance (West, Ansberry and Carr, 1957).

Phonation

Many studies confirm that the laryngeal note is affected as distinct from resonance (McWilliams, Lavorato and Bluestone, 1973). In these cases the vocal folds are adducted in order to provide adequate valving and prevention of nasal escape of air, especially in production of plosives and fricatives requiring adequate build-up of oral air pressure. This strong and frequent adduction of the vocal folds in order to prevent nasal air leak may result in vocal abuse and vocal nodules (Leder and Lerman, 1985; Wang, Yeung and Chen, 1986). Greene (1960) in a consecutive series of 300 cases of repaired cleft did not encounter a single case of vocal nodules. Renfrew (C.E., 1988, personal communication), however, reports instances of vocal nodules in some of her cases of repaired cleft palate. She confirms that further surgery must be considered to establish a competent palatopharyngeal sphincter. Leder and Lerman (1985) produced spectrographic acoustic evidence of vocal abuse in cleft palate individuals with hypernasality due to compensatory laryngeal valving activity.

Another commonly encountered symptom may be phonasthenia. The voice is breathy and not loud enough due to the child attempting to reduce nasality and avoiding being conspicuous by a vocal strategy of self-effacement (McWilliams, Morris and Shelton, 1984). Effortless speech, however, is the most effective way of reducing hypernasality and nasal escape in cases of palatopharyngeal deficit and is used in therapy (Greene, 1957).

Objective assessment: instruments

Spectrography

Spectrography analysis provides information concerning the formant structure of nasality. The predominant characteristic is generally accepted to be a loss of intensity in the vowel formants, especially the first formant, coupled with shifts in frequency (McWilliams, Morris and Shelton, 1984). In other words, the harmonics are thrown out of balance but retain the basic structures which retains their recognisable phonemic identity. Individual spectrograms are so variable that it is difficult to arrive at a definitive picture of nasality which can be used as a standard rule in assessment.

Oronasal sound pressure levels

Probe microphones can be introduced into the nose and mouth so that the acoustic ratio of oral and nasal contributions can be measured during speech. The Nasometer produced by Kay Elemetric Corporation provides a microcomputer system which measures pressure levels and displays the ratio immediately both graphically and statistically on a screen. This instrument has been designed by Fletcher and replaces the TONAR (Fletcher, 1970). An anemometer has been devised at Exeter University and is described in the chapter on instrumentation (p. 113) (Ellis *et al.*, 1978; Selley, 1979). These instruments offer useful information concerning hypernasality and are useful in biofeedback teaching but do not correlate perfectly with what is perceived subjectively (Edwards, 1980; McWilliams, Morris and Shelton, 1984).

Speech therapy

The child with nasal escape should be given speech therapy early and as soon as aberrant articulation, speech delay and excessive nasality are detected (Bzoch, 1979). This may be successful in correction of deviant articulation, muscular tension and vocal misuse. Hearing training and testing can be integrated into treatment and contact with mother and teachers also established. This preparation will guarantee a more immediate speech improvement after secondary surgery which is generally left until the age of 6 years or much later (Greene and Canning, 1959; Greene, 1960).

The assessment by the speech therapist and results of speech therapy are crucial in the planning of surgical and orthodontic strategies throughout the years of management.

Secondary Surgery

Assessment of palatopharyngeal mechanism

Hypernasality indicates incomplete or insufficient closure of the nasopharyngeal tube. A gap may be apparent when an isolated vowel is produced but the necessary closure effected by pharyngeal and palatal muscles may not be sustained in connected speech. Modern techniques of assessment permit a comprehensive view of the mechanism in action during speech from above the palate by a fibreoptic nasendoscope introduced through the nose. Pigott (1974, 1980) lays great emphasis on the thorough assessment of palatal sphincteric and valvular closure, using the most modern instrumental equipment, prior to choosing the type of secondary surgery to close the nasopharyngeal gap. Surgery must be adapted to suit the individual nasopharyngeal defect. There is no single surgical solution for all cases as there was in the past when knowledge was more limited (Morley, 1980).

Three-dimensional assessment

A three-dimensional concept of the pharyngeal isthmus is needed. This is obtained by the following procedures. A fibreoptically lighted endoscope is passed through the nose into the nasopharynx which permits viewing of the isthmus during continuous speech (Pigott, Bensen and White, 1969). This is coupled to a lateral X-ray image intensifier behind the patient and linked with a videotape recording system. Two planes at right angles are thus simultaneously recorded with sound. Radiographic screening through the floor of the mouth and the cranial vault and a lateral view by videofluoroscopy is carried out by Skolnick (1970) and Skolnick and McCall (1973) for examination of patients with persistent hypernasality following pharyngeal flap surgery and pharyngoplasty.

Lateral X-rays

The traditional lateral X-rays with barium outline can be misleading since the barium can pool or coat surfaces intermittently. Also they at best reveal the length and elevation of the palate in relation to the pharyngeal wall for one speech episode or syllable. The lateral barium outline gives no information concerning the width of the pharynx and the possible existence of unilateral or bilateral defects in closure such as lateral 'gutters' which allow nasal escape while central closure is complete. The fibreoptic nasendoscope view is therefore much superior (Figure 12.2).

Lateral barium contrast X-ray views are still useful in certain circumstances to check the basal X-ray (Pigott, 1977). It is also used when nasendoscopy is rejected by nervous patients and small children who object to the fibreoptic bundle being pushed up the nose and also to the taste of local anaesthetic. Moreover, insertion can be difficult and painful in cases of deflected nasal septum which is not uncommon in cleft palate.

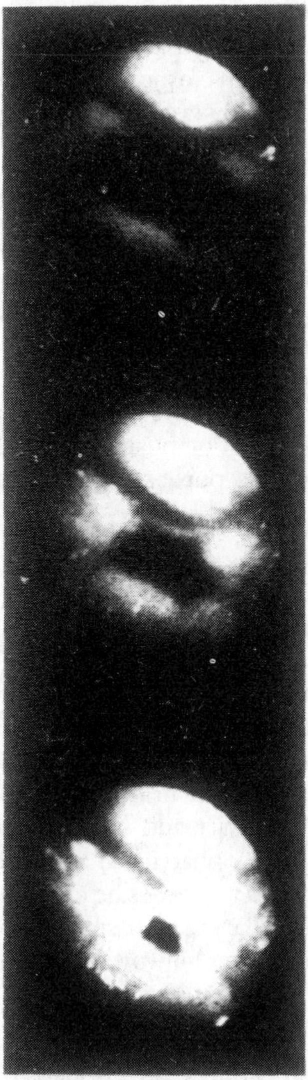

Figure 12.2. The fibreoptic nasendoscopic view of the palatopharyngeal isthmus (cleft palate). Three frames from 16 mm Ektachrome EF 1742 colour film at 25 frames per second. Recorded via a Storz teaching attachment. Despite marked degradation of the image, the essential diagnosis of failure to close is easily made. (By courtesy of R.W. Pigott, 1977, with kind permission of the author and publishers.)

The lateral X-ray with barium outline is still used routinely in plastic surgery units with or without the nasendoscope when financial considerations do not permit purchase of all the sophisticated equipment described above, nor the employment of technical staff to operate it.

Oral panendoscope

An alternative to the nasendoscope but seemingly less popular is the oral panendoscope designed by Taub (1966). This instrument causes the patient less discomfort and is easier to operate. The orally inserted 'telescope' restricts the speech-testing sequence and as many patients can obtain closure on a single 'pah' but cannot sustain closure in connected speech the results can be misleading (Pigott, 1977). However, Willis and Stutze (1972) explain that it is easily used, the scope being placed over the back of the tongue with the viewing window just behind the uvula. A clear view of the velum, pharyngeal walls, nasal conchae and orifices of the eustachian tubes is obtained. The instrument can be linked to video-tape and a permanent record obtained. Young children may not tolerate introduction of the panendoscope without gagging but Boone (1977) states that children of 9 years accept it.

Zwitman, Sonderman and Ward (1974) have described variations in velopharyngeal closure observed with the laryngeal telescope on 34 subjects. Movement of the lateral walls of the pharynx, if present, can be seen. Contact of the velum with the posterior pharyngeal wall may be visible but leaving lateral 'gutters' patent, or a purse-string type of closure when sphincteric closure is obtained.

Pharyngoplasty

The function of the pharyngeal isthmus has been described in detail by Pigott (1980) and the many methods of investigation it is possible to carry out simultaneously. He notes that no single mode is entirely reliable and therefore as many as possible are needed in order to arrive at the best surgical solution. The ultimate aim of secondary surgery is to reduce nasal escape and provide a seal which can maintain adequate oral breath pressure in connected speech. A complete seal is not necessary and some normal, non-cleft palate English speakers exhibit a slight velopharyngeal aperture in the endoscopic mirror. This articulatory manoeuvre increases head resonance or brilliance of tone to the voice when oral and pharyngeal harmonics are in tune. A relaxed tongue and oropharynx contribute to improved tone in cleft palate patients.

Surgical strategies

Numerous surgical procedures are available for improvement of velopharyngeal competence (Pigott, 1974; Randall, 1980; Bumstead, 1982). These comprise palatal pushback and superiorly and inferiorly based pharyngeal flaps. The choice of pharyngoplasty depends upon the nature of the pharyngeal incompetence. The palate may appear short in relation to a capacious pharynx or meet the posterior pharyngeal wall but exhibit lateral 'gutters' or gaps. Bumstead (1982) tabulates the surgical procedures possible with indications of advantages and disadvantages which provide a useful summary and source of reference. Powers (1986) indicates that the pharyngeal flap operation is the most commonly performed in the USA. A flap of tissue is taken from the pharyngeal wall and attached to the soft palate forming a permanent bridge. Ideally the lateral walls move in to meet the flap when palatopharyngeal closure is needed, thus preventing nasal escape laterally. The principle is that of a prosthetic bulb. Excellent results can be achieved but the bridge may shrink or be too wide and cause nasal obstruction.

Complications following surgery are fistulae in some cases but more frequently over-correction of the palatopharyngeal isthmus leads to nasal obstruction. Bzoch (1964) found this to be a greater problem than hypernasality due to insufficient closure. Tonsils can cause obstruction after pharyngoplasty and for this reason are generally removed before pharyngoplasty (Randall, 1980). As long as nasal breathing is not totally occluded (obstructed) the situation will improve in time as the pharyngeal flaps shrink after 3–6 months and as the pharynx increases in size as part of normal body growth.

Speech Therapy after Pharyngoplasty

It is anticipated that if speech therapy has been given preoperatively and the pharyngoplasty is successful, little or no speech rehabilitation will be necessary. When cleft palate speech persists therapeutic intervention becomes necessary.

Blowing exercises to exercise the palatopharyngeal muscles and eradicate nasal escape were for many years thought to be essential. However, it is now recognised that the mechanics of blowing are not those actually used in speech (McWilliams, Morris and Shelton, 1984) and that the manifestation of palatopharyngeal incompetence are more effectively treated through speech-related tasks (Kunzel, 1982). Practice in breath direction is necessary when nasal emission persists and when glottal stops and nasopharyngeal fricatives are substituted for plosives and fricatives. It is best tackled by gently blowing through pursed lips and by teaching correct articulation and use of the tongue (McDonald and Baker, 1951; Goda, 1966).

If the voice is hoarse or husky and lacking projection, a regimen of breathing and vocal control along the lines recommended for rehabilitation of vocal misuse (Chapter 9) will be necessary.

There are three general approaches to treatment: relaxation, hearing training and biofeedback.

Relaxation

The need for relaxed speech mechanism must be emphasised from the outset and specific exercises for relaxation of lips, tongue, jaw and throat given when necessary. A quiet voice and slow speech free from all tension and stridency should be encouraged. Most patients put far too much effort into speech production in their anxiety to be understood. Van Thal (1934) in her practical book on cleft palate speech is found cautioning the patient over the dangers of trying too hard.

Hearing training

All cleft palate patients should have a hearing test and, if there is a hearing loss, referral to an otologist must be made. The therapist must know the extent and severity of the deafness. Conductive hearing loss follows the same pattern as that of the 'catarrhal' and adenoidal child (p. 130).

Hearing training precedes all aspects of therapy. The patient has to discriminate and identify normal speech patterns if appropriate articulation and resonance are to be produced successfully. All teaching of vowels should be prefaced by hearing training, contrasting nasal and non-nasal vowels until the patient can clearly discriminate the difference. Hearing training lays the foundation for correct imitation of sounds and is especially necessary in reduction of nasality in vowel sounds, which these patients at first find more difficult to appreciate than consonants which provide stronger kinaesthetic and tactile feedback. Hearing training must include audiotape recording.

Vowel sounds must be contrasted until the patient can clearly differentiate between normal and hypernasal resonance in the therapist's voice and his own. Consonants must also be contrasted in the same way. The therapist presents the correct form and then the patient's substitution so that deviations can be readily detected.

Biofeedback

The use of instrumentation to provide biofeedback during treatment sessions and for practice accelerates treatment progress in many cases (see Chapter 7).

Remediation strategies

Therapeutic procedures are directed at correcting hypernasality and deviant articulation. These two areas are not discrete; they overlap and influence each other.

Correction of hypernasality

Following hearing training the therapist should encourage relaxation of the patient's mandible, tongue, faucial pillars and pharynx for the production of vowel sounds with normal resonance. This ensures an increase in the total volume of the oral and pharyngeal resonators.

Some vowels are more nasalised than others. For instance, /u:/ and /i:/ are often markedly hypernasal because the back of the tongue is necessarily moved upwards and forwards in order to produce these vowels. This creates a large pharyngeal resonator with a small oropharyngeal opening which favours nasal resonance as air is forced through the valve.

The vowels /ɑ:/ and /ð/ on the other hand may be little nasalised because the tongue is flat, the pharyngeal resonator small and the oropharyngeal orifice wide. The non-nasal vowels can be used to decontaminate the nasalised vowels in exercises such as the following:

1. /ɑ:,i:,ɑ:/ /ɑ:,i:,ɑ:/ – isolate i:
   /i:,ð,i:/ /i:,ð,i:/ – isolate i:

2. /uː,ɑː,uː,ɑː/ - isolate uː
/ð,uː,ð,uː/ - isolate uː

Non-nasalised consonants may also be used with the same purpose of reducing nasality in vowel tone. If /p/ and /t/, for instance are produced with no audible nasal escape it will be found helpful to practise exercises such as:

/puːp/ /tuːp/ /tuːt/ /tuːtuː/ etc.

The /uː/ is then isolated and incorporated into words.

Correction of articulation

The correction of audible nasal escape, breath direction and articulatory deviations is achieved most successfully when these aspects are dealt with concurrently. The articulation exercises are used as a means of directing air through the mouth rather than the nose.

Reduction of audible nasal emission
Nasal escape of air is accepted as unavoidable and no attempt is made to prevent it and no palate exercises are given. If there is nasal grimace this must be corrected and the patient instructed not to try to prevent air coming down the nose. It does not matter that there is some nasal escape; the goal is for it not to be audible. Mirror practice encouraging observation and elimination of excessive muscular tension may be helpful.

Breath direction
The patient is asked to:

- Blow softly through the lips then practise interrupting the breath stream by gently closing the lips with a soft /p,p,p/. Follow this with the voiced counterpart /b,b,b/. Elicit each 'new' consonant from one already mastered whenever possible.
- Practise blowing air through the upper teeth and lower lip, then interrupt with /f,f,f/. Follow with/v,v,v/.
- Sigh breath over the tongue between the teeth and obtain /θ/. Follow with /ð/.
- Control nasal escape on /t/ by prefacing with /b/.
- Produce /s/ and /ʃ/ ensuring that the air flows over the tongue tip.
- Sigh a prolonged /ʃ/ and interrupt with /t/ to improve /tʃ/.

As in the case of vowels it is also found that some consonants are produced with less nasal escape than others. The principle of decontamination can again be used to improve consonants by placing well-produced consonants adjacent to those with marked nasal emission. If, for example, fricatives are within normal limits but plosives remain abnormal exercises such as the following can be devised:

- /sp-sp-sp/ - isolate /p/
- /st-st-st/ - isolate /t/
- /spæt/pæt/ /spɪt-pɪt/, spaɪ-paɪ /
- steer-tear, store-tore, stow-toe

Consonant facilitation

In many cases where therapy directed at consonant production is required, glottal substitutions for plosives and pharyngeal fricatives for lingual fricatives have been used. The tongue tip is used minimally in speech and it is necessary to encourage its use as soon as possible. The acquisition of correct consonant articulation and elimination of glottal and pharyngeal substitutions is essential. McWilliams (1954) noted that there is a positive relationship between consonant articulation errors and nasality ratings as well as intelligibility ratings.

1. Velar plosives: /k/ and /g/ are the most difficult phonemes to achieve and are substituted by glottal stops. They can be produced more successfully if contact is made by the tongue against the palate further forward than in the normal speaker. The gesture is best accomplished by holding the front of the patient's tongue down firmly with a tongue depressor; the patient is asked to say /t/ or /d/ according to whether /k/ or /g/ is required.
2. Consonant clusters: the transition from eliciting these phonemes and then incorporating them into consonant clusters may present considerable difficulty in some cases. The glottal substitution previously used may be apparent although /k/ and /g/ are produced correctly in isolation. It is therefore important that the speech therapist should present tasks in a hierarchy of gradually increasing difficulty if the patient is not to become discouraged and lose heart. For example, it is usually much easier for the individual to produce /k/ following /ŋ/, as in 'think', when the articulators are in a position of readiness for producing /k/, than after /s/ as in 'skin'.
3. Alveolar plosives: it is frequently difficult to inhibit the use of a glottal stop when plosive phonemes are required. In order to obtain plosion with the correct placement for /t/ and /d/ it may be helpful to imitate spitting out pips with a firm contact of the tongue against the upper teeth. Alternatively small pellets of paper may be used. The sucking sound as the tongue tip pulls off the alveolus in the interjection of impatience /tʃ / - / tʃ / may also succeed in producing the correct results. /t/ may be elicited from /s/ after /θ/ has been mastered by the patient producing a long /s/ and stopping the air-stream with the tip of the tongue against the alveolus or teeth intermittently.
4. Nasal continuants: it is best not to introduce /m/, /n/ and /ŋ/ too early in treatment as this may disturb the new and unstable patterns of auditory and kinaesthetic feedback. Attempts at eliciting vowels with normal nasal resonance following nasal continuants, e.g. /ma:/ or /ni:/ is inadvisable until hypernasality is considerably reduced in other speech activities and

auditory monitoring is well developed. Then such exercises may be used effectively with others used in establishing improved voice production.

The speech therapist must bear in mind that the competence of the palatopharyngeal sphincter mechanism is chiefly the concern of the plastic surgeon. The patient should be treated as an individual with disorders of articulation and voice and not one in whom nasal escape is the over-riding factor.

'Speech should be improved by horizontal strata rather than vertical sections' (Greene, 1960). It is a mistake to concentrate too long upon one aspect of treatment and to concentrate on perfecting one sound after another.

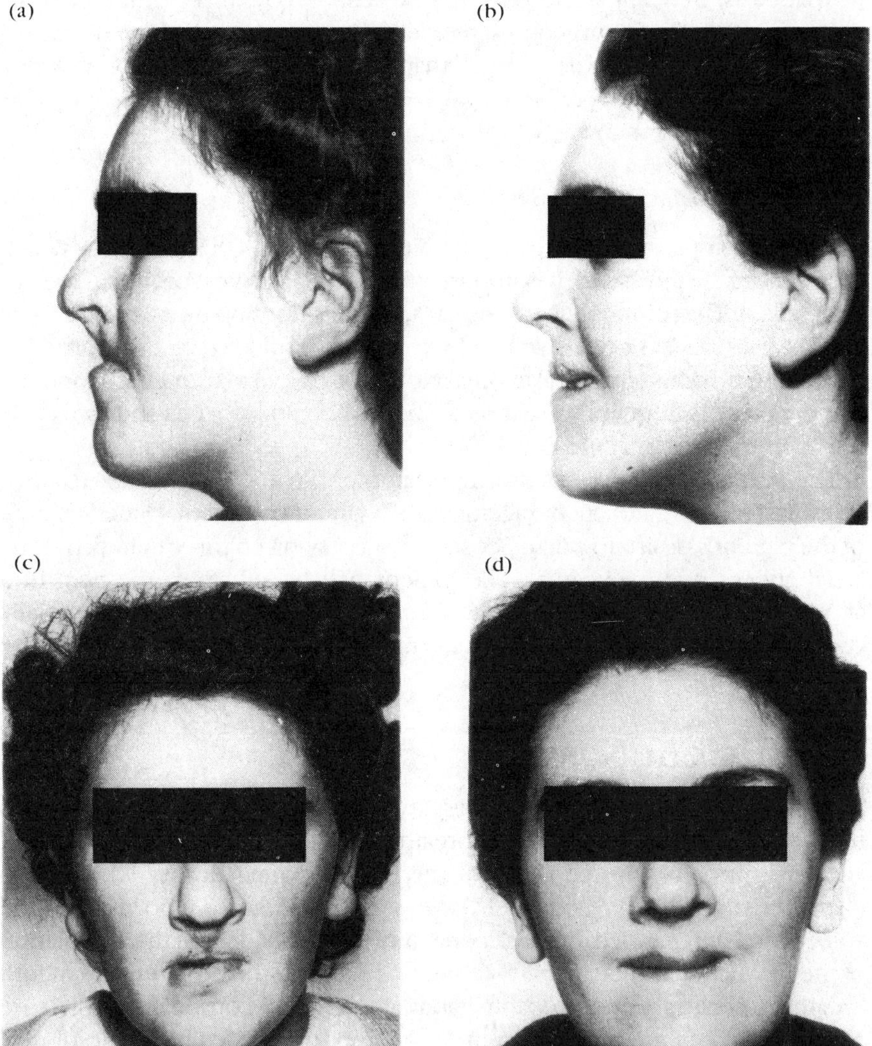

Figure 12.3. Photographs pre- and postsurgery to improve facial appearance (cleft palate). (a) Profile – preoperatively; (b) profile – postoperatively; (c) full face – preoperatively; (d) full face – postoperatively.

The improvement of resonance can proceed concurrently with correction of articulation, forming two separate lines of work at each treatment. The consonants can be taught in isolation one after the other in rapid succession, while those mastered first can be in the process of inclusion in all positions in words. It is important to give patients over the age of 10, who are generally very depressed and hopeless about their speech, a sense of achievement and progress.

Intensive therapy

Intensive speech therapy should be considered on both an in-patient and out-patient basis. In hospital, patients may be seen two or three times a day for short periods with the surgeon's agreement. Therapy along the lines described here requires less muscular activity than the patient usually employs when speaking and may therefore be started as early as a week after secondary repair of a palate or pharyngoplasty.

Psychological factors

Although cleft palate is an organic condition and the speech problems which arise are organically based, it is important that psychological problems are not overlooked. The response of the vocal tract to emotion and the effects on voice in all individuals has been discussed earlier and should not be disregarded in those with obvious structural anomalies. Although maladjustment may not be present there is frequently great sensitivity concerning speech and especially facial appearance in adolescence.

The speech therapist has an important role in the cleft palate team in providing support and encouragement throughout treatment. Understanding of the patient's desire to pursue cosmetic surgery when this can improve the facial appearance is essential. The patient will benefit from the help of a specialised beautician if there is facial scarring. Unless the patient is socially confident and determined to lead a normal life speech improvement may be disappointing.

Insufficient Nasality

The voice suffers from insufficient nasality when there is an obstruction of the nasal airway which renders nasal breathing difficult or impossible. Lack of adequate nasal resonance destroys the bright ringing quality which is so characteristic of head resonance. Vowel sounds are far from normal and the voice is dull and muffled, but lack of nasality is most evident in the articulation of the nasal consonants. Inability to breathe through the nose renders mouth breathing necessary and probably habitual. The nasal consonants, which are continuants, cannot be adequately maintained but resemble their plosive counterparts /b/, /d/ and /g/ on account of the precipitate release of the organs of articulation.

As the nasal consonants are frequent in the English language, their denasalisation renders speech distinctly abnormal and even unpleasant to the listener who rightly associates the lack of nasality with nasal obstruction. Severely denasalised speech is fortunately rare and a certain degree of nasality is possible for most speakers even when considerable obstruction of the nasal airway exists, provided the airway is not entirely closed. An individual is frequently able to compensate for lack of nasal resonance by increased pharyngeal constriction and deliberate prolongation of the nasal continuants.

Causes of hyponasality

Deflected septum

This is a common cause of reduced nasal resonance. It may be a congenital malformation and often occurs in association with cleft palate. Acquired deflected septum may occur if a broken nose is not surgically repaired successfully before healing takes place.

Pharyngoplasty

Nasal obstruction after pharyngoplasty and pharyngeal flap operations has already been described in connection with surgical correction of velopharyngeal incompetence.

Neoplasm

Nasal and nasopharyngeal tumours in adults are rare and require immediate investigation and treatment by surgery and/or radiotherapy if malignant.

Polypoid growths in the nasal passages sometimes occur and may be related to conditions of chronic allergic rhinitis. Polyps should be removed surgically in order to facilitate nasal breathing and improve resonance. They tend to recur and may also occur in the larynx.

Adenoids

Hypertrophy of the nasopharyngeal adenoid most frequently occurs between the ages of 3 years and 7 years. The tonsils are generally also enlarged. Inflammation of the nasal mucosa (rhinitis) accompanied by constant nasal discharge (rhinorrhoea) is a common and troublesome cause of insufficient nasality. Mouth-breathing results from the nasal obstruction and the child may present with the typical adenoid facies of pinched nostrils and prominent incisors in the later stages (Ballantyne and Groves, 1982). Inflammation may involve the laryngeal and pharyngeal membranes and produce chronic hoarseness. Adenoids alone do not cause complete nasal obstruction and mouth-breathing. Rhinitis and sinusitis may persist after adenoidectomy unless appropriate medical attention is given to an infection remaining after the operation. Hyponasality when there is no nasal obstruction can sometimes persist through force of habit until speech therapy is initiated.

Vasomotor rhinitis

Many patients complain of suffering from 'catarrh'; their symptoms may include nasal obstruction, postnasal discharge, rhinorrhoea and sneezing. These occur in reaction to certain stimuli although there is no identifiable allergic cause. The basis of this condition may be multiple. Causes include hereditary factors and infection while there is also evidence that the condition may be related to stress. Endocrinological influence is apparent with vasomotor rhinitis occurring frequently at puberty and during menstruation and pregnancy. A damp atmosphere, air pollution and alcohol intake will affect the response of the nasal mucosa in the vulnerable individual (Ballantyne and Groves, 1982). The mucous membrane of the nose is prone to produce nasal polyps in these patients.

Allergy

Another form of rhinitis which is most intractable is due to perennial nasal allery which assails the sufferer at all times of the year (perennial allergic rhinitis) and is not confined to the seasonal exacerbation of 'hay-fever' (seasonal allergic rhinitis). The condition is often associated with asthma and eczema in the individual or in members of the family; there appears to be a marked hereditary tendency to allergic conditions. Allergic substances (allergens) include pollens, fungal spores, feathers, dust, the house-dust mite and the fur of certain animals. Certain foods, particularly dairy products, nuts and seafood, can cause a reaction. Some nose drops also increase the severity of the symptoms when used over a prolonged period. In these patients the nasal mucosa becomes oedematous and there is a watery nasal discharge. There is a tendency to develop nasal polyps. The general psychological and physical health of the patient appears to be of some importance, sudden attacks of sneezing with streaming nose and eyes, and headaches, being reduced in time of fitness and well-being.

Systematic skin tests may trace the substance to which the individual reacts so that it can be avoided where possible. Injections of unavoidable inhaled substances may be administered for desensitization. Antihistamine preparations alleviate the symptoms in some individuals although they may cause drowsiness. Other treatments include administration of various nasal sprays.

The psychogenic contribution to nasal allergy and vasomotor rhinitis is well recognised. It is probable that in many individuals hypersensitivity to certain substances is the primary cause of disorders of the respiratory tract. Emotional factors later become attached to the original physical reaction and conditioning takes place. Many individuals appear to exhibit more severe reactions when they are under stress.

The numbers of sufferers of allergic rhinitis are apparently increasing. This appears to be due to the mounting stresses in society besides a range of synthetic materials, preservatives and colourings in food, cosmetic substances and chemical pollutants. However, the psychogenic aspect may require psychological adjustment and psychotherapy for some individuals.

Rhinitis can be invoked in some individuals by deliberate lack of sympathy on the part of the interviewer in a clinical situation and in the absence of the allergen. Similarly it may be allayed by an atmosphere of ease and sympathy even when a high concentration of the allergen is present (Wolfe, 1952).

Effects of nasal obstruction on resonance

Hyponasality is not entirely related to the degree of nasal blockage. Obstruction always causes the voice to be deficient in nasal resonance but does not necessarily exclude the possibility of nasality, which is dependent upon the size of the nasopharyngeal resonator and the relative sizes of its orifices. If the resonator is not properly adjusted to produce nasality, insufficient nasality may persist after removal of nasal obstruction by force of habit.

Case notes

1. The voice of a man of 18 years, for instance, continued to be denasalised after the complete removal of a large tumour which extended from the nasopharynx into the nasal cavity. His speech responded rapidly to speech therapy.
2. It is noticeable also that many of the children with cleft palate who exhibit insufficient nasality due to nasal obstruction and malformation of the septum, still continue to speak in the same way when the septum has been straightened and the airway freed.
3. A further illustration is that of a child who suffered from severe audible nasal escape after adenoidectomy. As movement of the palate developed she gradually reverted to her habitual denasalised speech although she could now breathe through her nose without difficulty.

In these instances of habit the individual continues to apply the same auditory patterns to speech production after the removal of the cause of the hyponasality and obstruction in the nasal resonator. The habitual sounds are produced, probably unconsciously and at a reflex level, but effectively adjust in articulation and resonance to compensate for lack of the nasal obstruction. This pattern will continue unless speech therapy is given.

Remediation

Cases of hyponasality should be fully investigated by an ear, nose and throat specialist in order to determine the aetiology of the obstruction. Speech therapy should not be attempted until appropriate medical or surgical treatment has been initiated.

Nasal hygiene

As a large number of cases of hyponasality involve nasal congestion, even after adenoidectomy and tonsillectomy, it is important to ensure that the nasal passages are clear of mucus particularly at the beginning of therapy sessions. Decongestant nasal drops, antibiotics and steam inhalations with Friar's

Balsam may be prescribed by the GP or laryngologist but it may be necessary for the speech therapist to teach the child how to blow the nose efficiently.

Nose blowing

The child's ability to nose blow should be tested at the beginning of treatment; many children only sniff or wipe the nose even when using a handkerchief. The sound effects may be convincing but it is necessary to check that the blow has been productive. In some instances the inability to nose blow efficiently may be due to lack of early training by the mother, but it seems that some children have coordinaton problems or dyspraxia which make it a genuinely difficult task. For this reason, it is not easy to teach but perseverence usually results in success and greatly improves the health of the nasal mucosa.

Method

1. Tell the child to keep the mouth closed. Close one nostril by applying pressure to the lateral wall. With a tissue ready at the other nostril, encourage the child to breathe out or to sniff in and puff out. Only one nostril should be blown at a time as this avoids excessive air pressure accumulating in the nasopharynx and consequently driving mucus into the eustachian tube.
2. Working with one nostril at a time ask the child to sniff in three times, then to puff out three times. The child then begins to feel and hear air circulating.
3. The child holds the handkerchief and practises the above exercises independently with the mouth closed.
4. A nasal manometer can be used in practice once the child has learned to nose breath.

Mouth-breathing correction

Breathing through the mouth can persist by habit after adenoidectomy and also because of persisting congestion. After carrying out the above procedures for removal of nasal obstruction, habitual nasal breathing can be established in the following way.

Method

1. With the child seated before a mirror contrast the appearance when mouth-breathing and when breathing with the mouth closed.
2. The child practises sniffing and puffing with the mouth shut, with a finger over the lips as a tactile reinforcer.
3. Seated in front of a mirror the child aims to keep the mouth shut while being read a story. A score is kept of the time for which the closure can be maintained and the number of mouth openings.
4. Games of any sort are played while the child endeavours to keep the

mouth closed throughout; any mouth opening is monitored and a system of marks, rewards and penalties can be used.

5. Parents and teachers are asked to remind the child.

Case history
A boy of 8 years from an uneducated and neglectful family attended a speech and language unit. His speech was unintelligible and he was severely retarded educationally although of average intelligence. His voice was husky and speech denasalised due to a constant cold and nasal blockage. When tested he was quite unable to blow his nose, only sniff, and shied away from a handkerchief like a nervous pony. Under instructions several times a day from the speech therapist he learned to blow his nose and to clear the nasal airway. At first, he removed large quantities of mucus; paper towels were used as tissues were inadequate. He cooperated well after a while because he said his nose felt better and his ears 'didn't pop'. Alertness improved. He had been referred to the hospital ENT department originally by the school doctor, but when he was given an appointment 2 months later his ears, nose and throat were clear and hearing was normal.

Remediation strategies

Hearing training

The principles and methods of application are similar to those described in the treatment of hypernasality. The patient is encouraged to discriminate between nasal and denasalised phonemes by identifying those sounds which 'come down the nose' and those which 'come out of the mouth':

- /m, n, ŋ/ contrasted with /p, b, t, d, k, g/.
- Contrast in syllables, e.g. /ma:,pa:,ba:/.
- Contrast in words and sentences, e.g. mad-bad, not-dot.

Development of nasal resonance

- Humming on /m/, /n/ and /ŋ/ feeling the lips tingle when relaxed and feeling vibrations when hands are placed on either side of the nose. Cup palms of hands over ears and hum listening to increased resonance.
- Practise singing syllables starting with /m/.
- Sentences and verse, and with children composing nonsense verse, containing as many nasal continuants as possible.

Establish in spontaneous speech the common negative abbreviated verbs, e.g. can't, don't, won't etc.

Case history
C.Z. a girl of 9 years exhibited severe hyponasality as a result of chronic rhinitis since the age of 2 years. /b/ /d/ and /g/ were substituted for /m/ /n/ and /ŋg/. Adenoidectomy at 6 years had not made the

slightest difference to the catarrhal condition or to her speech. Extensive examinations had been made without revealing the cause of the rhinitis and the speech therapist was the last in a long line of specialists who had endeavoured to help the child. The oral structure was normal, but the nose and cheek bones were flattened, exhibiting the typical skeletal structure of the adenoidal facies. The soft palate surprisingly showed no movement at all during the articulation of vowels. The child kept her nose clear by constant blowing and did not breathe through her mouth. She was tense, holding her thin little shoulders high, and her breathing involved the upper thorax almost entirely. She was nervous and so conscious of her speech that she was unable to read aloud in class without stumbling over every word, although in clinic she could read adult material fluently. Although not an only child she was extraordinarily staid and polite, and so quaintly old-fashioned that the school staff invariably referred to her as 'great-grandmother'. Her speech, which was precise and clipped, was in keeping with her personality.

Despite the rhinitis, which did not improve during treatment, she was from the beginning able to hum with normal nasality and to produce normal nasal consonants in isolation. She enjoyed humming tunes and practising 'playing on her trumpet', as we called it, with hands over the nose or ears. Great difficulty was experienced in obtaining normal nasal sounds in nonsense syllables and speech. Her auditory discrimination was good and she was able to discriminate correct and incorrect resonance accurately and was distressed by hearing a recording of her speech. Speech suddenly improved when it was suggested that she should relax and not try so hard with nonsense syllable execises but speak lazily and easily, drawling and prolonging the nasal continuants instead of producing them briskly so that plosives resulted. Not only did nasal consonants now become normal, but head resonance and voice quality improved so that speech became melodious and pleasing to the great joy of the child.

Chapter 13 Laryngeal Structural Anomalies, Infection and Trauma

Congenital Structural Anomalies

Congenital abnormalities causing stenosis of the larynx are mainly a matter of theoretical interest to the speech therapist since the condition either results in stillbirth or is alleviated in infancy or early childhood.

Arnold (1958) in discussing 'dysplastic dysphonia' and congenital cases of hoarseness, describes various abnormalities found in adult larynges which may be familial and associated with hoarseness in childhood. Laryngeal anomalies may also occur in conjunction with other physical deformities. Possible laryngeal anomalies producing hoarseness are sulcus of a vocal fold, one placed higher than the other, one fold broader than the other, and one ventricle may be larger than the other. The arytenoids may pass one in front of the other upon adduction in paralysis. Differences in the size of the wings of the thyroid cartilage or an abnormal bilateral protuberance of the thyroid cartilage extending into the vocal fold can create obstruction. Subglottic anterior deformity of the cricoid cartilage may also cause stenosis and abnormal thickening of the lateral walls of the subglottic space (Holinger, 1979).

Another congenital deformity concerns the epiglottis. In place of the usual flattened structure, it is folded in such a way that its lateral walls almost approximate (Wilson, 1952). The aryepiglottic folds offer considerable resistance to the air stream in inspiration and cause a vibratory stridor which is always present, but grows alarmingly louder upon exertion and especially when the infant cries, when it is said to resemble a crowing cock. There is no serious cyanosis although dyspnoea may be present and the child remains comparatively healthy. The condition requires no treatment and there are no symptoms by the third year.

Congenital Laryngeal Web

Congenital webs of mucous membrane may arise in the larynx across the anterior portion of the vocal folds leaving the airway patent posteriorly. There is a hereditary incidence in some cases. Baker and Savetsky (1966) reported congenital laryngeal web occurring in four members of the same family.

Symptoms include hoarseness in most cases with inspiratory stridor when the web is large. However, the web may be attached in such a way that it causes no severe atresia or breathing difficulty. The condition, in fact, can go unsuspected until puberty when a boy's voice may fail to break. Girls' voices remain childish on account of the diminished length of the vocal folds capable of vibration. Acquired laryngeal web may occur after trauma and certain specific infections such as healed diphtheria or tuberculosis (Ballantyne and Groves, 1982).

Snipping of the thin membranous web frees the vocal folds and the free edges of the membrane retract into the membranous cover of the folds. If the web is small it may be decided that surgical intervention is inadvisable as hoarseness will not necessarily be resolved and there is a possibility of formation of a fibrous band in healing.

Laryngeal webs vary in nature and degree (Holinger, 1979). The anterior muscular edges of the folds may be fused together with fibrosis extending below the glottis. In this event the surgical procedure consists of a thyrotomy, division of the folds and insertion of a tantalum plate until healing has taken place. Just splitting the web can result in stenosis due to the raw edges healing together. When cartilage extends into the web surgical intervention has to be carefully considered and is best avoided.

The voice will probably be hoarse immediately postoperatively and voice quality will subsequently depend upon the state of the folds after surgery. Speech therapy may be necessary to break entrenched habits of phonation. A course of hearing training and vocal exercises will improve pitch and reduce patterns of forcing which might have evolved in an attempt to achieve maximum loudness while the web was *in situ*.

> Case note
>
> Miss A. underwent an indirect laryngoscopy on account of an infective laryngitis and voice loss. Her normal voice was high-pitched and thin, but she was not concerned about this. The laryngologist diagnosed a web situated in the anterior commissure which he persuaded her could be rectified and her voice improved. On exploration he found a cartilaginous projection under the web and decided to go no further. After this the patient was angry because her perfectly satisfactory voice was now hoarse and weak. She was referred for speech therapy belatedly but this calmed her and also restored her 'normal' voice which her friends rather liked, especially her boyfriend who admired the childish quality.

Inflammatory Conditions

Speech therapists are so familiar with laryngitis due to vocal misuse that there is a tendency to overlook the possibility of the pathologies causing inflammatory diseases of the larynx (Vrabec and Davison, 1980).

Acute non-specific laryngitis

An acute inflammation of the laryngeal mucosa may be associated with viral infections or exposure to a polluted atmosphere as well as a period of vocal fold irritation such as shouting as described in connection with vocal abuse (p. 120). The voice will be hoarse and aphonia may occur. The condition usually improves after 2 or 3 days although in some cases of infection the dysphonia may continue for up to a fortnight. Voice rest is important.

Acute laryngitis may be followed by functional dysphonia and can frequently be identified as a 'trigger' in cases of psychogenic voice disorders.

Chronic non-specific laryngitis

Kleinsasser (1968) described the confusion of terms and conditions associated with the collective term 'chronic laryngitis' and remarked that every laryngologist has a different concept of the clinical picture presented by such terms as pachydermia, keratosis, leucoplakia, polyp, papilloma etc. We have already run into this difficulty in discussing contact ulcers and pachydermia, not to mention vocal nodules and polyps. It is with some trepidation that we embark upon description of chronic laryngitis and chronic hyperplastic laryngitis. Vrabec and Davison (1980) resolve the problem by advocating the term 'chronic non-specific laryngitis' to include a variety of long-standing inflammatory changes (laryngitis) in the laryngeal mucosa. Then subdivisions can be apportioned to chronic laryngitis, chronic hyperplastic laryngitis and differentiations made between each and other conditions such as Reinke's oedema and various specific infections.

Chronic laryngitis

This form of laryngitis can follow an acute infection but more commonly becomes established slowly with the ciliated mucous membrane being replaced by squamous epithelium. Long-term vocal abuse is regarded as the most important cause by Ballantyne and Groves (1982) with infections of the teeth, tonsils and sinuses and related coughing also being major factors. Air pollution and very dry indoor atmosphere, such as in central heating, are probably also important causes. Dehydrated air dries out the mucous membrane and arrests the ciliary movement. This permits infective organisms to penetrate the mucosa and set up inflammation. Laryngitis is thus established. Allergic responses to certain drugs may be contributory. Nevertheless, atmospheric pollutants are a prime cause. Men suffering from chronic laryngitis working in the cement works in Buckinghamshire, England, were given voice therapy in a trial instigated by the laryngologist. In some cases the inflammation appeared to be slightly reduced and less discomfort was reported when speaking. The chronic laryngitis was not cured, however, nor was the attendant dysphonia.

The chief characteristics are viscid mucus, chronic inflammation and epithelial thickening. Vrabec and Davison (1980) reviewing the literature, quote the possible aetiology:

- Repeated acute bouts of laryngitis.
- Debilitated health.
- Irritations from smoking and chronic use of alcohol.
- Pollutants of dust and fumes.
- Dry atmosphere.
- Climatic extremes.
- Chronic mouth breathing (in children).
- Vocal abuse.

Aerosol corticosteroids, which are used to relieve bronchial asthma, are also recorded as giving rise to phonatory abnormalities following prolonged use (Watkin and Ewanowski, 1985).

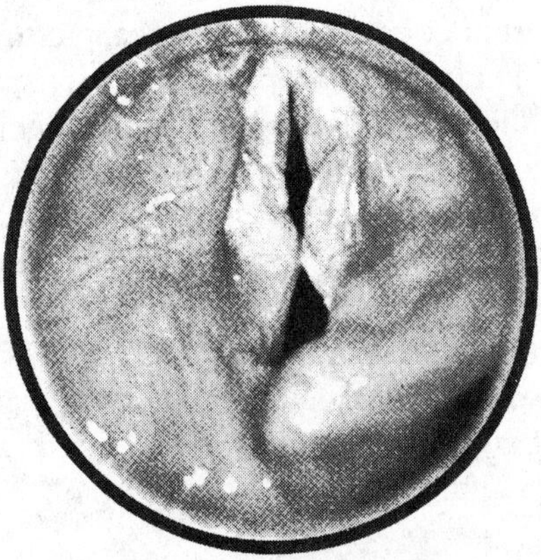

Figure 13.1. Chronic hypertrophic laryngitis.

In chronic laryngitis the vocal folds may be:

- Hyperaemic (pink or red according to the severity of the condition).
- Hypertrophic (thickened; possibly associated with thickening of other areas of the larynx).
- Oedematous (swollen and pale).

These symptoms are usually bilateral and symmetrical.

Treatment will consist of voice conservation and re-education, with removal of vocal tract irritants and the prescription of antibiotics when necessary.

Chronic hyperplastic laryngitis

Chronic hyperplastic laryngitis is characterised by a diffuse inflammatory process that extends over a wide area of the laryngeal mucosa (Kleinsasser, 1968). It is usually highly developed on the cords and eventually leads to epithelial hyperplasia, characterised by white raised patches on the vocal folds called leucoplakia.

The condition, unlike acute and chronic laryngitis, does not heal when infection or irritants are removed and it is a potentially pre-cancerous

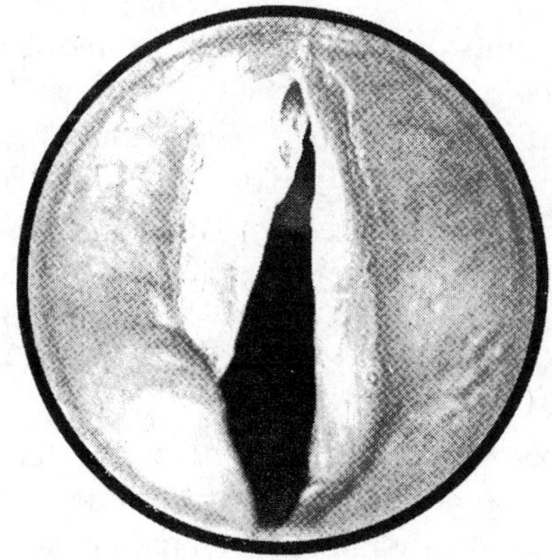

Figure 13.2. Leucoplakia (left vocal fold).

condition. Kleinsasser recommends stripping of the cords (decortication) and removal of the thickened epithelium since it arrests the disease and achieves voice improvement. It may also prevent malignancy developing. The new epithelium that forms after stripping of the vocal folds remains thin, smooth and non-inflamed for years afterwards in the majority of patients according to Vrabek and Davison (1980). On the other hand, Ballantyne and Groves (1982) report that recurrence is usual.

It is necessary to remove all possible irritants to the larynx including vocal abuse (Shaw and Friedmann, 1964). This develops as a result of the phonation difficulty and hoarseness which is secondary to inflammation. Most of these patients are or have been heavy smokers and they must be warned of the dangers of smoking and advised to stop. Air pollutants such as dust or fumes which may be inhaled regularly at work or in other situations should be avoided and masks worn.

Postoperatively voice rest is recommended but if the patient must talk the use of gentle normal voice is less harmful than whispering. Only when the vocal folds have fully healed and re-epithelialised, usually after 3–4 weeks, is speech therapy prescribed if necessary. It is remarkable how much voice improvement can be achieved in a short time if the patient is cooperative and carries out instructions for better voice production. In the cases we have treated the voice has improved but never recovered entirely normal quality, retaining a slight huskiness.

Hypertrophic posterior laryngitis

This is another term for pachydermia and interarytenoid pachydermia which was discussed in connection with contact ulcers and intubation granuloma (see Chapter 8). The condition shown on indirect laryngoscopy is a mass of grey tissue in the posterior commissure extending forward over the arytenoids and usually symmetrical. No conclusive aetiology has been decided but in the past the irritants of smoking, alcohol etc. were thought to be the chief factors. Delahunty and Ardran (1970) produced evidence of acid laryngeal and gastric reflux with oesophagitis occurring at night resulting in reflux pachydermia. Attention to diet, elevation of the head at night, and medication to reduce stomach acidity are recommended. Spicey and fried foods which cause 'heartburn' are especially to be avoided. Delahunty (1972) reported good results after 6–8 weeks on this regimen. Goldberg, Noyek and Pritzker (1978) describe a case of laryngeal 'granuloma' on two-thirds of one vocal cord attributed to gastro-oesophageal reflux which appeared to be identical with reflux pachydermia when histological structure was examined.

The speech therapist should not be daunted by a confusion of terms but if confronted with these conditions must consider the site, the histological report and judge from the dysphonia presented what therapeutic strategies, if any, may be effective.

Tuberculosis of the larynx (phthisis laryngea)

This is a secondary complication of pulmonary infection. Tuberculosis is highly infectious especially among children but it is almost unknown in affluent societies due to improved health and living conditions and treatment with antibiotics. Travis, Hybels and Newman (1976) reported 13 cases of tuberculosis over a period of 15 years. They warn that initial infiltration of the laryngeal mucosa can be misleading and mistaken for chronic laryngitis. In recent years there has been a resurgence of respiratory tuberculosis in the elderly over 65 years and we have had two patients referred with laryngitis attributed initially to vocal misuse. Further tests led to correct diagnosis.

An early report of the initial symptoms and progress of this laryngeal disease is of interest since in areas of the world deficient in medical services untreated phthisis laryngea is not a rarity. Smurthwaite (1919) noted that in the early stages of infiltration an adductor paralysis (myopathic paresis) may appear before any positive signs of inflammation are visible and that asthenic voice may be incorrectly diagnosed as an 'hysterical' disorder with bowing of the vocal folds (see p. 172). If infection progresses, ulceration of the fold can develop but antituberculosis chemotherapy results in a rapid improvement in the laryngeal condition (Ballantyne and Groves, 1982).

Complete vocal rest is essential and this must be strictly observed. Scarring and irregularity of the folds may occur during healing with resultant impairment of the voice dependent upon the degree and site of the damage. Thickening of the mucous membrane cover of the vocal folds may remain along their length or in the arytenoid region. The voice is characteristically deep and husky with a rather hollow tone (Turner, 1952).

Case notes

1. A female patient of 60 years was referred for speech therapy after treatment and cure of tuberculosis. She had developed considerable anxiety over her health and economic situation besides tension in trying to obtain a louder voice. She responded well to relaxation, breathing exercises, hearing training and raising the vocal pitch.

2. Another patient had recovered from tuberculosis some years previously and had not been anxious about her impaired voice until domestic difficulties produced a functional aphonia. Vocal exercises and discussion of her difficulties brought her voice back. She said it improved in clarity and strength during treatment and was better than it had been since her tubercular illness. In neither of these cases did the huskiness and 'veiling' of the voice disappear completely, since permanent changes and thickening of the vocal membrane had taken place.

Syphilitic inflammation and ulceration of the larynx

Syphilis of the larynx may occur as a congenital infection or as an acquired condition, secondary to primary infection. The disease may produce acute inflammation of the larynx with similar involvement of the pharynx and in advanced stages of the disease, ulceration occurs. The symptom of hoarseness is a prominent feature of syphilitic laryngitis, the voice is strong with a distinctive rough quality and generally causes no discomfort (Turner, 1952). In the early stages the intractable laryngitis and pharyngitis can be easily mistaken for a simple infection. In very advanced stages the formation of syphilomata may resemble cancerous tumours. Ballantyne and Groves (1982) note that syphilis can mimic all other laryngeal diseases and for this reason may cause diagnostic problems. Accurate diagnosis depends upon a positive Wassermann reaction being obtained from a test of the patient's serum, but in a small proportion of cases in the tertiary stages of syphilis a positive reaction is not obtained. Fortunately this is no longer encountered in Western countries.

Scarring of the vocal folds following ulceration is generally severe and may cause stenosis of the larynx and breathing difficulty (dyspnoea). Treatment must obviously be directed to the cure of the disease, and only after this has been achieved and the laryngeal symptoms alleviated can any attempt at improvement of the voice be undertaken. The patient may now be helped to make the best use of his voice. Prognosis is unfavourable unless cicatricial tissue is minimal or can be removed surgically, so that the vocal folds present even edges in adduction.

Fungal infection

Although rare, fungal infections of the larynx occur and result in hoarseness and laryngitis which may be indistinguishable initially from other causes of laryngitis. Isolated laryngeal candidiasis gives rise to intense pain in the oropharynx and if allowed to progress will cause breathing difficulties or systemic fungal disease. Patients who already have significant underlying disease and who are receving broad-spectrum antimicrobial therapy are particularly vulnerable to candidiasis. If hoarseness and dysphagia occur in this patient group, laryngeal candidiasis should be considered as the cause (Tashjian and Peacock, 1984). Granulomata of the vocal fold may also occur secondary to fungal infection. Although also rare these have been recorded in individuals dealing with plant matter such as sphagnum moss (Agger and Seager, 1985).

Biopsy and cultures of the affected area will indicate appropriate treatment. Hoarseness may remain if the infection has been extensive. Speech therapy is indicated in order to correct any patterns of vocal abuse which might have made the larynx particularly vulnerable to fungal infection when the spores were initially inhaled.

Laryngeal rheumatoid arthritis

Laryngeal arthritis involving the cricoarytenoid joints is another condition which causes aphonia or dysphonia according to the degree of immobility imposed upon the folds. Traditionally, it has been considered a comparatively rare condition with various studies suggesting clinical signs of arthritis on laryngoscopy being found in 17–33% of patients with rheumatoid arthritis. However, more recent studies using low voltage radiotherapy reveal that 45% of patients with rheumatoid arthritis have erosions and destructive changes of the cricoarytenoid joints (Jurik, Pedersen and Norgard, 1985). In the early stages of invasion of the larynx by the disease there is acute local inflammaton and extraordinary pain upon phonation. Great difficulty is experienced in moving the folds and there is pronounced hoarseness. Laryngeal stridor may also occur.

The principal treatment is medical, directed at alleviating the arthritic disease which can be widespread throughout the individual's system before the larynx becomes involved. Steroid injection into the cricoarytenoid joint to relieve acute inflammation may be prescribed and have good results (Habib, 1977). Local short-wave diathermy may also be helpful. Aspirin reduces pain and inflammation, also gentle massage with a soothing embrocation (Aronson, 1980). Severity of symptoms varies, a 'flare up' of symptoms can occur, especially with a respiratory infection, and subside spontaneously (Wolman, Dorke and Young, 1965).

During the acute stage there is red swelling over the arytenoids but the vocal folds may appear normal or only slightly oedematous. The throat feels tight and painful in swallowing, coughing and speaking and there is acute pain on palpation of the arytenoids, with pain radiating up to the ear (Montgomery, 1963). The voice is hoarse due to inflammation and swelling causing sluggishness in adduction and abduction of the vocal folds and should be rested.

When the acute stage of the arthritis subsides and normal movement is again possible voice therapy may be helpful in some cases. The importance of gentle onset of phonation and adequate breath support should be emphasised. Over-exertion should be avoided as this can aggravate any remaining inflammation but discomfort monitors speech output.

Williams, Farquharson and Anthony (1975) describe a patient with generalised rheumatoid arthritis who developed hoarseness but whose larynx was pronounced normal when examined by indirect and direct laryngoscopy.

A fibreoptic laryngoscopic examination with stroboscopic flash showed that the larynx was injected, although minimally. The folds moved abnormally in phonation with unequal and non-synchronous vibrations. This ruled out the suspected psychogenic factor and indicated speech therapy might be helpful.

When rheumatic laryngeal arthritis resolves before occurrence of ankylosis of the joints, the folds sometimes remain sluggish in movement and the voice is hoarse or breathy. This condition can be improved by voice therapy.

> Case note
> A female patient's voice was severely hoarse following a brief attack of arthritis of the larynx which rendered adduction of the folds difficult; she quickly developed a normal voice through the practice of voice exercises. Movement of the folds was stimulated by attempting their rapid adduction and abduction in quick succession. The patient was instructed to drink a gulp of cold air to obtain full abduction and then to shout a vowel to promote full adduction. Relaxation and diaphragmatic breathing exercises were necessary preliminaries.

Arthritic ankylosis

In a small proportion of cases, however, total fusion of the cricoarytenoid joint (ankylosis) takes place, in which case there is no chance of recovery. The position of the vocal fold in unilateral ankylosis of the arytenoid joint resembles that of the abductor paralysis of the recurrent laryngeal nerve with the fold fixed in the paramedian position (see p. 298). Rarely it is held in a position of extreme abduction by the fibrous bands which form through arthritic changes in the arytenoid joint. Should compensation by the opposite fold be impossible, a stronger voice may be obtained by a 'reverse King operation' and the fold transplanted to the median position. The most common form of laryngeal arthritis is, however, bilateral with both folds immobilised in the mid-line. If there is difficulty in breathing a tracheotomy will be performed. If the condition is not alleviated by medication and both folds remain permanently fixed in the mid-line, a Woodman operation can be performed (Woodman, 1946) or a Langnickel (1976) (see p. 301). It is doubtful whether speech therapy will help the voice postoperatively since the fold not operated upon remains immobile. Operation may not be feasible if the patient is aged and fragile. A tracheotomy and use of a 'speaking valve' tracheostomy tube will be the preferred choice of the medical adviser in such cases.

Laryngeal Trauma and Stenosis

Direct injuries

Direct trauma to the larynx can be classified into compression injuries, such as those caused by a blow to the larynx or attempted strangulation, and penetration injuries which can be caused by stabbing and gunshot wounds.

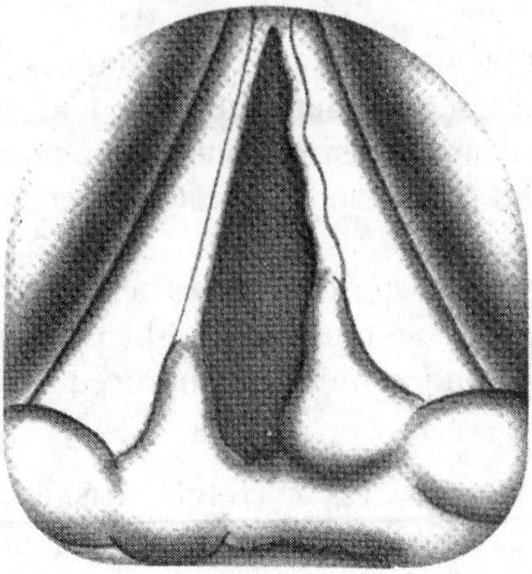

Figure 13.3. Dislocated right arytenoid cartilage.

They may be extralaryngeal, intralaryngeal and involve fractures of the laryngeal cartilages, particularly the thyroid. Fracture of the cricoid cartilage is usually fatal because of subglottic swelling (Ballantyne and Groves, 1982). Submucosal haemorrhage may occur in any part of the larynx with stenosis and infection also being major problems. In addition to respiratory and voice problems dysphagia and pain have to be dealt with.

Blunt trauma tends to result in more severe injury to the airway and voice than penetrating trauma probably because of the greater force needed to damage a larynx by a blow or compression (Cantrell, 1983). A penetrating laryngeal wound which is clean and localised may heal without damage to the vocal folds but it is also much more likely to be fatal.

Blows to the larynx are most commonly due to road traffic accidents (RTAs) when the body of the driver is thrown forward during sudden braking or on impact with another vehicle. The larynx is usually protected by the overhanging jaw and the forward thrust of the chest but may be exposed if the chin is forced up. Wearing of seat belts does not always provide protection but saves life and, paradoxically, increases the number of victims with laryngeal trauma (Cohn and Peppard, 1979). Severe laryngeal fractures occur when the larynx hits the steering wheel and the vocal folds may be torn and the arytenoids dislocated (Harris and Ainsworth, 1965). The adjacency of the recurrent laryngeal nerve to the cricothyroid articulation renders damage to the nerve and vocal fold paralysis likely. In cases of extreme damage to the larynx with resulting severe stenosis of the airway, laryngectomy may be necessary eventually.

The immediate need is to attend to the respiratory condition of the patient and obstruction of the laryngeal airway. A tracheotomy will be necessary if damage is extensive and emergency treatment vital. There may be other injuries, head and limb injuries engaging the services of orthopaedic and neurological specialists. Under such stress, treatment of the fractured and contused larynx may be postponed but it is vital that a laryngologist be called in to assess the damage to the larynx and take immediate steps to realign fractured parts, dislodged arytenoids and torn muscles. Delay in stabilising the cartilage and prevention of webbing can jeopardise the end result (Duff, 1968). Endolaryngeal stenting should be carried out as soon as practicable.

The state of the voice once healing has taken place depends on the condition of the larynx and the laryngological description. Stroboscopic examinaton will help in the detection of the extent of scar tissue. EMG evaluation is also useful in some cases (Hirano, Shigejiro and Terasawa, 1985). The recurrent laryngeal nerve may recover from bruising and compression in time as may the mobility of the cricoarytenoid and thyroarytenoid msucles. This may take many months and the patient remain hoarse with easy fatiguability of the voice and considerable laryngeal discomfort as would follow any injury to muscular tissue, ligaments and synovial joints. There is evidence to suggest that initial vocal fold paralysis indicates a poorer eventual voice and airway result than where the folds are mobile in the early stages of recovery (Leopold, 1983).

Speech therapy may prove helpful but post-traumatic shock must be taken into account with its attendant anxiety and depression. In the case of injury to others guilt may exacerbate the psychogenic disturbance.

In road accident injuries it is well to remember that litigation and claims for damage are often in progress. In this case, if the patient can claim for loss of voice and damage to career prospects, this will be taken into account in settlement of compensation. Full potential recovery may be deliberately delayed until compensation has been settled.

> Case note
> A young man whom we treated suffered from intermittent stammer and dysphonia following an RTA in addition to whip-lash injuries. The voice and speech disorder vanished as soon as the litigation and claims for compensation were settled and the patient failed to attend for further treatment.

In the case of associated head injury the speech therapist will also consider the possibility of aphasia, dysarthria and dyspraxia militating against communicative effectiveness.

Laryngeal burns

Burns to the laryngeal mucosal lining may be both thermal and chemical as with the inhalation of scorching air and fumes in a fire. Inhalation of caustic fumes from acids and swallowing of acids causes laryngeal burns though most damage may occur in the oral cavity, pharynx and lungs on account of the natural protective valvular mechanism of the larynx. Cohn and Peppard (1979) review the possible sites of damage and the medical treatment for surface burns. Sloughing of the mucosal lining of the larynx and adhesion in healing, forming webs, may develop but this is rare with careful medical treatment. Oedema can cause difficulty in breathing and intense irritation causes coughing. The voice will be hoarse until healing is complete and complete vocal rest must be observed during this period. Shock from the accident may result in psychogenic voice problems rather than mechanical dysphonia.

Laryngeal abrasion

Endotracheal damage to the laryngeal mucosa and resulting granuloma are well recognised and have been described already in connection with contact ulcers. Intubation injuries are frequent in patients who have required prolonged care in an intensive care unit. Any procedure which necessitates the prolonged presence of a tube between the vocal folds renders the patient liable to laryngeal trauma. Kirchner (1983) explains that the inspiratory activity of the posterior cricoarytenoid abolishes the phasic respiratory movement. The longer this lasts the more difficult it is to recover abductor action.

Damage may also occur during rough intubation and when an excessively large tube has been used. Arytenoids can be dislocated in this way. The intubation damage is not necessarily readily apparent on extubation. In some cases it is not until approximately 3 days later that inflammation and oedema of the arytenoids can be seen in association with limitation of vocal fold movement and incomplete adduction of the posterior portion (Whited, 1985).

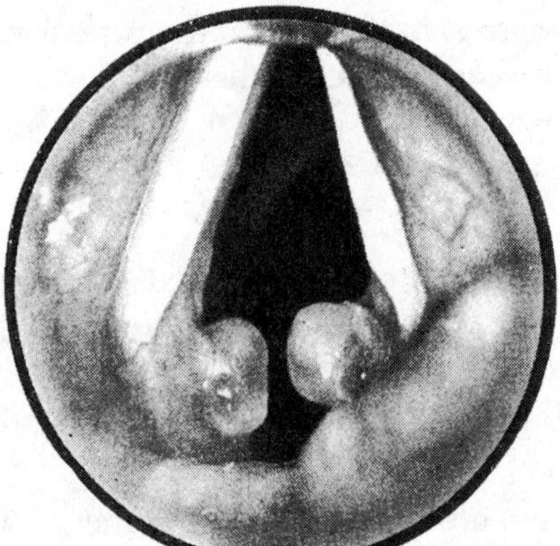

Figure 13.4. Intubation granulomat

Intubation can also cause superficial abrasions and granulomatous formation in the area of the arytenoids; this causes hoarseness and, sometimes, dyspnoea. In cases of associated granulomatous formation, which might impair the airway and the voice, carbon dioxide laser can be used for its removal without damaging the underlying mucosa (Gussak, Jurovich and Laterman, 1986).

The speech therapist may be asked to see these patients if the dysphonia does not improve. It is important to be aware that vocal abuse or a psychogenic overlay may contribute to prolongation of the voice disorder.

Neoplasm

Laryngeal neoplasms may be benign or malignant. This section is confined to benign growths. Malignant tumours are discussed in relation to laryngectomy (see Chapter 17).

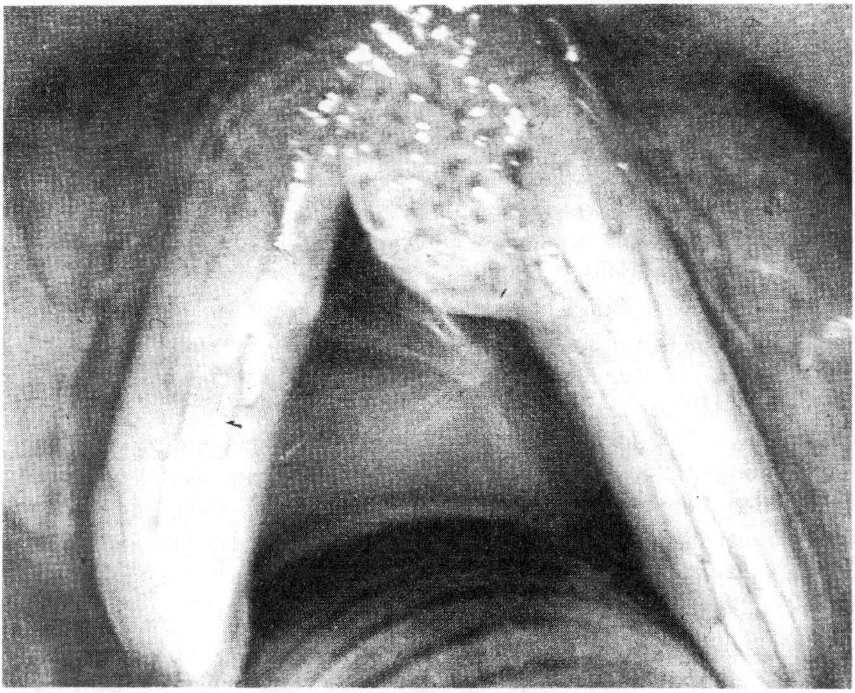

Figure 13.5. Early papillomatosis involving the right vocal fold and anterior commisure.

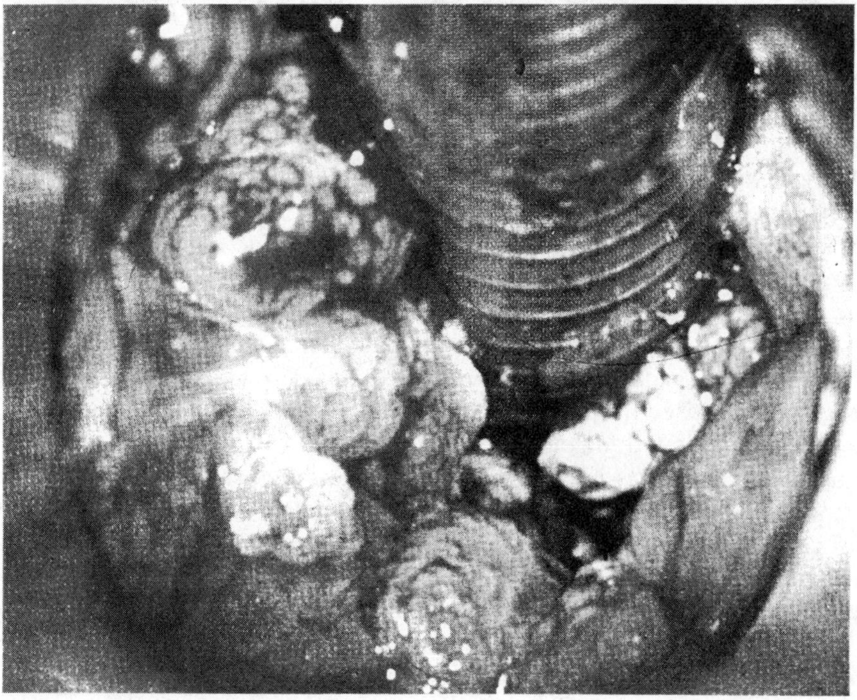

Figure 13.6. Advanced papillomatosis.

Papilloma

Papillomata are benign neoplasms consisting of a vascular connective tissue core, which may have several subdivisions, covered by stratified squamous epithelium. They are sessile or pedunculated and are attached to the mucous membrane of the respiratory tract. They occur mainly on the vocal folds but can invade the trachea (Dekelbaum, 1965).

Papillomata are pinkish red in appearance and translucent; they are easily recognisable since multiple lesions form in clusters like warts. Indeed, they have long been attributed, like warts, to virus infection (Bone, Feren and Nahum, 1976). The specific virus, however, has not been identified.

Juvenile papillomata are the most common laryngeal tumours in children (Robbins and Howard, 1983) and occur most frequently between the ages of 4 and 6 years (Kleinsasser, 1968). Multiple laryngeal papillomatosis is more likely to occur in the child than in the adult. The condition usually involves the vocal folds and the ventricular bands but may extend to the trachea, bronchi and epiglottis. They rarely make their first appearance later in childhood. In some children there is recession at 11 years of age (Senturia and Wilson, 1968) but regression may be delayed until puberty (Robbins and Howard, 1983). A distinction is made between juvenile and adult papilloma by some authorities, not so much by reason of their histological structure but by their clinical performance (Bone, 1986). Single papilloma occurs more frequently in adults and is rare in children.

Varying degrees of hoarseness are present whenever the vocal folds are involved. In many cases there is also a pattern of vocal abuse which arises as the child attempts to increase the loudness and carrying power of the affected voice.

Despite the assumption of viral infection, there is a hormonal influence. Holinger, Schild and Mauriz (1968) drew attention to the fact that papilloma occurs more frequently in the male than female adults although there is an equal distribution before puberty. Recession often occurs at puberty and during pregnancy but the disease recurs later. Cook *et al.* (1973) reported papilloma incidence to be in the ratio of two males to one female. Recurrence may occur at the menopause.

The depressing feature of papillomatosis is that despite the several forms of treatment practised there is rarely a cure and recurrences occur at frequent intervals in childhood and often after long intervals of remission, in adulthood. It must be regarded as a potentially lifelong condition (Brondbo, Alberti and Crowson, 1983). The efficacy of treatment can only be judged by immediate dispersal of papilloma, but long-term follow-up is required in assessment of real curative therapy. Some treatments seem to achieve longer intervals of remission than others.

Treatment of papilloma

Numerous treatment procedures have been tried in an attempt to remove the papillomata efficiently while, if possible, reducing the recurrence rate.

Methods include carbon dioxide laser surgery, ultrasound, cryosurgery, hormones, steroids, antibiotics, chemotherapy, forceps removal, cauterisation and vaccine (Robbins and Howard, 1983; Abramson, Steinberg and Winkler, 1987).

In children the primary concern is to preserve the respiratory airway from obstruction (Holinger, 1959). Holinger, Schild and Mauritz (1968) advocated forceps removal and no tracheotomy which presents problems with wearing the cannula and renders the child susceptible to respiratory infections and bronchitis. On the other hand, persistent recurrences cause anxiety concerning sudden onset of dyspnoea. Forceps removal also endangers the surfaces of the vocal folds and adjacent laryngeal structures. The development of microendoscopy has largely reduced the possibility of damage and greatly improved the accuracy of the surgeon's scalpel. Laser surgery (Andrews and Moss, 1974) has been found to be more successful than excision in that it provides longer periods of remission (Brondbo, Alberti and Crowson, 1983). There are some hazards attendant upon laser surgery since it requires great expertise to achieve absolute precision of the burn and quickly. However, there is no bleeding and immediate coagulation occurs so that logopaedic intervention can start a day after surgery (Sorensen, 1982). Laser surgery is the preferred treatment for adults but in childhood excision may be preferred depending on the laryngologist's assessment.

Papilloma does not become malignant at any stage although this was though possible at one time. It was found, however, that irradiation of the larynx to disperse the growths of childhood led to later malignant degeneration (Rabbett, 1965; Vermeuling, 1966) or to damage of the laryngeal cartilages. Cauterisation is rejected on the grounds that it can cause scarring and stricture of the vocal folds (Abramson *et al.*, 1987).

Whatever surgical procedure is used it is likely that it will be necessary to perform it on many occasions because of the frequent recurrence of the papillomatosis. In very rare cases of great severity in which obstruction of the airway is a major problem, laryngectomy may be necessary. Robbins and Howard (1983) record that out of 63 patients over 24 years of age with papillomatosis, two patients were treated with laryngectomy because of severe disease.

Drug therapy

The most encouraging development in treatment of papillomatosis of the larynx is the administration of leucocyte interferon therapy. Haghund, Lundquist and Cantrell (1981) noted regression of plantar warts in a woman being treated with interferon for cervical cancer and carried out a study of seven patients suffering from laryngeal papilloma. A further study was carried out by Bornholt (1983) which confirmed temporary regression of the growths. As Bone (1986) points out in his concise and valuable review of papillomatosis, the palliative effect of interferon appears only to work while the substance is being administered. This and the fact that interferon is exceedingly expensive means that the treatment cannot be generally applied as yet. Much ongoing research is necessary. Interferon was discovered by Alick Isaacs and Jean Lindenmann in Oxford in 1957. It interferes with virus infection by stimulating the natural biological manufacture of antigens in the cells of vertebrate animals. It is known to be effective against many viral diseases including hepatitis B, and it arrests growth of malignant cells. It does not have the toxic side effects of chemotherapy.

Voice therapy

Hoarseness is the first sign of papilloma recurrence and may remain a problem after successful removal and arrest of neoplasm. The efficacy of remediation procedures depends upon the existing surface structure of the vocal folds and the correction of misuse arising out of the recurring periods of laryngeal obstruction and hoarseness.

The efficacy of voice therapy for children while suffering from papilloma of the larynx is not generally recognised. Boone (1971) stated categorically that such cases were not candidates for therapy for hyperfunction, a view which is omitted, however, in the second edition (1977). Cooper (1971) on the other hand is of the opinion that vocal rehabilitation can reduce or even eliminate papillomata. In a study of eight cases of biopsied papilloma, four out of five who cooperated in treatment improved. Three who refused treatment made no improvement. Vocal abuse may well act as an irritant and help the spread of papilloma. Rabbett (1965) has drawn attention to the need to cure infections and to restore the larynx to health quickly as this renders the mucosa less susceptible to invasion by virus.

Taking into account the resemblance papilloma bears to warts, which are known to be contagious and prone to spread from one site to another, it seems feasible that hyperkinetic laryngitis and vocal abuse may well promote spread of papilloma in the larynx. Furthermore, since warts may be charmed away by suggestion, the belief that a speech therapist is going to cure the papilloma may be a potent factor in their disappearance. Who knows?

Case histories

1. A case confirming Cooper's view that speech therapy can reduce or even eliminate papillomata in children was encountered by Greene in Auckland. She was asked to examine a boy aged 9 years who had become hoarse and papillomata had been diagnosed. He was under periodic review by the laryngologist and dreaded his visits and feared an operation. The speech therapist in charge wanted to know whether voice therapy was advisable as his voice production was very strained. She had told mother and child of the visiting therapist from England and both were much impressed by the honour, especially the child who thought she must have Royal connections. Assuming an authoritative and omniscient role, the need for quiet speech and no shouting was emphasised. The importance of relaxation and central breathing was made clear. A happy and much less anxious boy and

mother departed home. Two weeks later the speech therapist telephoned Greene in Dunedin to say that the laryngologist had seen the boy again and had been amazed to find that the clusters of papillomata were reduced in number and much smaller. He sent a message to the effect that the Queen's representative must be congratulated upon the 'magic' she had worked.

2. Mr F., 67 years, had had laryngeal papillomatosis for many years and had undergone various procedures for removal of the papillomata. Eventually he had undergone successful laser surgery which left only a small 'tag' of papillomatous tissue in the anterior commissure. The laryngologist referred Mr F. for voice therapy in order to improve vocal efficiency and the patient's awareness of vocal hygiene and conservation.

Mr F. was a cheerful and sociable person who talked incessantly in the clinic. His wife died a year earlier; it had been a very happy marriage and he missed her company acutely. There were no children and he lived alone with his dog. His philosophy was that no-one liked a miserable person and so he made great efforts to be cheerful and friendly. He had established a circle of acquaintances at his local pub; acted as a good neighbour to a number of people he regarded as less fortunate than himself; and went for long walks with his dog.

His voice was inappropriately high pitched and its production was obviously effortful with visible tension of the external laryngeal muscles and a markedly raised larynx. Breathing was clavicular with noisy intake. Although listeners supposed that phonation must cause discomfort he was adamant that this was not so.

Mr F. was not particularly concerned over his dysphonia but was prepared to cooperate with therapy because his surgeon, in whom he had great faith, had thought the referral was necessary. The therapeutic approach was based on helping the patient to have insight into his present method of voice production and why this might exacerbate laryngeal dysfunction, in addition to outlining ways of conserving the voice. The problem of the raised fundamental frequency was tackled early in treatment with a combination of relaxation and a firm, but gentle, cough to establish the natural pitch. The effects of grieving were gradually discussed when the occasion was appropriate. The responses of the vocal tract when the individual is under some stress but remaining stoical were also explained in relation to phonation.

Mr F. responded positively to treatment although he found it difficult to talk less when he had the opportunity to be with other people. Pitch became more appropriate and phonation was less effortful. Initially, he attended for weekly treatments which were reduced over a period of 9 months as the voice improved. At this time he was discharged when the laryngologist pronounced satisfaction with the larynx. There was no sign of inflammation and the voice was satisfactory although it remained breathy.

Laryngeal Cysts

Cysts of the vocal folds occur rather rarely but are especially common on the false vocal folds in persons over 50–60 years of age (Kleinsasser, 1968). Almost all are retention cysts and develop secondary to degenerative process in the ductal system of the mucous gland network. They may be multifocal and bilateral. They may hang from the inlet to the ventricle and obstruct the airway or may be situated deep within the false vocal fold, but are not painful. Surgical treatment presents no problems; the cysts are opened up, drained and the mucosa sutured thereafter. Lymphatic cysts also occur on the free edges of the aryepiglottic folds and epiglottis but generally are so small that they need not be removed.

Although the removal of cysts on the false folds and ventricle should not disturb the voice cases of dysphonia are sometimes referred for speech therapy postoperatively.

Case notes

1. A woman of 70 years developed a severely deep and broken voice after removal of a cyst situated on the false vocal fold. Although the larynx presented an entirely normal appearance it was some months before vocal rehabilitation restored a normal voice. In this case there were no obvious anxiety symptoms and, in fact, the patient, who was very active and young for her age, was impatient with therapy but her husband did not like her changed voice, which had been very pleasing and musical.
2. A woman of 45 years developed, besides hoarseness, an anxiety state after the fright of a sudden enlargement of a cyst which obstructed breathing. She began to have difficulty with breathing on exertion after discharge from hospital, and then an inspiratory stridor developed in speech. She was given relaxation and diaphragmatic breathing exercises and was treated as a case of anxiety state and hyperventilation since there was no impairment of the vocal fold movements. Delay in being admitted into hospital for surgery and the subsequent delay in obtaining speech therapy had upset her.

Chapter 14
Neurological Dysphonias

Dysarthria is a disorder of articulation due to neurological lesions causing paralysis and paresis of the muscles of articulation and deglutition. Dysarthria affects articulatory, phonatory, respiratory and phonological aspects of speech. Peacher (1949) suggested the term 'dysarthrophonia' to denote neurological dysphonia accompanied by dysarthria in order to distinguish this condition from nuclear and peripheral lesions in the lower motor neurone pathway. These dysphonias do not include dysarthria but are confined to palatal paralysis and laryngeal paralysis. It can, however, be argued that hypernasality and devoicing of phonemes is an articulatory disorder and therefore dysarthric. Such hair splitting is beyond our scope. It explains why 'dysarthrophonia' has never been generally accepted and the cover term 'neurological dysphonia' is preferred.

The dysarthrias are now most commonly described in accordance with the Mayo Clinic classification based upon the research of Darley, Aronson and Brown (1975). Their classification given below provides broad guidelines in the tangled web of sensory and motor pathways which constitute the nervous system (Sherrington, 1947). We wish to emphasise that no part of the nervous system is self-contained nor able to function independently of any other. Discrete symptoms do not actually exist but may predominate in a complex of

Table 14.1 Classification of neurological dysphonia

Site of lesion	*Myopathy*	*Neurological condition*
1. Upper motor neurone	Spasticity	Pseudobulbar palsy
2. Lower motor neurone	Flaccidity	Bulbar palsy Laryngeal palsy
3. Cerebellum	Ataxia	Cerebellar ataxia
4. Extrapyramidal (striatal)	Hypokinetic Hyperkinetic – quick Hyperkinetic – slow	Parkinsonism Chorea Athetosis (Dyskinesia) (Dystonia)
5. Mixed lesions	Mixed symptoms	MND, MS

After Darley, Aronson and Brown (1975).

dysfunctions. The site of lesions also may be obscure as in the case of tremor or dyspraxia.

Assessment of neurological dysphonia needs to be detailed and encompass intellectual, emotional, articulatory, phonatory and respiratory functions. On the basis of what is lost, what is impaired but can be improved, and what remains intact, therapy has to be pragmatic. It aims at restoring and retaining intelligible communication often in cases where damage appears irreparable and disease is tragically progressive. (See Table 14.1 for a classification of neurological dysphonia.)

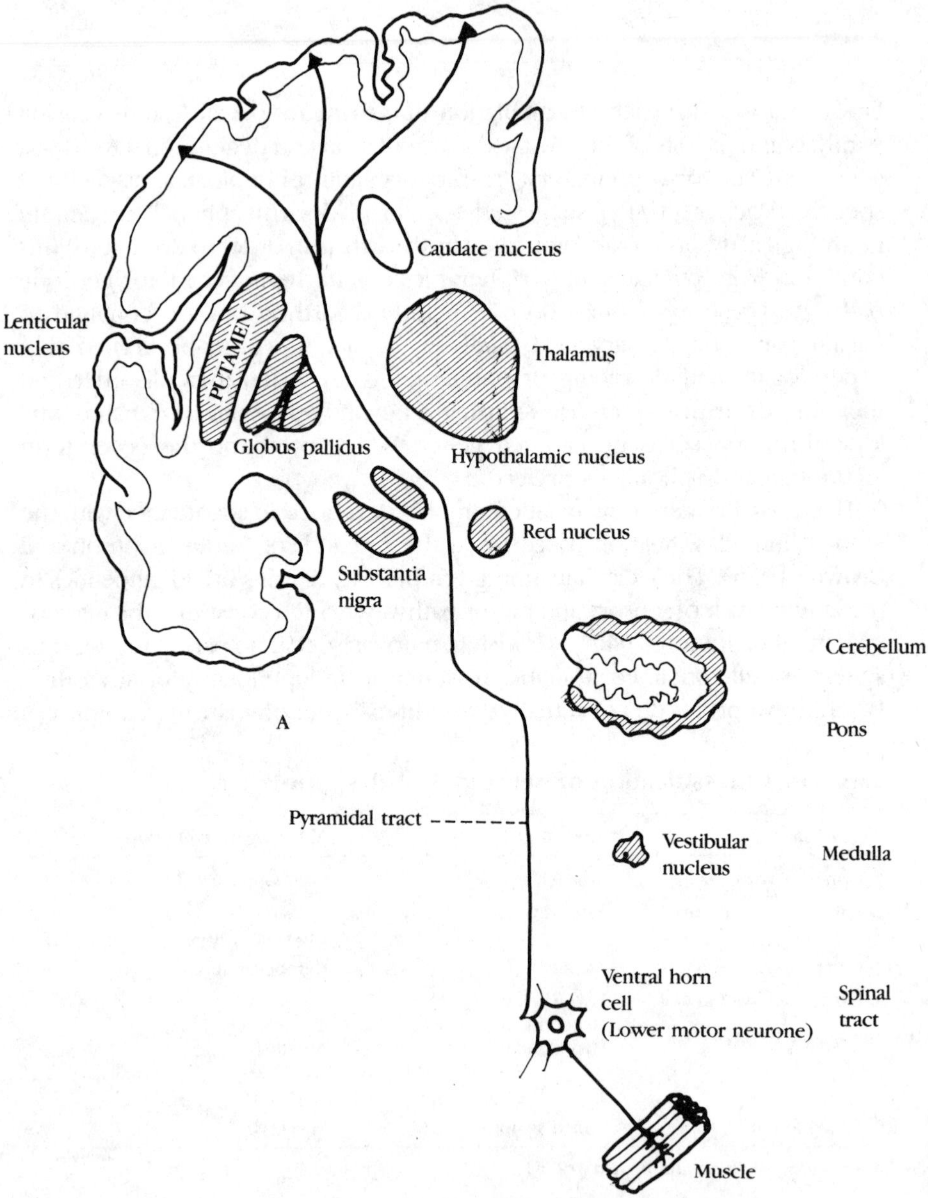

Figure 14.1. Upper motor neurone pathway (corticospinal tract).

Lesions of the Upper Motor Neurone (Pyramidal) System

The upper motor neurone (UMN) pathways arise in the motor cortex (precentral gyrus) of both cerebral hemispheres and form the corticobulbar and corticospinal tracts. This is the pyramidal system, also called the 'direct activation' tract.

Some fibres of the pyramidal system, the direct pathway, remain on the same side of the body throughout their route, synapsing with the cranial nerve nuclei and, subsequently, with the lower motor neurones without interruption. The fibres of the indirect pyramidal tract decussate (cross-over) and change sides at the bulbar level then join the fibres of the direct pathway at the nuclear synapse. The conjoined fibres descending from the cranial nuclei form the lower motor neurone pathway.

The indirect neurones of the pyramidal tract have multiple off-shoots and synapses with the basal ganglia and reticular formation of the brainstem. They appear to contribute to temporospatial orientation while the direct system is related to skilled discrete movement. The upper motor neurones do not govern isolated muscles, but groups of muscles. The frontobulbar portions of the pyramidal tracts connect with the nuclei of the ninth to twelfth cranial nerves (besides of course the first to eighth), thus controlling articulation, phonation and respiration.

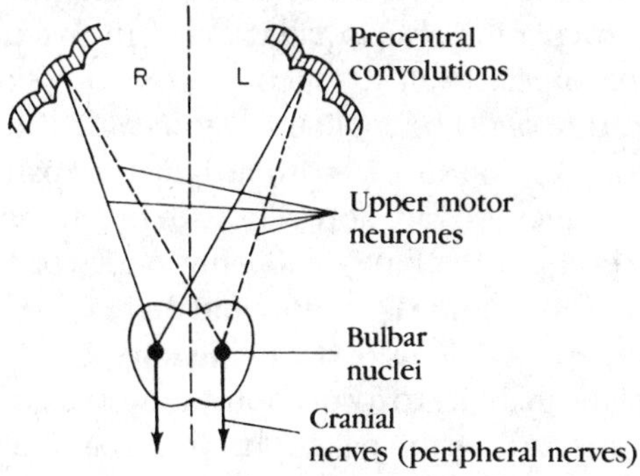

Figure 14.2. Double connection, from both hemispheres, of upper motor neurones with bulbar nuclei.

Causes of UMN lesions include multiple cerebrovascular accidents (CVAs), cerebral trauma, cerebral tumours and multiple sclerosis. Affected musculature is hypertonic (spastic) with associated weakness. Movements are slow and are reduced in range. In pseudobulbar palsy these effects are apparent in the tongue, face, larynx and palatopharyngeal sphincter with the result that, in addition to speech production difficulties, the face may be expressionless. Swallowing is always affected. There is emotional lability, due to the lack of cortical inhibition of laughing and crying which results in emotional outbursts or excessive reactions which are not indicative of the true emotional state.

This lack of control does result in very real distress in the individual, however, on account of being aware of its unsuitability.

Pseudobulbar (spastic) dysphonia

It is important to stress that the spastic dysphonia associated with pseudobulbar palsy has to be distinguished from psychogenic spastic dysphonia and spasmodic adductor dysphonia (also referred to as spastic dysphonia) which are described elsewhere.

Due to the bulbar nuclei receiving innervation from both hemispheres, lesions of the UMN pathway must be bilateral in order to produce vocal fold paralyses. A unilateral UMN lesion produces a spastic hemiplegia which affects the contralateral side. Impairment of the bulbar sited cranial nerves is not severe. Although there may be facial and lingual weakness on the affected side, with the further complication of aphasia in the case of a left cortical lesion, there is no unilateral vocal fold paralysis.

The bilateral lesions resulting in pseudobulbar dysarthria cause severe speech problems. Excessive effort is used in an attempt to counteract the resistance of the hypertonic speech musculature. Articulation is slow and laboured. Phonation has a distinctive 'strained-strangled' quality (Darley, Aronson and Brown, 1975) as air is forced between the hyperadducted vocal folds. Pitch is monotonous (monopitch) and low, and the voice may be overloud and lack volume variation.

Although there may be reflex elevation of the soft palate and symmetrical elevation on articulation of an isolated vowel, the excursion of the velum to the posterior pharyngeal wall is incomplete and slow. Hypernasality is a prominent feature of pseudobulbar palsy because the palate moves too slowly and inefficiently to coordinate with articulatory patterns.

Respiratory difficulties are apparent with breathing often out of phase with phonation (reverse breathing) and only one word, or short phase, being uttered at a time. Breathing is shallow and there is a decrease in airflow rate. To some extent these problems of breathing for speech arise as a result of loss of air because of the inability to form appropriate and coordinated closures in the larynx, oral cavity and at the palatopharyngeal sphincter. Similarly, maximum phonation time is greatly reduced from normal due to the inability to coordinate diaphragmatic and intercostal mechanism with closure of the laryngeal valve. Normal prosodic features are absent and in combination with severely distorted articulation, speech becomes unintelligible.

Lesions of the Lower Motor Neurone System

The fibres of the lower motor neurone (LMN) constitute the final common path travelling from the cell bodies in the bulbar medulla and anterior horns of the spinal cord to the muscles. This tract, the motor unit, consists of the motor neurone cell bodies, axons, the myoneural junction and the muscle fibres. A lesion occurring at any point on this pathway results in the loss of voluntary, automatic and reflex movement. Lesions may be bilateral if a lesion in the medulla affects both nuclei, or they may be unilateral.

Causes of LMN lesions include cerebrovascular accident (CVA), viral infections, tumours, trauma, toxic chemicals, poliomyelitis and myasthenia gravis, all of which affect various parts of the motor unit. Lesions may involve individual cranial nerves, and therefore individual muscles, or be extensive with widespread dysarthric symptoms.

Myasthenia gravis

Myasthenia gravis is a disease resulting in generalised muscular flaccidity due to a lack of the neurotransmitter acetylcholine at the myoneural junction. This deficiency prevents the conduction of neuromuscular contraction impulses. General bodily weakness and extreme fatigue occur on any effort and the palatopharyngeal and laryngeal valves may be affected early: hypernasality and asthenic voice are frequently the first diagnostic symptoms. Reversal of the condition can be obtained by regular injections of neostigmine compounds or by thymectomy in severe conditions. It is essential for the patient to avoid exertion and to rest in order to conserve energy. Voice therapy is therefore contra-indicated as in health the voice is normal.

Bulbar palsy dysphonia

Lesions in the bulb produce a flaccid paralysis with reduced muscle tone (hypotonia). There is atrophy (muscle wasting) and fasciculation (twitching). If a lesion occurs at a point where sensory fibres are associated with the lower motor neurones, sensation will also be affected.

The cranial nerves involved are:

Trigeminal	(fifth) -	face
Facial	(seventh) -	face and lips
Glossopharyngeal	(ninth) -	tongue, pharynx, palate
Vagus	(tenth) -	larynx, respiratory muscles
Hypoglossal	(twelfth) -	tongue

Typically, when the lesion is bilateral the phonatory characteristics of bulbar palsy include breathiness, possibly with stridor, as a result of the vocal folds only partially adducting and abducting. Monopitch and monoloudness are common features in addition to hypernasality with audible nasal escape. The inability to produce competent closure of laryngeal, palatopharyngeal and articulatory valves exacerbates the underlying respiratory difficulties. Respiratory movement is shallow and more frequent than normal in compensation for reduced vital capacity; clavicular breathing develops in an attempt to enlarge the thoracic movements and capacity. Short phrases are used because of the reduced vital capacity and the inability to control exhalation. Attempts to phonate on residual air occur frequently. The inadequacy of vocal fold movement, combined with poor respiratory function, makes the build-up of sufficient subglottic air pressure for coughing extremely difficult. The voice frequently has a 'wet', bubbly quality arising from the collection of secretions in the glottis.

Articulation resulting from bilateral lesions is affected by poor lip seal and limited tongue tip elevation arising from the hypotonic and wasting musculature. Tongue protrusion may not be possible. In some severe cases there is great difficulty in raising the mandible to the closed position (Darley, Aronson and Brown, 1975) and therefore in producing labial and lingual consonants. Unilateral lesions are apparent in the lips drooping on the affected side. The tongue may fasciculate and be wasted on the paralysed side, deviating to the affected side on protrusion. Intelligibility is poor as a result of the involvement of all parameters and the subsequent effect on prosody.

Peripheral lesions: recurrent laryngeal nerve lesions

In the case of peripheral lesions of the vagus nerve recurrent and superior laryngeal branches, the voice alone is impaired. There is no associated neuromuscular involvement of articulation. The laryngeal and palatal palsies are accordingly described in a separate section (see Chapter 15).

Cerebellar Lesions

The cerebellum has an integrating and controlling role over movements which arise in other parts of the motor system. It regulates the force, speed, range, timing and direction of movements so that excesses are inhibited. The regulation of equilibrium, posture and gait is undertaken by the cerebellum. It seems that it does not control patterns of movement but acts as a processing centre for motor activity (Darley, Aronson and Brown, 1975).

Lesions of the cerebellum occur as the result of tumours, multiple sclerosis, Wilson's disease, trauma, excessive alcohol intake, degenerative conditions and hereditary conditions such as forms of Friedrich's ataxia. Cerebellar signs are also evident in some victims of Legionnaires' disease, but although there is disruption of respiratory, laryngeal and swallowing mechanisms, the overall pattern of dysarthria is unlike the typical ataxic dysarthria (Mackenzie, 1987).

Muscles are hypotonic. A conspicuous feature of cerebellar damage is inaccuracy in targeting movements, as when a patient is asked to stretch out the arm and then touch the nose with the forefinger. The basic movement pattern is intact but the target is over- or undershot. Intention tremor appears at the end of movements and static tremor may be present if attempts are made to maintain a limb in a steady position. Patients suffering from cerebellar ataxia are frequently accused of being drunk on account of slurred speech, wide gait, impaired balance and general incoordination.

Ataxic dysphonia

For speech to be affected the cerebellar damage must be bilateral and widespread. The speech musculature is hypotonic and movements are slow and inaccurate.

Unpredictable movements of articulation, phonation and respiration occur. Articulation is jerky and inaccurate with exaggerated excursions of lips, jaw and tongue. There is obvious incoordination in integration of all speech parameters. Speech is slow; syllables may be attempted individually with equal stress which results in the characteristic scanning speech of ataxia. Grewel (1957a) in his classifications of dysarthria describes this as bradylalia or bradyarthria using European terminology.

The voice is explosive and staccato at times, then hoarse, harsh and breathy at others. The lack of coordination between respiration and phonation results in reduced maximum phonation time and pitch breaks. Control of pitch and loudness is impaired and the ataxic speaker frequently speaks loudly. The presence of severe dysrhythmia disrupts normal prosody but speech, although bizarre, remains intelligible.

Extrapyramidal Lesions

The extrapyramidal system consists of the basal ganglia in the cerebral hemispheres and the substantia nigra and subthalamic nucleus in the upper brainstem. The basal ganglia consist of the corpus striatum and its associated nuclei, the caudate and the lenticular nuclei. The latter is divided into the putamen and the globus pallidus. Lesions in the corpus striatum are sometimes referred to as 'striatal lesions' (Walshe, 1952). The extrapyramidal tract influences the pyramidal, or direct, pathway the function of which is to regulate the muscle tone required for posture and for changing position. In addition it is involved in the automatic component of skilled voluntary movement.

Extrapyramidal lesions result in hyperkinesia (excessive movement) or hypokinesia (reduction of movement). Darley, Aronson and Brown (1975) distinguish between quick and slow types of hyperkinesia, also known as dyskinesia or dystonia (Aronson, 1980).

Quick hyperkinesia

Chorea is characterised by rapid jerky movements. The muscles of face, lips, tongue, palate and larynx are involved producing a quick hyperkinetic dysarthria. Sydenham's chorea (St Vitus' dance) is caused by acute rheumatic fever in children. It can occur, but rarely, in pregnancy. Huntington's disease is a hereditary form developing at about 40 years of age with choreiform movements, ataxia and progressive mental deterioration. There are irregularities in the respiratory and laryngeal movements which produce irregular pitch and volume changes and speech arrests. These interruptions and repetitions may resemble cluttering or stammering.

Slow hyperkinesia

Athetosis produces a slow hyperkinetic dysarthria and occurs in children suffering from cerebral palsy. There are involuntary random and writhing movements of the body and orofacial grimacing. Rounding and pursing of the lips, involuntary tongue movements and laryngeal and respiratory spasms occur which can render speech unintelligible. The voice may be overloud at times and then fade to a whisper due to spasmodic movement of the respiratory and laryngeal muscles. Difficulty is experienced in sustaining phonation and the habitual pitch may be high and strained but drops to a groaning quality (Mecham, 1987). At rest, the patient may make disturbing grunting sounds.

Tremors

Individuals in normal health have a physiological tremor of small amplitude. A fine tremor of 8–12 vacillations per second is continuous both at rest and in movement (Lippold, 1971). It is imperceptible but accounts for the vibrato distinguishable in the singing voice although an excess becomes a disagreeable tremolo.

Familial tremor (essential tremor)

This tremor occurs in childhood and before 25 years of age. It may occur in more than one member of a family and in successive generations (Critchley, 1949). The tremor of 4–8 vacillations per second is generalised but most conspicuous in hands, tongue and lips. It is not progressive but is aggravated in voluntary movement and by emotion. It must be distinguished from functional (conversion) tremor. The distinction is based upon the history which will confirm the familial origin. Patients may be referred with diagnosis of functional dysphonia in which case the tremor is audible in the voice and is of long standing. This cannot be cured but the reason for the individual's sudden concern over the voice must be dealt with.

> Case note
> A woman employed at a hospital as a cleaner was referred complaining of voice tremor which she said had been the cause of losing her job after being absent from work with 'flu. When the reason for being sacked was investigated and a request for reinstatement made by the speech therapist a different interpretation of the situation had to be made. The woman had been sacked for stealing from elderly patients' lockers. The vocal tremor was a congenital neurological disorder which had never worried her until she thought she could use it to advantage.

Senile tremor

Tremor occurs not infrequently in old age. It is not present in the limbs at rest. It is most marked in the hands and head and can be heard in the voice. Hyperthyroidism is often accompanied by a fine rapid tremor.

Toxic tremor

Toxic agents can cause fine tremor, especially alcohol, barbiturates, cocaine and mercury poisoning.

Neurological lesion

Tremor is also associated with neurological disease and is encountered in bulbar and pseudobulbar palsy, besides parkinsonism. The nervous system acts as a whole and although neurologists attribute distinct features of muscular disorder to localised parts, there is uncertainty about the discrete functions of the basal ganglia. As Brain (1985) remarks, many theories concerning functions of the corpus striatum (caudate and lenticular nuclei) are debatable and do not explain all the symptoms in extrapyramidal syndromes. Damage to one cluster of cells is not discrete and any pathological damage has diffuse effects particularly in this concentrated area of the nervous system. A lesion in one group of cells is inextricably linked with adjacent parts besides the corticospinal paths.

Hypokinesia (parkinsonism)

Parkinson's disease is the epitome of hypokinesia. The disease is due to a deficiency of dopamine produced by the substantia nigra. Normally, dopamine, which is a neurotransmitter, has an inhibitory or monitoring effect on the release of acetylcholine which excites muscle activity at the normal synapses. The essential maintenance of muscle tone is impaired with dopamine deficiency so that regulation of all movement including posture, locomotion and changing from one position to another is affected.

The smooth, automatic coordination and flow of movement is disrupted by hypokinesia so that movement is slow, rigid and markedly limited in range as if a brake were imposed on the muscles. There is a general loss of vigour. Muscles relax in jerks which can be felt if wrist or elbow are manually flexed by the examiner. This is known as cog-wheel rigidity or rachet joint. Accompanying the rigidity is a regular coarse tremor of between 4 and 7 vacillations per second. This tends to subside in voluntary movement and is arrested in sleep.

Although the aetiology is still not fully understood, various forms of parkinsonism are recognised. The illness starts generally after 40 years of age. The idiopathic form (paralysis agitans) has a familial basis, otherwise the cause is unknown. There is also an arteriosclerotic form which produces degeneration of cells in the basal ganglia. A postencephalitic parkinsonism can follow encephalitis lethargica as long as 20 years after the illness. An epidemic of sleeping sickness after World War I resulted in many cases of Parkinson's disease in the 1930s. The incidence of sleeping sickness has decreased in the Western World and is now rare.

Psychopharmacology can induce parkinsonian symptoms; reserpine and phenothiazine have these side effects if doses are excessive or taken for prolonged periods. Damage may be irreversible but if drugs are withdrawn in time the parkinsonian symptoms will disperse although this period of recovery may take up to 2 years (Williamson, 1984; Scott, Caird and Williams, 1985).

Medical treatment

Chemotherapy reduces parkinsonian symptoms. The aim of therapy is to compensate for the absence of dopamine with the drug levodopa. This damps down the unleashed effect of acetylcholine with anticholinergic drugs (Hildick-Smith, 1980). There are side effects and dosage has to be carefully monitored. Approximately 10% of patients fail to benefit from this treatment.

Patients who are helped by drug therapy enjoy a marked reduction in symptoms and a great improvement in the quality of life for some 7 years' duration. A slow progressive decline in benefits from drug therapy is inevitable however after this. Frequently, death finally occurs as a result of respiratory infection. In some cases there is intellectual decline and confusion and, more rarely, dementia. There is great variability in progression of the disease and in some fortunate patients parkinsonism is arrested (Hildick-Smith, 1980).

Research prospects

Research into development of other neurotransmitters continues in the hope of discovering better therapeutic drugs. In its infancy is the experimentation with brain cell transplants of healthy dopamine-producing cells from aborted fetuses. These transplants have an immediate beneficial effect but the long-term result is debatable.

An interesting, if little relevant, item of information pertaining to the disease is that cigarette smoking appears to prevent development of Parkinson's disease. A lower incidence has been recorded in heavy smokers (Scott, Caird and Williams, 1985).

Symptoms

The disabling effect of rigidity, tremor, lack of range of movement and arrests in movement produces clear diagnostic perceptual characteristics. There is great difficulty in rising from a chair or bed and in turning in the horizontal position. Walking is greatly impaired, the patient loses balance and can fall due to steps becoming smaller on account of rigidity impeding range of movement. Unaided, the patient totters forward with increasing speed (festinating gait) until support of wall or chair is reached. When changing direction, turning or attempting to start walking the patient may become transfixed on the spot and involuntarily beat a tattoo with the feet.

Manual skills are impaired. Tremor often produces a 'pill rolling' movement between thumb and forefinger at rest and tasks such as fastening buttons are severely affected. Writing is also handicapped by the tremor and reduced range of movement so that letter formation becomes increasingly small and

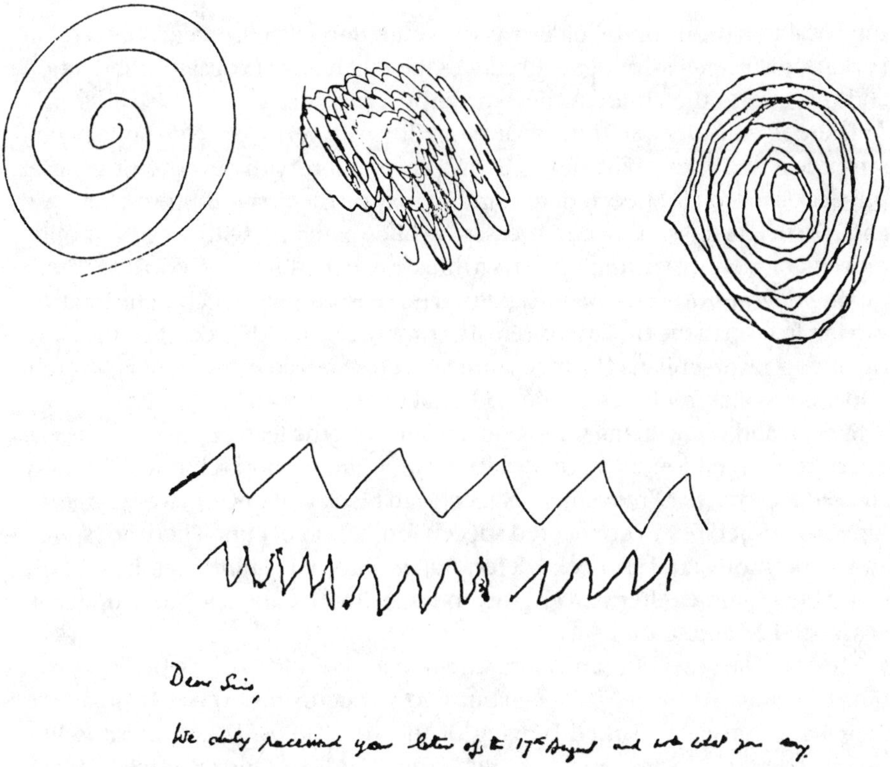

Figure 14.3. Example of writing and copying of patterns of patient with Parkinson's disease.

illegible. The cog-wheel rigidity affecting smooth rotation of the wrist gives rise to further problems. Posture is typical with head, neck, trunk, hips and knees slightly flexed.

Paralinguistic communication

Paralinguistic communication is severely affected. Facial expression is absent or markedly reduced with a resulting mask-like expression. This will appear unfriendly and make the listener withdraw from the individual with parkinsonism. It has to be understood that the refined muscular control of expression is not possible but that, internally, emotions are viable. The social handicap is further compounded by the fact that laughter and gesture are not initiated spontaneously. Inability to smile, laugh and use hand and head gestures is real handicap (Brown *et al.*, 1988).

Speech symptoms

Speech and voice are eventually involved in the progressive decline in all motor activity. It is estimated that approximately 50% of parkinsonian patients have speech and voice problems. Weismer (1984) suggests that phonatory characteristics are similar to the vocal behaviour of the aged, with a relatively high fundamental frequency and some vocal roughness. A further similarity to the vocal behaviour of the elderly is the reduction of the voiceless interval in parkinsonism; excessive rigidity reduces the efficiency of vocal fold abduction and this affects the ability to devoice appropriately.

There is considerable individual variability in severity of voice and speech symptoms and these have little, if any, correlation with severity of general physical symptoms. Speech deterioration may be the first symptom of disease and particularly in unilateral cases, while patients with severe bodily movement may have minimal dysarthria. Speech does not correlate with varying degrees of tremor and rigidity. The reasons for speech deterioration varying from patient to patient remains obscure when degree of tremor and rigidity appears similar. Of course, in advanced stages all movement is severely impaired, which includes eating and swallowing as well as speech.

Speech and voice characteristics correlate with the features of hypokinesia. There is reduced loudness, bradylalia, tremor and monopitch due to rigidity and reduced range of movement. Speech can be clear if one or two words at a time are uttered but in connected speech festination occurs. There are spurts and repetitions and speech deteriorates into an unintelligible, almost inaudible mumble. Alternatively, the body can 'freeze' and speech propulsion is arrested (akinetic mutism).

The voice lacks volume and pitch variation in addition to being breathy or, at times, rasping (Aronson, 1980). Breathy voice occurs in severely hypokinetic patients because of marked bowing of the vocal folds. When there is less rigidity better closure may be achieved (Ludlow and Bassich, 1984). Respiratory movement is reduced in range and regularity. Phrases are short and there are frequent aphonic episodes as respiratory support ends and attempts at restarting voice are made. Articulation is imprecise and phonemes may be repeated. The most prominent impairment is that of prosody with pitch, volume and temporal rhythmic features being disorganised.

Mixed Lesions

Mixed dysarthrias are the result of multiple lesions throughout the central nervous system and occur in conditions such as motor neurone disease (amyotrophic lateral sclerosis), multiple sclerosis and Wilson's disease. The speech deficits exhibit the characteristics of the different types of dysarthria.

Motor neurone disease (amyotrophic lateral sclerosis; progressive muscular atrophy)

Motor neurone disease (MND) is a degenerative condition which presents in various forms and affects upper and lower motor neurones. In the initial stages of the disease the predominant symptoms may be bulbar, limb or a combination of limb and bulbar symptoms, but as it progresses there is general involvement. Flaccid or spastic features may predominate at different stages of the disease (Aronson, 1980). The patient remains intellectually and linguistically normal and can communicate by writing until generalised weakness eventually makes an alternative method of communication essential. Dysphagia of increasing severity eventually necessitates feeding by nasogastric tube.

The cause of MND is unknown and it is irreversible. Death is usually caused by respiratory failure and may occur within 2–3 years of diagnosis, although in some patients progression of the condition is more delayed. A genetic abnormality was for long thought to be a cause of MND. However, research by neurotoxicologists now points to plant toxicants in food. A study of the Chamorro people of Guam in the Marianas islands has thrown fresh light on the mystery. The 'Guam disease' which is associated with motor neurone disease, parkinsonian dementia and Alzheimer's disease has a 50–100 times higher incidence than in the rest of the world. People begin to develop neurological symptoms much earlier between 20 and 30 years and have a longer life expectancy. A link has been found between the diet of the Chamorro and the diet of some peoples of India who suffer from lathyrism, a form of motor neurone disease. The Chamorro eat large amounts of flour made from the fruit of the cycad (sago palm) and the Indians consume quantities of chickling peas. Both peas and cycad contain a toxin of complex chemical composition known as L-BMAA. It is to be hoped that the solution to prevention of the three degenerative diseases MND, PD and Alzheimer's lies in the further research of toxicologists (Spencer *et al.*, 1987; Goldwyn, 1989). Further evidence compounding the Guam saga was the discovery of two other localities where MND is prevalent. In the Japanese Ki peninsula, cycad is dispensed as a herbal medicine by pharmacists. In New Guinea, tribes along the Ia river use cycad poultices on septic wounds. A great problem in tracking down toxicants is the latency of disease; years elapse between exposure and illness.

The mixed dysarthria of MND is a combination of bulbar and pseudobulbar palsy which impairs all parameters of motor speech production and eventually results in unintelligibility. The speech musculature is markedly spastic, phonation is effortful, with a harsh, strained–strangled quality and hypernasality. Typically the voice is low pitched and limited in range. In the early stages of the disease some patients complain of raised pitch which is apparently the result of hypertonic supraparyngeal muscles elevating the larynx and increased tension of the vocal folds.

Multiple or disseminated sclerosis

Multiple sclerosis (MS) is another disease of unknown origin although there are suggestions that it is caused by a virus. Demyelination of the nerve sheaths occurs randomly in the cerebral hemispheres, spinal cord and cerebellum. It occurs in youth and rarely after 40 years and is progressive, although there are remissions frequently lasting for years. Early symptoms may include impaired vision. Subsequently ataxia, nystagmus, intention tremor and dysarthria develop. Speech is slow and hesitant with impaired articulation and hypernasality. Respiration is diversely affected in a minority of patients.

Wilson's disease

A similar picture is seen in Wilson's disease which is a progressive hepatolenticular degeneration starting early in life and often familial. The illness starts in adolescence and is a genetic metabolic disorder preventing processing of copper in food resulting in copper deposits in the liver, brain and kidneys. Treatment is by introducing a diet low in copper and by appropriate chemotherapy. Speech is affected on account of muscular rigidity, tremor and ataxia; dysphagia may be a concomitant problem.

Apraxia and Dysprosody

Apraxia of speech presents an interesting neurological problem. There is impairment of the voluntary ability to organise the correct positions of the articulators in production of phonemes and phoneme sequences in the absence of paralysis. Controversy concerning the site of the lesion is continuously argued in the literature and is well reviewed by Buckingham (1979) and Edwards (1984). The focus of contention is whether verbal dyspraxia involving speech and phonation is a disorder of motor programming solely, or whether it is always associated with language disorder, i.e. dysphasia (Martin, 1974).

The Mayo Clinic team (Darley, Aronson and Brown, 1975) are unequivocal in their view that apraxia of speech is due to a left cerebral hemisphere injury. These authors believe that there is no impairment of muscle function (paresis or paralysis) and no disorder of comprehension or language formulation. The central language processor they aver is intact but the motor programming centre, possibly at the vestibular and reticular level, is impaired. The dysprosody which accompanies the disorder is considered, by Darley, Aronson and Brown, to be secondary to apraxia of speech and to arise as the result of impaired sequential organisation.

It is, however, widely observed by experienced speech pathologists that dyspraxic dysprosody is a linguistic suprasegmental manifestation. This view regards the dysprosody as a primary feature and considers apraxia of speech to be a disorder involving the breakdown of the inextricably linked motor and linguistic processes (Kertesz, 1983). It is considered to be an impairment of higher level planning and not only a neuromuscular disorder. The dyspraxic errors are regarded as similar to, or indistinguishable from, paraphasic errors of aphasia. Anomalies of voice onset time (VOT) result in inappropriate voicing and devoicing so that, for example, 'pan' becomes 'ban'.

The difficulty in sequencing articulatory gestures correctly results in phonemic errors including substitutions, omissions and additions. There are characteristic groping movements of the articulators and errors are inconsistent and unpredictable. The patient is aware of mispronunciations and struggles to correct them. Intonation is abnormal while voice quality remains normal (Deal and Darley, 1972).

Bridgeman and Snowling (1988) in a study of twelve dyspraxic children found some evidence of difficulty in perception of phoneme sequences.

The perceived speech characteristics of apraxia of speech have been clearly defined by Kent and Rosenbek (1983) in an acoustic analysis using a SonaGraph. Seven dyspraxic patients without severe aphasia or agrammatism produced 'higher order' errors of articulation, metathesis and segmental additions besides incoordination. The acoustic visual displays showed acoustic, segmental and prosodic abnormalities. These included:

1. Slow speaking rate; prolongation of phonological transitions; lengthening of steady states and intersyllabic pauses (syllable segregation).
2. Reduced intensity variation across syllables; slow, inaccurate articulatory gestures, inconsistent errors.
3. Incoordination of voicing in both vowels and consonants and difficulties in initiation.
4. Errors in selection of sequencing segments.
5. Overall difficulty in motor control of spatiotemporal schema.

Speech may give the impression of a broad dialect or a foreign language. The famous case reported by Monrad-Krohn (1947a) is often quoted. A Norwegian lady made a good recovery from stroke and dysphasia but was left with an altered melody of language – a 'broken accent' similar to that of German. This caused her some distress and embarrassment at that time of being at war with Germany. Monrad-Krohn, not a linguist but a neurologist, defined the prosodic features of speech as 'that faculty of speech which conveys different shades of meaning by means of stress and pitch, irrespective of the words and the grammatical construction'.

Dyspraxia is not confined to speech and other performances are disrupted. Ideational dyspraxia allows the patient to carry out a task effortlessly, but with the component actions in the wrong order. Ideomotor apraxia retains the underlying programme of the task intact but spatial and temporal errors occur. There are problems in dressing and using everyday objects. Limb kinetic dyspraxia suggests loss of kinaesthetic memory for specific parts of the body and speech organs (Brain, 1985).

> Case note
> A patient who was later diagnosed as having suffered a stroke in her sleep was rushed into hospital after being found by her husband in hysterics in her bathroom. She explained later that not only could she not speak but she became terrified when she 'could not think what to do' with a toothbrush and tablet of soap. The situation must indeed be traumatic when unable to organise the necessary actions.

Careful assessment of language function reveals deficits. In assessing numerous cases after stroke and brain surgery on a busy neurosurgical unit over a period of 10 years Greene found that all patients with apraxia of speech had dysphasic deficits of varying degree.

Edwards (1984) has made the interesting suggestion that hypernasality and unexplained fluctuations in soft palate elevation during speech may be due to dyspraxia. This appears to be the explanation for the excessive nasality in the speech of the dyspraxic herdsman described on p. 289.

Developmental childhood dyspraxia

In concentrating upon dyspraxic adults it must not be forgotten that children suffering from severe speech and language handicap can also be dyspraxic in the absence of paralysis. Morley (1957) in her survey of 100 families in Newcastle-upon-Tyne, England, selected for detailed study 164 children with defective speech. Among these she described 12 children with a specific articulatory disorder which she termed 'developmental articulatory dyspraxia'. Clumsiness and poor coordination are present but inability to organise sequences of actions is evident in many everyday activities - in play, feeding and dressing. Miming, telephoning, manipulating knife and fork, for example, are bizarre and disorganised. The Illinois Test of Psycholinguistic Abilities (ITPA) expression tests show up dyspraxia very clearly (Greene, 1976; Edwards, 1984).

The child's crying and babbling develop normally but speech inception is very late, not until 3 or 4 years of age if then, and consonant and vowel production is grossly deviant. The child cannot imitate phonemes and words in the normal way and has to be helped by manipulation of lips and tongue reinforced by visual clues (lip-reading) as for the hard of hearing. Oral gestures have to be taught in order to elicit consonants and vowels. Intelligence of these children is normal and speech comprehension is usually good.

Greene (1967) in describing the predicament of such children in her paper 'Speechless and backward at three', emphasises the stress suffered by the child and the family if not given speech therapy early. As speech develops, severe deficits in language acquisition become apparent confirming the link between language and praxis. When speech is sufficiently fluent dysprosody becomes conspicuous. There are attendant learning difficulties once education starts and children suffer from dyslexia and dyscalculia to the despair of parents, children and teachers. Special educational facilities must be provided besides intensive speech therapy (Greene, 1983a).

Aphonia following Closed Head Injury

In some cases of severe closed head trauma, patients are mute during the early stages of recovery and remain aphonic or dysphonic even when articulatory movements recover and laryngoscopy reveals normal vocal fold movement. Hartman and Von Cramon (1984) in their acoustic analysis study of these patients found that recovery of phonation fell into two subgroups. The first presented with voice quality with breathy and tense components which gradually became more normal during the follow-up period. The second group initially had normal or lax, breathy voice which became more tense.

The differential diagnosis of aphonia following closed head injury in the absence of laryngological signs may be complex. Sapir and Aronson (1985a) suggest three possible causes. The frontal lobes and limbic system are important in the regulation of affect, emotion and the vocal expression of emotion. Damage to these areas may reduce the drive and controlling mechanisms of phonation. The resulting disorder of affect is characterised by the 'flatness' of facial expression and general lack of drive which is reflected in the aphonia or quiet voice with reduced intonation patterns. However, the symptom may also have a psychogenic basis and be part of the emotional response to brain injury. Recovery is frequently accompanied by depression and feelings of hopelessness so that the neurological problems give rise to psychological symptoms (Sapir and Aronson, 1987a). Finally, as discussed in the previous section, apraxia of phonation should also be considered as a possible cause.

Spasmodic Adductor Dysphonia ('Spastic Dysphonia')

This voice disorder (SAD) must be clearly distinguished from psychogenic spasmodic dysphonia and from the dysphonia associated with spastic dysarthria. The site of the neurological lesion causing the bizarre adductor action of the vocal folds is so far uncertain but the condition seems to originate in the extrapyramidal system. The vocal folds suffer involuntary spasms somewhat similar to those of chorea. Frequently there is tremor in the vocal folds and in head, neck and hands. In many cases, however, these overt neurological signs are not present (Greene, 1983b).

Traube in 1871, according to Arnold and Heaver (1959), first described a spastic type of hoarseness of nervous origin characterised by a choking or strangulated type of dysphonia. Critchley (1939a) attributed spastic dysphonia to a neurological disorder having cranial nerve symptoms with a resemblance to facial tics and spasmodic torticollis. Thomson, Negus and Bateman (1955) compared spastic dysphonia to writer's cramp. Others have compared the vocal spasms to those encountered in severe stammering. All observers are agreed that the condition is incurable and highly resistant to all forms of treatment - psychiatric, pharmaceutical and vocal rehabilitation.

However, these early neurological comments were forgotten and the disorder of spastic dysphonia continued to be attributed to hysterical conversion symptom (Luchsinger, 1965b). In 1960, Robe, Moore and Brumlik published a study of 10 patients suffering from spastic dysphonia whose encephalograms revealed central nervous system damage with abnormal paroxysmal discharges in the right temporoparietal region. These findings have not been duplicated according to Schaeffer (1983). The possibility, however, that a condition previously thought to be psychogenic could be neurological created great interest. Research now transferred to location of the lesion in the nervous system and more appropriate forms of treatment.

Neurological aetiology

Aronson *et al.* (1968a,b) published two surveys: the first was concerned with neurological and psychiatric aspects of spastic dysphonia, and the second drew a comparison between essential voice tremor and spastic dysphonia.

Twenty-seven patients out of a group of 34 suffered from essential tremor and other neurological signs. These included involuntary twitching of face and tongue accompanied by head and hand tremor. Seventeen patients had abnormal EEGs and some complained of difficulty in swallowing, pain in the neck and throat, and tightness in the chest. The tightly squeezed and strangled dysphonia was common to all.

Aronson and Hartman (1981) postulated that essential voice tremor is the definitive diagnostic sign of true adductor spasmodic dysphonia and distinguishes the condition from psychogenic spastic dysphonia. Schaeffer (1983) asserts that positive evidence of tremor is difficult to prove in cases of severe paroxysms of vocal fold adduction. Tremor is most apparent in mild cases. Dedo (1976) attributes the disorder to neurotropic viral infection which attacks the sensory fibres of the vagus and spares the motor fibres.

The description of hyperkinetic dysarthrias and extrapyramidal disorders (Darley, Aronson and Brown, 1975) which are characterised by abnormal involuntary movements, bears some resemblance to the symptoms exhibited by sufferers from spasmodic adductor dysphonia. The organic cases of voice tremor described by Aronson *et al.* (1968b) had more regular voice arrests due to the hyperadduction of the vocal folds than the spastic dysphonia cases in whom spasms occurred irregularly.

Schaeffer *et al.* (1983a,b) have found brainstem conduction abnormalities in spasmodic dysphonia. Schaeffer (1983) has described very fully the neuropathology of spasmodic dysphonia. Brainstem responses were tested in 29 patients and abnormal responses were found in the auditory, cephalic–gastric and cephalic–cardiac reflex systems. Vocal tremor and the number of associated neurological findings correlated positively with the severity of impairment registered in the brainstem tests. Schaeffer (1983) produced conclusive proof of laryngeal somatic and visceral nervous system damage. He proposes the hypothesis that this occurs in the brainstem nuclei and motor pathways.

Abductor spasm

An abductor form of spasmodic dysphonia has been described by various authors. Aronson (1973) in his audio seminars on psychogenic voice disorders included examples of abductor spastic dysphonia. In a revised account of clinical voice disorders, Aronson (1980) gives brief mention of an abductor voice arrest which can occur in conjunction with the adductor type or as an isolated symptom. Aphonia and breathy voice intersperse speech.

Zwitman (1979) dealing with bilateral vocal fold dysfunction and abductor type spastic dysphonia recognises that involuntary parting of the vocal folds does occur and states that the neurological term 'spastic dysphonia' is inappropriate in connection with this symptom. Wolfe and Bacon (1976) compared two types of spastic dysphonia with two patients, using spectrographic analysis and concluded that the abductor symptom could be psychogenic. The existence of a neurogenic abductor spasmodic dysphonia is also questioned by Ludlow and Connor (1987) whose research suggests that only the muscles involved in vocal fold adduction are involved in this condition. Schaeffer (1983) describes various strategies assumed by patients to avoid and replace the adductor spasms. These are breathiness and aphonia, which seems a rational explanation of observed abductor movements in the larynx in cases of spasmodic adductor dysphonia. The diagnosis and existence of abductor spastic dysphonia is speculative and in the unquestioned existence of adductor spasm, pursuit of another hare seems irrelevant.

Vocal characteristics of SAD

The spasmodic adduction of the vocal folds during phonation (laryngospasm) produces the characteristic strangulated voice which is immediately recognisable. This has been described by Dedo and Shipp (1980) 'as though the individual is speaking while trying to lift an immovable object'.

The typical pattern of development is that initially the patient notices an occasional 'catch' in the voice which gradually becomes hoarse and develops pitch breaks. The onset of the disorder is slow with progressive deterioration, stabilising after 3–5 years' duration. Respiratory viral infection or trauma to the head or neck may precede the onset or there may be no obvious related factors.

As the struggle to phonate progresses, facial grimaces including eyeblinking and eyebrow twitching (blepharism or blepharospasm) become established. Voiceless sounds may become voiced if the vocal folds remain adducted during the voiceless segment (Dedo and Shipp, 1980). Prosody is disturbed and symptoms such as vocal tremor and stuttering may be concomitant features. Breathing patterns are exaggerated in some patients as they try to overcome the strongly adducted vocal folds. Laryngospasm is particularly marked if phonation on residual air is attempted. Some patients complain of chest and throat pain. Dedo and Shipp (1980) note that all symptoms of the disorder become more severe as the day progresses and when the individual is using the telephone. Fibreoptic laryngoscopy may reveal a degree of laryngeal spasm occurring irregularly even when the vocal folds are at rest. Tremor of the palate, tongue and neck is frequently visible. These are positive neurological signs.

Vegetative functions such as coughing, throat clearing and laughing may be normal. The patient may also be able to produce isolated vowels and to sing without spasm. Another feature is alleviation of symptoms with change of therapist. Symptoms are exacerbated under stress; inconsistencies occur, the speaking voice apparently improving for short periods and then deteriorating again. In some cases the voice may stabilise at a mild stage of the disorder and the patient adjusts to the symptoms although they are always present. This is especially the case if speech therapy is given early.

Age of onset

The onset of spasmodic adductor dysphonia is usually in middle age with a greater incidence in females. There is some disagreement concerning the sex ratio with Dedo and Shipp recording two females for every male and Aronson (1980) noting a male to female ratio ranging from 1 : 1 to 1 : 18.

Wilson (1987) also refers to the condition in teenagers in whom he notes early symptoms which include moderate stridency, harshness, breathiness and slight vocal tremor. There is no sudden aphonia but hoarseness sometimes accompanied by visible tightening of the external laryngeal muscles and elevation of the larynx during phonation. Wilson records some therapeutic success when the disorder is in the incipient stage but confirms the general opinion of poor prognosis at the advanced stage. We have no experience of such cases in childhood.

Psychological aspects

Psychological disturbance, such as anxiety and depression, is only to be expected from a crippling social and occupational handicap which inevitably has dire socioeconomic consequences. A marked feature of the dysphonia is lack of conversion symptoms and evidence of evading voice recovery. There is an unfailing determination to overcome the handicap, to seek treatment and to lead a normal life. This aspect induced Dedo (Dedo, Urrea and Lawson, 1973) to operate upon his first patient, Mrs Mildred Younger.

Treatment

The resistance of this condition to treatment is notorious and has included psychiatric intervention and hypnotherapy. Trials of injection of primidone, which has been reported as being effective in reducing benign essential tremor, have been conducted without success (Hartman and Vishwanat, 1984). Voice therapy never effects a cure but in all cases can help to alleviate the symptoms by giving the patient insight into the condition and encouraging relaxed, breathy phonation which reduces the strength of the laryngospasm and may in some cases prevent further vocal deterioration.

Botulinum toxin injection

Studies using injection of botulinum toxin into the thyroarytenoid muscle unilaterally are taking place in the USA and the UK (Garfield Davies, 1988). The effect of injecting the sterile substance is that of chemical denervation. Early results are encouraging in producing fluent voice, but the technique is still in its infancy.

Recurrent laryngeal nerve section

Dedo first reported his procedure for recurrent laryngeal nerve (RLN) section for the relief of spasmodic adductor dysphonia in 1976. Unilateral section of the RLN paralyses the vocal fold in the paramedian position. The healthy fold, although continuing to exhibit adductor spasm, is unable to make closure of the same force with the paralysed fold across the mid-line.

Prior to surgery a lignocaine (lidocaine) injection into the RLN is given to immobilise the fold temporarily so that patient and laryngologist can assess the probable effect the surgery will have. The patient must understand that voice after surgery will not be perfect and that relapse can occur. Recordings must be studied by the patient and assent to surgery obtained.

Postoperative voice therapy

Speech therapy is considered essential postoperatively because the voice will be breathy in the early stages of recovery and diplophonia may be present for 6–8 weeks. The spasmodic features are greatly reduced which is a great relief to the patient. Tremor with synchronous head, neck and jaw tremor will persist and is not relieved by surgery but may be diminished (Dedo and Shipp, 1980; Dedo and Izdebski, 1983b).

Recurrence of SAD

Unfortunately, the good results obtained by RLN section do not last indefinitely. Izdebski, Dedo and Shipp (1981) reported 15 cases who had benefited and retained significant reduction of symptoms over a period of 3 years. Dedo and Izdebski (1983b) reported intermediate results of 306 RLN sections for spastic dysphonia. Although 4 years postoperatively 90% of the patients judged their voices to be 'easier' than preoperatively, some voices lacked volume due to atrophy and shrinking of the paralysed fold. This was treated with Teflon injection. Another problem occurred with adduction of the paralysed fold to the mid-line and the return of spasticity.

Spasmodic dysphonia returned in 10–15% of Dedo and Shipp's patients (1980) from as early as 1 month postsurgery to 2 years later. In cases of recurrence Dedo and Shipp advocate debulking the paralysed vocal fold by cup forceps or carbon dioxide laser to produce an air leak, along a 2 mm wide strip after a period of 1 year or more. Similar procedures are advocated by Forder (1983) and Isshiki (1980).

Aronson and de Santo (1983) reported disappointing results in follow-up of 38 patients after surgery. They found that 64% had voices which were worse after 3 years lapse than preoperatively. Failure among women was considerably higher than among men. In the whole group only one patient whose voice improved had normal voice. Improved voices were breathy, hoarse, falsetto or diplophonic. Pitch breaks occurred and tremor was evident on prolonged vowels. These authors confirm that surgery has long-term limitations.

Fritzell *et al.* (1982) described experience with four subjects (three female and one male) who had RLN section for spastic dysphonia. Two patients who had voice therapy did not relapse but two who did not receive therapy suffered return of spasmodic dysphonia after 3 months. Electromyography indicated re-innervation of the vocal fold on the paralysed side. One patient's voice recovered with lignocaine (lidocaine) injection and was, as a result, operated upon again with good effect. The other patient also underwent surgery but it was impossible to locate the nerve and the voice was no better after surgery.

Wilson, Olding and Mueller (1980) reported a case of return of spastic dysphonia 6 months after RLN section. Nerve section was performed again and during this operation the nerve was tested and found to be intact.

In conclusion, it can be assumed that both conversion and organic (neurological) types of spasmodic adductor dysphonia occur. The 'spastic' (conversion) type can be cured by appropriate therapy. The neurological type is due to some indeterminate damage to the nervous system, possibly at the vestibular reticular motor processing level (Darley, Aronson and Brown, 1975). As with many neurological disorders impairment is of variable degree and adductor spasm can be mild in which case nerve section is probably best avoided. If severe, the relief provided by surgery is perhaps the best, though imperfect, solution.

In the final analysis, differential diagnosis of this puzzling condition depends on whether the adductor spasm vanishes with therapy or remains for life. Careful assessment and follow-up of a large number of sufferers over a period of many years is necessary to clarify the situation.

Case histories

The following histories demonstrate clearly the difficulties in diagnosis and the need to take care and time in assessment. A psychogenic history can be constructed of the personalities of most individuals, and patients with true adductor spastic dysphonia are no exception. The psychosomatic aspect in the diagnosis must not throw out of focus the possible presence of neurological symptoms.

1. Mr S. (53 years) was referred for speech therapy suffering from slight laryngitis and hoarseness following a severe attack of influenza, laryngitis and aphonia some 4 weeks before. The continuing mild laryngeal inflammation was thought to be due to vocal strain. The vocal folds adducted strongly in phonation.

   The voice was hoarse and produced with excessive force. Traditional speech therapy was given, i.e. relaxation, breath control and soft attack. After 4 weeks, review by the laryngologist reported a healthy looking larynx and improvement in phonation but need for extended speech therapy.

   Mr S.'s voice, now that the laryngitis had resolved, was stronger and not breathy but an adductor spasm was clearly present. Spastic dysphonia was diagnosed.

   There were indications of a conversion symptom in Mr S.'s history. He had joined the staff of a bank on leaving school and had soon been called up to serve in the Navy. He had a good record for courage and reliability in the Atlantic convoys during the war. On returning to the bank after the war he had good prospects of promotion and hoped to become a head of department if not a manager. As time went by his hopes faded. The bank's policy changed and instead of promoting older and experienced employees, bright and promising young people were selected and trained for the well-paid posts in higher management. Adding insult to injury, he had been delegated to lecture to these students occasionally on special courses. He had felt some tightness in the throat which he had put down to 'nerves'. He resented this disregard of his experience and ability exceedingly but became reconciled eventually to his job behind the counter as he enjoyed this and the contact with customers.

He was an extravert, talkative person and gave information about himself and discussed problems freely. He was happily married to a teacher and had two children both training to teach. He was a staunch Methodist and took a very active part in church activities: Sunday school, outings and holiday camps in which his wife assisted.

Speech therapy helped but did not eradicate the adductor spasm. His voice improved in the first months and then stabilised. He was a great talker and his voice was not an inconvenience. He enjoyed coming to speech therapy which he did regularly once a week on his way home. The satisfaction he felt in leaving work early and, as he said 'getting his own back' on the bank, contributed to his pleasure. He was not discharged as this was a rare case of 'spastic dysphonia' which could be followed for years. Eventually regular sessions were terminated upon his retirement. He was seen 6 months and a year later but there was no change in his voice.

This case postulates the possibility of a psychogenic dysphonia although Mr S. was a cheerful, well-adjusted individual and his reaction to the bank situation very understandable. A grievance does not explain spasmodic adductor dysphonia. In the absence of neurological signs, good health and abundant energy the adductor spasm could be attributable to a discrete lesion suffered during the viral invasion. Alternatively, the laryngospasm could be a habit spasm or tic arising out of the lecturing situation and comparable to blepharospasm.

2. Mr Y. (53 years) had been troubled by his voice 'trailing off' unaccountably when speaking. During this period he had had a number of laryngological and medical examinations which excluded any organic pathology. About the time his voice began to deteriorate he was experiencing stomach trouble which was diagnosed as psychosomatic. Six months prior to being referred for speech therapy he had suffered a coronary thrombosis and his voice had worsened after this.

   He was a clerk to the Electricity Board, married happily with two sons. One lived at home and was 'a problem'; the other was married and happily settled.

   He was a cheerful, cooperative and friendly person with a sense of humour, and appeared to be amused by his vocal symptoms rather as a spectator than a participant. On superficial acquaintance he was the last person one would suspect of suffering from psychoneurosis. His vocal and respiratory symptoms were exactly those of spasmodic adductor dysphonia described above. His voice, sometimes normal over a span of several words, would suddenly be interrupted by a laryngeal spasm and his thorax and abdomen become rigid. He complained himself of the abdominal tension. He ignored the failure of voice and continued to speak in a whisper or with choked and strained voice.

He was obsessional and anxious about his work. He had been happy in the electrical company's employ before nationalisation but thereafter he had always felt he was working under pressure. As he described it himself, his life was a 'perpetual fight against anxiety and the feeling that he could not cope with everything that had to be done'. He could never rest or be idle. He took on extra jobs at the office because he was interested and wanted to be helpful. He always took work home and when this was done he would be busy decorating his house, doing repairs or gardening.

He responded to relaxation and voice therapy and was able to obtain a normal voice in humming, vowel exercises and repeat reading. Sometimes his speech was free from spasm for a few minutes but this was never maintained. Sometimes he reported having had little trouble during the week and at other times, just like a stammerer, he would report a setback and be depressed over lack of progress.

A marked feature of his response to treatment was a distinct improvement in voice production when taken by another therapist in the department or by students. This was entirely due to greater attention to effortless phonation. Laryngospasm was reduced in force but always present. He increased in his ability to manage phonation consistently and no longer feared total breakdown in his speech. He was discharged after a year and followed up at 3-monthly periods for another year during which the spastic adductor dysphonia stabilised further.

3. Mr B. (52 years) was a telecommunications employee and a keen 'radio ham'. He had noticed his voice deteriorating 2 years prior to examination by a laryngologist. The larynx was free from disease and symptoms, except for the laryngeal spasm in phonation and he was referred for speech therapy. He was then referred to a psychiatrist who passed him on to a clinical psychologist who gave him relaxation therapy which resulted in minimal improvement. In all he had 24 hours treatment from the psychologist and 17 hours from the speech therapist.

He was an extremely voluble and forceful character and it was only his own conviction that he was not 'off his head', as people apparently thought, and his insistence that something must be done to relieve his condition, that eventually conveyed him to a specialist centre.

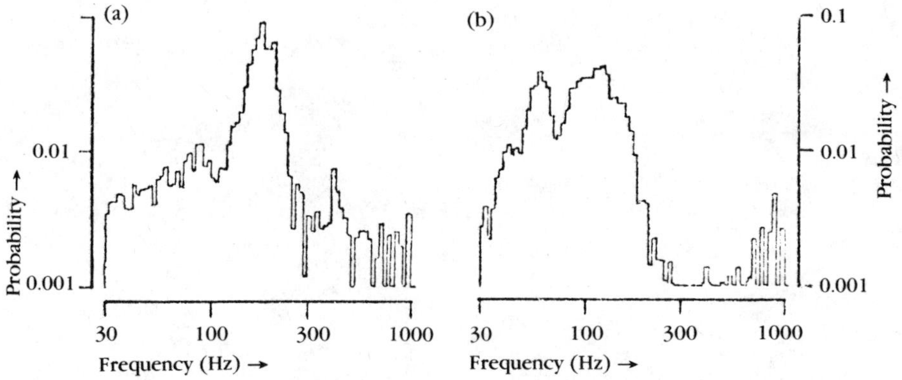

Figure 14.4. Spasmodic adductor dysphonia: electrolaryngograph analysis. (a) Before RLN section; (b) after RLN section. Professor A. Fourcin reported: 'The laryngograph records show a marked difference in ability to control *Lx* frequencies employed in phonation. There is a marked reduction postoperatively in the high frequency irregularity and a considerable increase in low frequency regularity. There is no doubt of course from the two distributions, as indeed is evident from listening to the tape, that his voice quality is still abnormal.' (By courtesy of Adrian Fourcin, University College, London University.)

He had all the typical features of SAD, with extreme laryngeal and pharyngeal tension and severely segmented vowels. He found it easier to communicate in a stage whisper and this he used habitually. He had not allowed his vocal disorder to interfere with his work and had kept going except for hospital treatments. He had other neurological signs: a marked regular tremor of the upper lip and tremor of the hands.

His voice responded well to the trial injection of lignocaine and immobilisation of the right RLN. He was overjoyed by the result and the great relief experienced in phonation, and agreed to the operation. This produced a considerable improvement in his voice which was further stabilised by a short course of speech therapy. Five months later, when reassessed, his voice appeared to have deteriorated a little. It continued to do so but remained much improved to the preoperative condition.

Chapter 15
Therapy for Neurological Dysphonias

Speech and voice therapy for patients suffering from neurological damage has primarily to be based upon the standard principles of normal voice production as described in Chapter 9. After careful assessment of a patient's voice, articulation, respiration, health and motivation, specific difficulties will emerge and realistic targets for improvement in communication can be envisaged. In the complex spectrum of dysfunction associated with neurological damage inflicted by the diseases already described, subdivisions of dysfunction such as hyper-, hypo-, slow and quick kinesia are largely irrelevant. A holistic approach is necessary. Current neuroscience emphasises the importance of neuronetwork systems running 'in parallel' or concurrently with many interconnections. This is not a new concept but a revival of old truths as described by Sherrington (1947) in *The Integrative Action of the Nervous System*. There are new technologies now which can quantify more accurately brain function, and knowledge acquired will be correlated with computer technology and improved communication aids.

Much depends upon the courage and spirit of the afflicted patient and the therapist can alleviate anxiety and depression in both patient and carers. Any improvement in communication, whether by speech and voice exercises or use of speech aids, is worth while since it improves the quality of life out of all proportion to the proof expected from scientific measurements.

General Principles

Compensatory techniques

The primary aim in therapy is to achieve intelligibility of speech by improving function or sustaining it by means of compensatory mechanisms. Therapy cannot reverse the underlying neuropathology. There is the possibility of some spontaneous recovery of function in certain cases but more possible are the compensatory functions remaining in less impaired pathways. In cases of degenerative disease, strategies and techniques can be learned in the early stages in order to deal with increasing difficulties as effectively as possible.

Holistic approach

In many instances of neurological dysphonia other speech parameters are involved; effective treatment must integrate all relevant features of communication. In addition, a particular aspect of dysphonia may predominate, in which case treatment will naturally have its bias, but this one symptom is never an isolated entity. Many features of neurological lesion cluster around a central theme and have to be taken into account.

Psychological encouragement

Early treatment is advisable so that the patient has objective goals to work for. An optimistic approach from the outset prevents deterioration and development of poorer standards of speech than are obtainable. This applies especially to progressive cases of motor disorder. There may be periods of remission or stability and the patient should be encouraged to make the best use of residual function.

The morale of the patient is all important. Encouragement and a positive and hopeful therapeutic approach bolsters up the spirits of both patient and family and does much to alleviate the natural despair and depression following neurological trauma. Early speech therapy is mandatory on both psychological and physiological grounds. The prevention of poor speech habits arising from the dulling of self-perception and self-monitoring, and the establishment of compensatory manoeuvres can preserve the voice and intelligibility in progressive disease.

A fighting spirit, well maintained, can achieve unexpected results even in crippling disease. The world renowned physicist Professor Stephen Hawking is such an example, continuing to postpone the effects of motor neurone disease on his exceptional research work by sheer force of spirit and intellect. When speech was lost, computerised communication came to the rescue and so the work of solving the riddles of the universe carries on while the thin thread of life runs out.

Practice

The reinforcement of motor, proprioceptive and kinaesthetic patterns achieved in exercises with the therapist should continue with practice outside the treatment session. If patients can be motivated to carry out regular practice, alone or with their carers, more benefit is derived from therapy than if it is forgotten once the patient has escaped from the clinic.

Biofeedback

The importance of biofeedback is discussed in relation to certain disorders in this chapter and this technique should be used whenever possible unless there is any danger of the patient being distressed by its use. Audio and video recorders, Visipitch and Visispeech, amplifiers, loudness indicators are helpful.

Organisation of treatment sessions

Neuromuscular disorders are particularly susceptible to the effects of fatigue. For this reason the length of treatment and time of day it is given should be considered. The success of an exhausted patient is low and strongly dispiriting.

Cooperation with other professionals

This is essential in order to facilitate a coordinated approach which does not conflict at any point.

Drug regimen

The therapist should be aware of the effects of medication on each patient and arrange treatments to avoid periods of the day when adverse reactions make maximum cooperation difficult.

Augmentative and alternative communication aids

Patients should be given the opportunity to use such equipment if functional communication is enhanced. Carefully considered introduction of alternative communication aids to patients with degenerative diseases before they really need them can be reassuring. Before such equipment becomes necessary, familiarity and proficiency are established.

Assessment

Assessment has been fully described in Chapters 6 and 7. Instrumental and informal and formal perceptual assessments of voice are appropriate. Some research suggests that acoustic analysis of voice may have a part to play in the early and differential diagnosis of patients with neurological disease and that it may contribute to the measurement of progression of the disease (Ramig *et al.*, 1988). In addition, evaluation of linguistic skills and general effectiveness of communication is essential. Where there is involvement of the articulators, in addition to laryngeal involvement, a dysarthria profile can be compiled using a formal perceptual assessment such as the Frenchay Dysarthria Assessment (Enderby, 1983) or the Robertson Dysarthria Profile (Robertson, 1982). These profiles indicate the relative severity of deficits affecting various speech parameters in addition to the areas of phonatory inefficiency.

Treatment

Respiratory and laryngeal deficits

These, and problems of incoordination, are treated using strategies described in Chapter 9. Robertson and Thomson (1986) list useful exercises for all aspects of dysarthria, including phonation.

Hypernasality

Hypernasality can be treated with exercises and prostheses. Surgical intervention in neurological palatopharyngeal incompetence is not successful (Johns and Salyer, 1978) and should be avoided.

Articulation and phonation exercises

These are directed at strengthening muscle movement initially, if necessary, with non-speech strategies aimed at increasing intraoral air pressure, e.g. closing the lips and puffing-up the cheeks. Coordination of palatal movement is encouraged by practising consonant–vowel (CV) syllables using plosives and gradually progressing to words and phrases. Hypernasality resulting from incoordination of the palatopharyngeal closure is frequently due to sluggish movement of the velum. Consequently, a slightly slower speech rate allowing time for closure, in combination with increased mouth opening, reduces the impression of hypernasality.

Palatal lift prosthesis

Palatal lift prostheses are widely reported to reduce hypernasality (Massengil, 1972; Wedin, 1972; Enderby, Hathorn and Servant, 1984; Rosenbek and LaPointe, 1985). Aten *et al.* (1984) reviewed the reported efficacy of palatal lifts in the improvement of resonance and carried out their own investigation. A group of 16 dysarthric patients with severe articulation, respiratory and voice problems were given palatal prostheses and then evaluated perceptually by a panel of judges. There was considerable disparity of opinion upon the improvement of speech intelligibility but general agreement that there was a reduction in nasality. These authors considered that palatal prostheses with wire connectors were better than the traditional solid acrylic bulb prosthesis.

Tudor and Selley (1974) described a palatal training device (PTA) and a visual speech aid for use in the treatment of hypernasality. The palatal device is a simple removable intraoral appliance not to be confused with a palatal lift prosthesis. The PTA is made for the individual patient by a dental surgeon. It consists of a 'U'-shaped wire with the open ends embedded in an acrylic dental plate. The wire has to be adjusted so that it only just touches the palate (Selley, 1979, 1985). This palatal training device is worn throughout the day and removed at night.

The Exeter visual speech aid (VSA) allows rapid visual feedback of soft palate movements. The patient can confirm visually that the soft palate is moving when phonating vowels and thus bring movement under voluntary control. The VSA, like the PTA, consists of a removable dental plate carrying a pair of insulated electrodes which just touch the soft palate in the region of the maximum lift. The wires from the VSA are connected to a control box with a small lamp which lights up when the palate is lowered and touches the wires, and goes out when the palate is raised. The VSA is used for periods of practice only and under supervision of the speech therapist, but the PTA is worn continuously during the day. The PTA and VSA provide very successful treatment for isolated cases of velopharyngeal malfunction (Curle, 1979; Selly, 1985).

Dysphagia

Swallowing problems arising in some patients with neurological dysphonia can be helped by the speech therapist following careful assessment of the oral, oral preparatory and pharyngeal phases of swallowing. Videofluoroscopy clearly images the movement of the bolus for assessment purposes. Encouragement is given in assuming correct posture, lip-closure, chewing and tongue movements. Advice concerning diet and the consistency of food can be given. This specialised management comes outside the problem of dysphonia. Suggested reading is an excellent article by Enderby (1984) and the book by Logemann (1983a).

The palatal training device already described can also improve swallowing and reduce drooling (Curle, 1979; Selley, 1985). It has been demonstrated over a period of many years that this treatment materially assists stroke patients with certain types of swallowing difficulties and drooling, besides hypernasality. The treatment also assists in the retention of dentures by strengthening the oral musculature. A stroke patient discharged from hospital, for example, was causing grave concern at home on account of swallowing difficulties and refusal of food. He was rescued by his speech therapist and transferred to Selley's care. With intensive use of PTA and VSA his swallowing improved and he was able to eat adequate meals and return home.

The rehabilitation of oral and palatopharyngeal musculature has a hope of success in restoring partial function and compensatory muscle movement in many acquired neurological conditions. In progressive disease such as amyotrophic lateral sclerosis it is doubtful whether swallowing strategies can delay the ultimate necessity for nasogastric feeding.

Parkinson's Disease: Speech Therapy

It has long been recognised that patients with Parkinson's disease can imitate and execute speech exercises under a speech therapist's supervision with success but that there is no carry-over in conversation (Greene and Watson, 1968). As a result, doctors and neurologists have regarded speech therapy as useless and have failed to refer patients for assessment. The situation has improved considerably since the foundation of the Parkinson's Disease Society and promotion of better understanding of these patients. The Society campaigns for services which improve the quality of life, including physio-, occupational and speech therapy. The funding of research which demonstrates the value of speech therapy has been a valuable contribution in creating a more positive attitude to therapy (Robertson and Thomson, 1984).

Speech festination and prosody

The voice of the Parkinson's disease patient is breathy and lacks volume. Articulation is affected by muscular rigidity; breathing is irregular and initiation of speech may be a problem. The analysis of such features is largely irrelevant when speech is severely impaired since the main obstacle to intelligibility is the festination of speech. A remark starts clearly but all motor aspects become limited in range, accelerate and trail into an almost inaudible mumble of poorly differentiated sound. It is now accepted that lack of rhythm, stress and intonation resulting in dysprosody is the most conspicuous handicap. If speed and rhythm of utterance can be controlled, other features also improve and fall into place (Mueller, 1971; Scott and Caird, 1981, 1983; Scott, Caird and Williams, 1984).

The preservation and retrieval of prosody therefore is a primary aim. To this end many visual feedback strategies are used: Visipitch and Visispeech present patterns of intonation and tempo.

Delayed auditory feedback (DAF) in selected cases was found to be efficacious in slowing festinant speech by two patients in a sample of 11 patients suffering from Parkinson's disease (Downie, Low and Lindsay, 1981). The constant use of a portable body-worn DAF device was necessary to sustain speech improvement and intelligibility.

Scott and Caird (1981, 1983) reported substantial improvement in vocal volume, quality and rate using the Vocalite training device. Prosody was little improved. The Vocalite only lights up when the voice is loud enough. It can be used for improvement of vocal strength and monitoring of rhythm and speed of vocalisation but not pitch change. The Voice Loudness Indicator described in Chapter 7 serves a similar purpose.

Auditory perception

Greene and Watson (1968) found that patients capable of operating the switch on a pocket amplifier were helped by amplification. One patient explained that he was able to hear himself better. This appears to be a crucial feature in parkinsonism. There is a fading of the proprioceptive, kinaesthetic and auditory feedback essential in automatic self-monitoring of speech production. The strategies found successful by Scott and Greene dealt with this failure in auditory perception.

Kinaesthetic perception

In this context the observation of Liberman (1957) in his research into how the individual perceives and discriminates speech signals are pertinent. Liberman found that in learning new and unfamiliar speech patterns the normal person has to say over to himself these patterns. Liberman states, 'Speech is perceived by reference to articulation, that is, that the articulatory movements and their sensory effects mediate between the acoustic stimulus and the event we call perception'. The individual mimes orally what is heard, then responds to the articulatory movements and the proprioceptive and tactile stimulus. Liberman reverses the long-accepted view regarding the primary importance of acoustic stimuli in recognition of speech and suggests that perception is actually more closely related to articulation than is the acoustic stimulus itself. The speech therapist who doubts this may recall the difficulty as a student in perceiving the unfamiliar sound combinations of the phonetics lecturer and the need to mime or repeat the necessary articulatory movements to be analysed. Visual clues from watching the phonetician's mouth were also important. The sight of students mouthing to themselves as they write phonetic transcriptions and descriptions recalls the oral gesture theory of the origin of language put forward by Paget in 1930.

Impairment of kinaesthetic feedback would account for the success of many different approaches to the improvement of prosody. Methods which succeed in the Parkinson's disease patient self-monitoring speech will bring about improvement.

Intensive therapy

The long-term benefits of instruction depend upon intensive courses of speech therapy. Robertson and Thomson (1984) arranged an intensive daily, 2 week course of speech therapy on a hospital out-patient basis. Group sessions were devoted to teaching respiratory capacity and control, voice production with emphasis on intonation, volume, rate and articulation. Video-recording was used and played back for comment and discussion among patients, which stimulated communication. In many cases this had been reduced to a minimum. Facial expression and social awareness improved. Patients became motivated as a result of group activity which was a strong determinant in their improvement. Most encouraging was the fact that improvement following this course lasted for 3 months and in some cases speech continued to improve without further speech therapy. Stones and Drake (1984) also reported the success of an intensive 2 week course of therapy for Parkinson's disease patients.

The importance of maintaining facial communication and correcting the mask-like expression of the Parkinson's disease patient is stressed by this study. Scott, Caird and Williams (1985) have described the beneficial effect of proprioceptive neuromuscular facilitation (PNF) in this respect (see p. 285).

Cerebral Palsy

The cerebral palsied child does not suffer from discrete symptoms related to any one form of neurological lesion. Diffuse cerebral damage produces composite forms of motor disorder although spasticity or athetosis, for example, may predominate. For this reason a general approach to therapy based on assessment of each individual child's difficulties is advisable rather than attempting the treatment of refined neurological symptoms of flaccid, spastic, hypo- and hyperkinetic, ataxic etc.

Treatment of dysarthria in children must differ radically from that of the adult with acquired neurological damage who has had established motor speech patterns pre-morbidly. The adult knows what speech movements are necessary and has the memory of old patterns against which to match the new. The child, however, has to learn from the beginning and by imitating what is heard learns to accommodate the motor deficiencies. On the other hand, time is on the child's side and great gains may come from maturation of the nervous system and the tide of growth and chronological development.

Team approach

The physiotherapist and speech therapist need to work together, literally side by side, establishing relaxation, the best posture and the respiratory coordination and controlled movements which form the basis of voice work. But how often is the ideal of physiotherapy and speech therapy and 'the team approach' stressed in teaching and how often neglected in practice? The cerebral palsied child requires assessment by neurologist and pyschologist, psychiatrist, paediatrician and otologist, whose explanations and advice need always to be available and give direction to the practical work of the physiotherapist, speech therapist and teacher. Too often ortho-education is practised in isolation by the experts, struggling in ignorance of the contributions made by other team members.

This team approach must include the child's parents as in the early years they are the prime movers – the chief teachers. They need enormous support, supervision and guidance so that they do not over-protect the child and reduce effort. Alternatively, unrealistic expectations aggravate the child's sense of failure and difference from normal children.

Realistic aims

Levitt (1962) in her realistic and practical book on physiotherapy in cerebral palsy advocates combining the best techniques from all the seemingly conflicting methods of physical treatment for cerebral palsy, most of which have value in some but not all conditions. She believes it is wrong to impose the aim of normalcy on children with incurable lesions. The aim is adequate function with as good a pattern of movement as is possible for each individual child. Levitt's remarks are as valid for speech and voice as for locomotion and posture. Insisting upon normality imposes anxiety on all concerned and introduces harmful emotional factors into the educational picture owing to discouragement due to failure and extreme frustration. Ingram (1960) also commented on the dangers of speech therapy with these children.

The child must receive encouragement and experience success. Guidance must be given in the acquisition of new speech skills, and help provided in the passage from one developmental milestone to the next when each particular child is physiologically ready to take the next step.

Infant development

With regard to voice and speech the encouragement of vocalisation and babbling in infancy is of prime importance. The speech therapist who is in touch with the mother or carer must emphasise the importance of the early developmental stages of vocalisation, the emergence of cooing and the melodic changes and importance of talking while playing with the infant.

Rehabilitation philosophies

There are various schools of thought regarding the best method of treatment for cerebral palsy and each claims to obtain the best results. Progress is dependent upon the severity of the condition, the intelligence and hearing both of which may be normal or impaired. Time and maturation are on the child's side and some severely handicapped children exceed all early expectations. In this the mother is really the key to success when given sensible guidance.

The Bobath method: reflex inhibition

The Bobath method based on reflex inhibition for eliciting speech has also been described by Marland (1953) and Mysak (1959b). Desensitisation of the oral zone is recommended. Facilitation of phonation follows with the child in a supine position with flexed abducted knees, with shoulders fixed on the therapist's arm and head prevented from falling back. Voicing is elicited by vibrating the chest with the therapist's other hand while the therapist vocalises the desired sound for the child to imitate. After a period, vocalisation follows. Efficient respiratory patterns must be developed. Facilitated babbling along the lines of motokinaesthetic speech training first described by Young and Hawk (1955) may be introduced.

Reverse breathing and inspiratory phonation are corrected by some physiotherapists by the following method which the speech therapist can adopt also. It comprises components of reflex inhibition and reflexology advocated by Mysak (1968).

1. Roll child over on back, giving support to neck and shoulders on therapist's arm. Knees are brought up to chest. Expiration takes place as diaphragm ascends under tensed and compressed abdominal muscles.
2. Child now on back, knees up, inhales as therapist extends child's legs.
3. Child rolls up again breathing out, straightens legs and inspires, synchronising respiration with movement and obtaining slow easy rhythm.
4. Vocalising on the expiratory phase follows, imitating therapist.
5. Next stage: place the child in rest position on couch, back, head and neck supported on cushions. While the therapist's hand on the lower chest guides respiratory movement, vowels are emitted.
6. Prolonged vowels, coos, glides and babbling in different rhythms are imitated.

The British Association of Bobath Trained Therapists (BABTT) was founded in March 1988 and can provide further information.

The Peto method: conductive education

Conductive education for cerebral palsied children was devised by Professor Peto of Budapest who founded the Institute for Conductive Education of the Motor Disabled and Conductors' College in 1945. An experiment using conductive education with a group of very severely athetoid children was carried out in 1966 at the Lady Zia Warner Centre in Luton, England, under the auspices of the Spastic Society and the Luton and Dunstable Spastics Group. Ester Cotton, physiotherapist, and Margaret Parnewell, occupational therapist, were in charge of the treatment (Cotton, 1965). The experiment lasted 9 months. Two psychologists who tested the children after 7 months did not note improvement in intelligence, which was never claimed, but Cotton and Parnewell noted considerable progress in functions not tested by the psychologists, i.e. self-help, communication, socialisation, general and fine motor control. The children had been selected on account of their failure to respond to traditional training and education in the nursery and school groups at the Centre.

Some of the Peto principles are observed in centres such as Cheyney Walk in London, England (Miller, 1972) but the great strength of the method is the concentration and cohesion incorporated in the Conductor herself who acts as physio-, occupational and speech therapist, and teacher and nurse to a small group of children. All activities are taught by the highly trained graduate Conductor so that no conflicting therapies are applied. The training and maintenance of an institute is, of course, very expensive hence the absence of such facilities and lack of interest in England and elsewhere. Recently, however, a group of British parents have been accepted for a period of instruction at the Budapest Institute.

To understand the Peto educational system, an excellent account is provided by Cottam and Sutton (1986) which also gives sources of present on-going research. The aim of conductive education is to enable cerebral palsied children to achieve total physical independence. It is based on the teaching of Pavlov and of Luria (1961, 1966) who described the connection between speech and active movement. A simple example of the principle involved is that a small child told to squeeze a bulb in his hand cannot do so, but can initiate the movement if he says 'go – go'.

Rhythmical intention is the method by which children perform movements in specific and general training programmes. Rhythmical speech and counting reinforce actions and new movement patterns are learned reflexly (Pavlov) in conjunction with the 'second signalling system', meaning speech (Luria). Treatment is functional in that it teaches repetitively and intensively and is intrinsic to all daily activities. The conductive institute accepts pre-school children and prepares them for normal school. Not all applicants are accepted. Children are resident and much of their exercise is executed on plinths, on which they sleep at night, as do the Conductors.

Proprioceptive neuromuscular facilitation (PNF)

Mysak (1968) it seems first drew attention to the therapeutic implications of oropharyngeal reflexology. In central and peripheral types of dysarthria the vegetative reflexes (swallowing, gagging etc.) may be diminished or exaggerated. The excitation of desired reflex actions which have disappeared can be developed in some cases by appropriate stimulation such as stroking the back of the tongue with a spatula. Mysak postulated that a particular chain of synaptic connections could be developed, established and brought under voluntary control.

Kabat and Knott (1953) further developed techniques for therapeutic reflexology and coined the term 'proprioceptive neuromuscular facilitation'. The account of PNF by Voss, Ionta and Myers (1985) is accepted as the standard reference on the subject. Knott and Voss (1968) produced a book on the philosophy and practice of PNF. Since then their methods have been used in treatment of neuromuscular disorders by physiotherapists and speech therapists in the UK. The basic principle is that of increasing the excitability of neurones by bombarding them with impulses which facilitate movement of paralysed muscles. A practising speech therapist's account of management of swallowing disorders using PNF methods is given by Langley (1988).

Stimulation is achieved by icing, brushing and manipulation of muscle stretch and resistance. 'Slow' icing, uses a slow, rhythmic stroking of lips and tongue to reduce spasticity. Sucking an ice cube before eating facilitates swallowing. Ice packs applied to the thyroid prominence can facilitate voice, the subject being exhorted to cough, to produce vowel sounds and to count.

'Fast' icing, in which flicks with an ice cube are administered, can be applied to lips or cheeks and is helpful in flaccid paralysis. The treatment may help parkinsonian patients (Scott, Caird and Williams, 1985).

Recourse to PNF techniques should not be instituted by therapists without the knowledge and acquiescence of medical and nursing staff. Ideally, treatment should be in collaboration with physiotherapists. Speech scientists state that there is no objective evidence of the beneficial results of PNF methods. However, this criticism is aimed at all types of alternative medicine. Experienced speech therapists and physiotherapists report that the method often produces improvement in muscle function. Therefore on pragmatic grounds no speech therapist should withhold PNF because of lack of scientific proof. If all medical treatment had to rely on evidence of cure, it would be a sorry outlook indeed for many patients.

Therapy for Spasmodic Adductor Dysphonia (SAD)

In view of the difficulties in diagnosis between spastic conversion dysphonia and spasmodic adductor dysphonia a course of speech therapy of no less than

3 months should be prescribed. The laryngologist's opinion and those of a neurologist and psychiatrist should be sought when speech therapy fails to cure the spasm and SAD needs confirmation.

In view, also, of the fact that many patients after RLN section are often not satisfied with their voices and also suffer recurrence of laryngeal spasm after some time, speech therapy is mandatory. The hope is that with reduction of involuntary adductor spasm, vocal efficiency will improve. The patient's comfort and confidence may so improve in communication that surgery will not be deemed necessary.

Voice therapy

The aim of therapy is to minimise spasm by relaxation of the mental set, general bodily tension and laryngeal tension.

1. Easy, relaxed and rhythmic breathing must be established. The respiratory muscles are generally involved with laryngeal spasm not necessarily as part of the neurological involvement but as a result of the endeavour to force air through the locked vocal folds.
2. A relaxed posture of the head, neck and shoulders must be established.
3. Laryngeal relaxation can be encouraged by gentle massage of the extrinsic laryngeal muscles. With finger and thumb placed on the thyroid wings and with lowered chin, gentle circular movements free tension in the hyoid region especially and relieve the aching throat (Aronson, 1980).
4. Phonation should be attempted on a sigh, /h/ plus vowels, e.g. 'ha-ho-hee', 'hm-hm' etc. Progress from one stage to another should not be made until the earlier exercise is achieved without laryngeal spasm. A soft breathy attack having been obtained, serial speech can be used to begin the process of generalisation.

Many patients, especially those who do not depend on speech in their professions, will be satisfied with the improvement in the voice. Rehabilitation appears also to arrest vocal deterioration and the dysphonia may remain static. On the other hand it is arguable that only those patients with a mild and stable form of adductor spasm benefit from speech therapy. The enigma of 'spastic dysphonia' is by no means solved and much further research and follow-up of patients over years is necessary.

Recurrent laryngeal nerve section

Serious discussion with the patient contemplating nerve section is necessary: the nature of the operation, the slight scarring of the throat, hospitalisation etc. must be explained. Also, the prospect of vocal recovery has to be discussed (Dedo and Shipp, 1980). No patient after operation has a completely normal voice although many patients think voice is normal. In many cases patients complain of vocal weakness and notice that they cannot raise vocal volume against background noise. Occasionally there is slight diplophonia or creak.

Dedo and Shipp regard postoperative speech therapy as essential. The speech therapist should visit the patient as soon as possible on the same day after surgery to give reassurance that all is well. The throat will be painful and pain may extend to the back of the neck and the chest due to insertion of the laryngoscope. There may be alarming difficulty in swallowing, and choking episodes aggravated by inefficient coughing due to adductor inadequacy. That this is a good sign for phonatory recovery can be explained. The voice may be very good or very poor at this stage; it tends to be at its worst on the second or third day after surgery followed then by steady improvement.

A vocal tremor is present in some 15–20% of patients and this may not be obvious before operation but more noticeable when the spasm is eradicated. The neurological symptom of tremor consists of minute fluctuations in vocal volume. It is not a very noticeable feature in speech. Tremor is mostly conspicuous on prolonged vowels and in singing which the patient is unlikely to accomplish with or without tremor when suffering from a paralysed cord.

In order to strengthen the voice, if phonasthenia after RLN section is pronounced, the forcing exercises described in Chapter 16 may be used in moderation. If these fail, Teflon injection can be given to increase the bulk of the operated fold. There is a danger that over-compensation will take place. Some Teflon can be removed by opening up the vocal fold and removal with a cusp or a laser beam may be possible. This is just as well, since in the case of recurrence of adductor spasm symptom, withdrawal of Teflon will alleviate the over-adduction of the vocal folds.

Throughout management of every case of SAD and at every stage of treatment, high fidelity voice and speech recordings should be made. These should follow a set format including vowel prolongation, counting, highest and lowest notes possible and reading of a set passage. The tape is used for assessment and treatment and is a very necessary permanent record of vocal history. Acoustic analysis, using the Voiscope and Sona-Graph if available, can support the perceptual assessments.

Apraxic Dysphonia

Laryngeal dysfunction is only one aspect of oral apraxia in which purposeful movements of tongue, lips, pharynx and cheeks may be affected. The patient is unable to execute learned, skilled movement although motor strength and coordination are adequate. Therapy, therefore, is based on a hierarchy ranging from reflexive laryngeal function, such as a cough or laugh, to exercises involving increasing laryngeal control (Halpern, 1981). Voluntary phonation is stabilised only gradually and treatment sessions should be frequent, possibly two or three times a day in the first days of treatment, for maximum effectiveness.

1. The patient who is unable to initiate phonation for speech because of apraxia should be encouraged to prolong a laryngeal sound as elicited by coughing or laughing. Involuntary adduction of the vocal folds, unaffected by dyspraxia, is achieved.

2. Imitation of the therapist saying /ɑː/ while sitting facing the patient should be facilitated by providing a clear visual and auditory model.
3. Kinaesthetic feedback can be provided by the patient feeling the therapist's laryngeal vibrations and then placing finger tips on his own larynx. The therapist may need to present the target sound repeatedly but must be careful to observe any sign of increasing frustration on the part of the patient if progress is slow.
4. Some patients are encouraged to phonate more easily by singing familiar songs and by imitating automatic and serial speech.
5. As laryngeal activity comes increasingly under voluntary control it is integrated into syllables and practised in a structural progression (Dabul and Bollier, 1976; Halpern, 1981). With improvement, the patient who is not voicing appropriately will frequently respond well to the therapist indicating the larynx when voicing is required.
6. Nasal consonants are elicited by placing the finger tips on the side of the nose, and fricatives by feeling the oral air stream on the hand. Comparison of vowels and diphthongs can be presented.

The presentation of target sounds should also have a hierarchical structure. A suggested pattern might be as follows:

1. The therapist says the sound or word; the patient and therapist repeat the sound in unison. When there is a high success rate the next step can be taken.
2. The therapist says the sound or word; the patient repeats it alone.
3. Following high achievement the target is presented in written form. Therapist and patient say the target together; with progress the therapist withdraws.

Audio tapes are helpful and allow the patient to work alone. In the early stages of treatment particularly, the patient will benefit from seeing the therapist's lip movement for articulatory placement. Articulograms (diagrams of articulatory positions) provide useful guidance.

Melodic intonation therapy (Sparks and Holland, 1976; Sparks, 1981) is another approach used successfully in the treatment of apraxia and for improving the prosodic aspects of speech. It is also used successfully in the treatment of cerebral palsied children (Alvin, 1961). A hierarchy of four levels beginning with humming the melodies of phrases and sentences accompanied by hand-tapping is clearly defined by Sparks. Dysprosody is improved by various strategies using musical instruments, especially drums, and audio tapes of rhythms and chants.

Visual presentation of intonation and rhythm on Visispeech, Visipitch and Voiscope (laryngograph) provide excellent feedback and monitoring of the therapist's patterns fixed on the screen (see 'Treatment of the deaf').

The complexities and divergence of opinion concerning apraxia of speech and the theoretical basis of treatment is too complex for extended discussion in a text on voice disorders. It is sufficient to say that apraxia, with or without laryngeal involvement, may occur and that for further information the reader should refer to the work of authorities such as Dabul and Bollier (1976), Rosenbek and LaPointe (1985) and Edwards (1984).

Case history

It is unusual to have referred an adult of almost 30 years suffering from congenital speech problems not previously assessed, diagnosed or treated.

A herdsman was referred by the laryngologist with the report that the patient suffered from injected vocal cords due to heavy smoking. The man's chief complaint was that he could not formulate his words properly and was embarrassed by the handicap socially. The laryngologist thought that the real worry was that it cramped the man's style with the ladies and perhaps he needed 'elocution' lessons, not speech therapy.

The herdsman was tall and good-looking, well-dressed and well-mannered. His speech came as a shock, totally out of keeping with his appearance. He spoke in a broad dialect reminiscent of a Buckinghamshire accent. As a boy, his family had moved from London to Cambridgeshire and later to Wiltshire. Perhaps he had picked up one of these regional accents or mixed up all three? He had been teased at school about his speech and had articulation difficulties. He was increasingly unhappy and self-conscious about his speech especially as he had become honorary secretary to the local National Federation of Young Farmers' Clubs. Having to speak at committee meetings was an ordeal. He loved animals and his job but thought that with poor pay and the speech of a yokel he would never get married. He was a sincere and stable individual with no 'psychogenic' reason for his speech disorder.

His speech was hypernasal. He spoke with closed teeth and tense jaws. Articulation of consonants was slurred, inaccurate and inconsistent, e.g. /b/ = /mb/ or /m/, /cʃ/ = /ʃ/ or /s/. Consonants in clusters were often omitted. Vowels were inaccurate and inconsistent, e.g. /i:/ might be /oi/ or /ɑi/; /oi/ might be /ɑi/ or /ou/ besides being nasalised.

There were no signs of language disorder; his grammar and choice of words were those of an educated man. He had been rather slow at school and had left at 16 years.

He embarked upon a weekly course of speech therapy with patience and dedication. A programme of hearing training, contrasting the therapist's pronunciation with his own and using practice tapes for work during the week. Perception was poor at first but rapidly improved. Relaxation of jaw, lips and tongue resulting in open articulation reduced nasality.

Work on articulation improved accuracy of single consonants but attempts at consonant clusters confused him and he was unable to produce these correctly, seeming not to know where to place his tongue. However, by listening at home to short phrases and repeating in a relaxed way, this aspect of speech also improved. Repetition of phrases with varied intonation and stress improved dysprosody.

After a year's hard work, speech was almost normal and his crowning success was the delivery of a talk on 'Recruitment and publicity' to the Young Farmer's Club which 'went down very well'.

Hearing Loss

Deafness in children is, in the UK, the province of teachers of the deaf. They are responsible for training mothers in the early months how best to stimulate speech development. Teachers of the deaf are also responsible for education of hard of hearing and severely deaf children when of school age.

Voice therapy

Latterly, speech therapists have been invited to help with the voice problems associated with severe deafness. The use of visual display instruments (Voiscope, Visispeech etc.) are invaluable in teaching self-perceptual skills and subsequently self-monitoring of prosodic patterns (Parker, 1974; Pronovost, 1977; Wirz, 1986) and arrest of monopitch. Once imitation of prosodic visual patterns can be imitated using biofeedback much time must be devoted to producing target responses without visual feedback. Over reliance upon the instrumentation may lead to failure in establishing good habits in spontaneous speech.

Individual vowels and diphthongs present clearly distinct differences in harmonic structure on the SonaGraph display. Vowel accuracy can be improved which is far more difficult than consonant production. Vowels and diphthongs present less distinct tactile, kinaesthetic and visual sensory feedback. Rhythmic improvement is also an important aspect of teaching and shown up on the screen. The linking of segments and their separation and timing in short phrases are further aspects necessary in remediation.

Hypernasality

The quality of the deaf voice is quickly identified and is sometimes described as hollow and harsh, but hypernasality is also a characteristic feature. This is due to formation of a cul-de-sac resonator by raising of the back of the tongue and excessive pharyngeal tension. Palatal movement is normal and there is no audible nasal escape.

Spectrography

Spectrography displays may be used since there are positive differences to be perceived between normal and deaf speakers. In the deaf there is amplification of the higher frequencies in speech (Wirz, Subtelny and Whitehead, 1979). The assessment of vocal quality at the laryngeal, supralaryngeal and subglottal levels using the Vocal Profile Analysis (VPA) is discussed by Wirz (1986). The analysis highlights the chief loci of tension.

Excessive vocal volume is another common fault in deaf speech. Volume meters have long been used by teachers of the deaf to monitor speech by watching a digital meter or a column of light.

Speech therapy must not rely entirely upon biofeedback techniques. Relaxation of the articulatory and laryngeal muscles may be necessary to improve vocal quality and reduce nasality. Breathing patterns may also need attention (Parker, 1974).

Delayed pubertal voice change, which is discussed in Chapter 11, is a problem in some male adolescents.

Cochlear implantation in deafened people

The cochlear implant procedure involves the implant of an electrode in the cochlear which creates a sensation of sound in severely deafened individuals with acquired deafness. It is unsuitable for children and for congenitally deaf adults. Success relies upon the survival of some nerve fibres in the cochlear, though the hair cells may have died. A microphone picks up noise at ear level and a lead transfers the stimulus to a sound processor box worn on the body. Sound is converted into a radio signal which is then transmitted to the single channel electrode within the ear.

The single channel system has been devised by Fraser (1987) in conjunction with the Department of Physics and Bioengineering and the Phonetics Department, University College, London, and the Royal National Institute for the Deaf, with financial help from the Sir Jules Thorn Trust. The system does not provide pitch discrimination but volume levels at a frequency of 500 Hz. The device costs £600. A four channel device which is capable of pitch extraction has been developed by Professor Adrian Fourcin in the Department of Phonetics, University of London. It is exceedingly costly and beyond the means of any National Health resource.

The single channel implant has proved to be of great benefit to carefully selected individuals. The age, alertness and ability to profit from the implant and make the most of limited restoration of auditory sensation has to be very carefully assessed. Support from the medical team, from otologist to social worker, teacher of the deaf and speech therapist is essential for successful rehabilitation. Fraser emphasises that cochlear implantation is 'more than just an operation'.

The improved hearing results in increased confidence as social interaction no longer relies on lip-reading alone and the individual is able to become part of the social scene. Self-monitoring of vocal volume is improved. Speech deterioration is arrested and in many cases speech improves considerably (Cowie, Douglas-Cowie and Kerr, 1982). The cochlear implant acoustic system is no benefit, however, in understanding speech against background noise which bombards the ears with unselected noise.

Heath (1987) has been active in publicising the needs of deafened individuals, some of whom have started going deaf in adolescence. Herself deafened in middle age, she has derived great benefit from a cochlear implant. The National Association of Deafened People (NADP) was formed in 1984 with Jack Ashley MP as President. This provides a support and information service. It is devoted to the promotion and development of better technical systems in rapidly developing technology.

Heath found from a questionnaire sent to members of NADP that many adults had received very little help when deafened in adult life. Speech therapists had not become engaged in pre- or postcochlear transplant rehabilitation. Thus we make a strong plea to therapists to seek out these people and give them the benefit of their expertise. Handling the depression and lack of confidence attendant upon hearing handicap is necessary. Making best use of the vestigial hearing restored to the deafened is important but not the only approach to rehabilitation.

For addresses of the British Societies for neurological disorders see Appendix III at the end of the book.

Chapter 16
Laryngeal Palsy

Vagus nerve pathway

The vagus (tenth cranial nerve), which supplies all the muscles of the larynx, has an interesting course which must be known if damage to the nerve pathways at different levels is to be understood in terms of laryngeal paralysis. Some of the fibres originate in the medulla in the nucleus ambiguus while others originate at a higher level. Fibres from the upper section of the nucleus ambiguus join the glossopharyngeal nerve (ninth cranial nerve) and those from the inferior portion join the accessory cranial nerve (eleventh cranial) (Gray, 1949). These nerves, the ninth, tenth and eleventh cranial nerves, are so intimately connected in the medulla that all the muscles supplied by them are frequently involved either equally or progressively in lesions of the medulla oblongata. For this reason Walshe (1952) groups them together in pathological conditions affecting the nucleus ambiguus in what he terms the 'glossopharyngeal-accessorius complex'. Nuclear lesions of the vagus must be associated, therefore, with paralysis of the palate, tongue and larynx.

Laryngeal innervation

The vagus forms a flat cord from its many united filaments and leaves the skull through the jugular foramen and passes vertically down the neck within the carotid sheath. The superior laryngeal nerve branches off from the vagus at the ganglion nodosum (inferior ganglion) below the level of the jugular foramen and subdivides into the internal and external superior laryngeal nerves. The internal branch of the superior laryngeal nerve consists of both sensory and secretomotor fibres. The external branch of the superior laryngeal nerve provides the motor supply to the cricothyroid muscle (see Chapter 3).

The left and right recurrent laryngeal nerves supply the rest of the muscles of the larynx. They differ significantly with regard to their origin and pathway (Figure 16.2). The right recurrent laryngeal nerve arises from the main trunk of the vagus in front of the subclavian artery. The left recurrent laryngeal nerve arises from the vagus at the arch of the aorta round which it winds before ascending to the larynx. On account of its extensive course the left recurrent nerve is more liable to injury than the right, and is especially vulnerable to

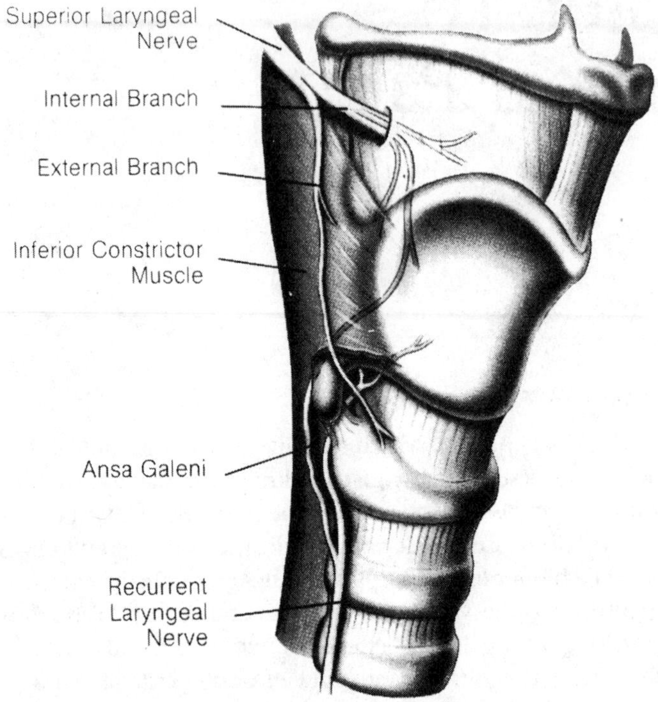

Figure 16.1. Distribution of recurrent laryngeal nerve (lateral view).

pressure from aortic aneurysm. The left vocal fold is affected twice as frequently as the right in laryngeal palsy.

The recurrent laryngeal nerves on both sides ascend the groove between the trachea and oesophagus for a variable distance in different individuals and then divide into anterior and posterior branches before entering the larynx behind the cricothyroid articulation. The recurrent laryngeal nerves are especially vulnerable in the operation of thyroidectomy below the level of their entry into the larynx.

On account of the distribution of the superior and recurrent laryngeal nerves the fact to remember is that in order to produce a total paralysis of the larynx on one side, the lesion must occur at, or above, the level of the ganglion nosodum before the superior laryngeal nerve branches off from the vagus. This means that in lesions involving the recurrent laryngeal nerves the cricothyroid muscle will be spared. Nuclear lesions of the vagus already described in connection with bulbar palsies are caused by a variety of pathological conditions: multiple sclerosis, medullary tumours, focal thrombosis, encephalitis lethargica, tabes dorsalis and chronic bulbar palsy. Poliomyelitis (Bosma, 1953) is also a possible cause of a lesion since it confines itself to focal infection of motor nerve cells in the brainstem and spinal cord. Damage to the nucleus ambiguus may result in complete laryngeal paralysis as it involves both superior and recurrent laryngeal nerves.

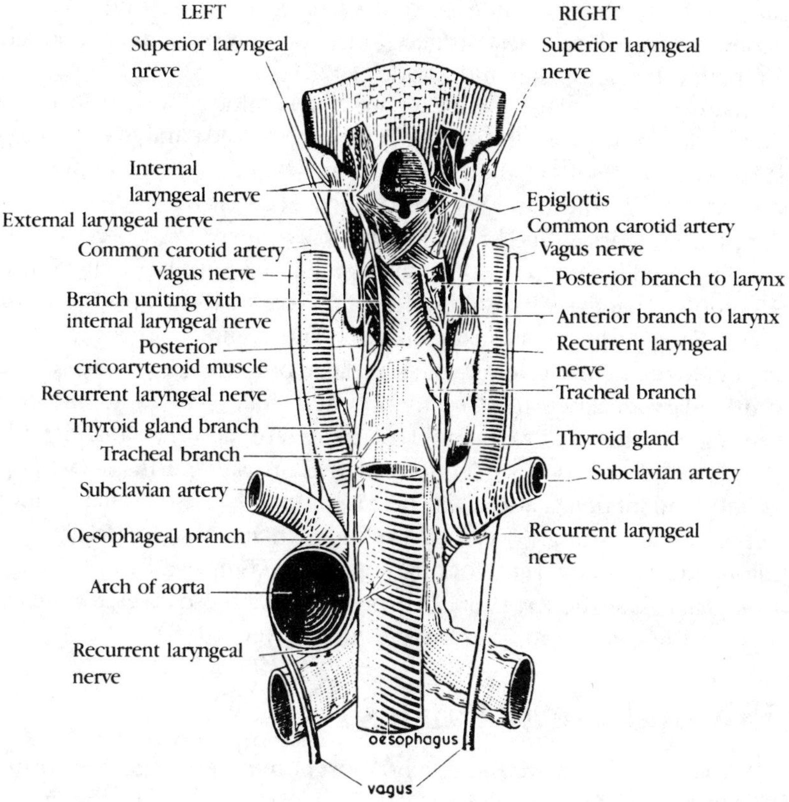

Figure 16.2. Posterior view of the larynx showing the distribution of the left and right laryngeal nerves.

Causes of RLN Damage

- Pressure from tumours in the neck or apex of the lungs, enlarged bronchial glands, enlarged thyroid gland, aortic aneurysm, mitral stenosis and enlarged left auricle. Enlargement of the thyroid gland and penetration into the retro-oesophageal and tracheal areas can create pressure on the laryngeal nerve and thus impair function of the muscles. This is of rare occurrence according to Sonninen (1960). He reported only one such case of laryngeal palsy due to compression preoperatively in a series of 131 patients. Patients may be referred with 'functional voice disorder' when suffering from real vocal weakness on account of organic diseases such as these.
- Trauma: external injuries such as gunshot wounds, or blows to the larynx in road traffic accidents. Lesions incurred during surgery, e.g. thyroidectomy.
- Endotracheal intubation, on account of the tube being too large or being left *in situ* for a prolonged period (Hahn, Martin and Lillie, 1970; Ellis and Pallister, 1975; Ellis and Bennett, 1977). Peripheral nerve damage may also occur when the RLN is compressed between the inflated endotracheal

tube cuff and the overlying thyroid cartilage (Cavo, 1985). Vocal fold paralysis may follow chest surgery but is probably due to endotracheal intubation (Hirano, Shin and Nozoe, 1977).

- Premature infants in intensive care are given endotracheal intubation and mechanical ventilation and can suffer from vocal fold paralysis and tracheal stenosis as a result of this life-saving procedure. (Cases of hereditary abductor vocal fold paralysis also occur - see below.)
- Peripheral neuritis and a temporary palsy may be caused by toxic conditions which prevent conveyance of nervous impulses to the muscles. A complete paralysis fixes the folds in the paramedian position in these cases. The condition is usually bilateral, and complete recovery is to be expected once the toxaemia subsides. Lead poisoning is a toxic condition causing laryngeal neuritis. Commonly cited examples of systemic disease causing neuritis and vocal fold paralysis are diphtheria and typhoid (Musgrove, 1952). Virus infections such as measles, pertussis (whooping cough) and influenza also cause neuritis. Acute localised inflammation in herpes zoster (shingles) can also reduce efficiency of the RLN.
- Idiopathic: congenital and/or unknown cases comprise 14% of all cases of laryngeal palsy (Tucker, 1980). It is possible that these cases are caused by a central lesion (Ward, Hanson and Abeymayer, 1985).

Childhood Vocal Palsies

Vocal palsies in children are the second most common laryngeal abnormality of the newborn (Swift and Rogers, 1987). Cavanagh (1955) reviewed the available literature on the subject and reported upon her personal examination of 107 children. Thirty-seven of these children had laryngeal paralysis, most were unilateral but 10 were bilateral, some were congenital and others were acquired. A wide degree of variation in improvement of the airway and recovery of the vocal fold movement was noted. Of interest are her observations on those children with unilateral paralysis in which the healthy fold was seen to abduct three to five times to one abduction of the recovering fold. In several babies with congenital laryngeal stridor, one arytenoid was placed further forward than the other while the aryepiglottic fold on the affected side was usually rolled towards the midline and seemed shortened. Greene examined a 7-year-old boy with this condition which was accompanied by a unilateral palatal palsy on the opposite side to that of the affected fold. He had an inspiratory stridor on effort and when speaking, but no hypernasality.

Van Thal (1962) reported an interesting case of familial laryngeal palsy with four generations of aphonia in the same family. This report appears to be unique in the literature on the subject of congenital laryngeal palsy. Gacek (1976) has also reported cases of hereditary abductor vocal fold paralysis.

Types of Vocal Fold Palsy

The aetiology and duration of a unilateral paralysis will affect the voice which varies according to the position of the paralysed fold and the effectiveness of compensation achieved by the mobile fold (Ward, Hanson and Abeymayer, 1985).

The inefficient closure of the glottis associated with most forms of laryngeal palsy naturally affects phonation, swallowing and coughing. The voice is breathy and weak, and the inefficient laryngeal seal can result in food and liquid being aspirated into the trachea. Maximum phonation time is usually abnormally short and the lowest notes of the vocal range can no longer be produced (Hirano, 1981).

Phylogenetic Theory of Laryngeal Paralysis

In the past, interest concentrated upon the positions assumed by the vocal folds in paralysis and endeavoured to relate these to neurological laws. Felix Semon propounded an evolutionary explanation concerning abductor and adductor action of the recurrent laryngeal nerves. Sir Victor Negus, the great authority on the larynges of all creatures great and small, meticulously examined the problem in his classic *The Comparative Anatomy and Physiology of the Larynx* (1949). The end result of this most scholarly research was that the evidence supported Semon's law (Negus, 1931).

Semon was a great laryngologist of his time also. He treated the Prime Minister, Gladstone, for hoarseness. Queen Victoria complained that the leader of her Government always addressed her like a public meeting, which probably accounted for his dysphonia . . . (Hutzinga, 1966).

A further historical vignette supplied by Greene is that Sir Victor, who was an assessor of her first edition of *The Voice and its Disorders* (1956) for the College of Speech Therapists Fellowship, discussed laryngeal palsy. He informed her that as regards voice therapy, which he administered himself to his private patients, he disregarded palsy and achieved excellent results with humming exercises.

A comprehensive review of old controversies concerning the phylogeny of neurological damage in relation to vocal fold position and paralysis and paresis can be found in Capps (1958) Semon Lecture, Arnold (1957) and Dedo (1976).

The accepted view presently is a pragmatic one - that vocal fold paralysis and position is determined by site of lesion in the lower motor neurone. In the case of neck injuries and peripheral nerve damage, whether the superior laryngeal nerve (cricothyroid tensor) and/or the RLN is involved, produces differences in position and mobility. Being a lower motor neurone (LMN) lesion, muscles atrophy and are flaccid. As a result of the loss of muscle stiffness the consistency of the mucosa and muscle are similar. The normal mucosal wave of movement as a separate entity from the underlying muscle movement is lost and these components of the vocal fold vibrate as one according to Moore *et al.* (1987).

Positions of Paralysed Vocal Folds

(After Thomson, Negus and Bateman, 1955.)

- Median (adductor, phonatory and mid-line are synonymous with median): the fold adopts a position in the mid-line.
- Glottic chink: the folds are adducted but slack allowing minimal separation during respiration.
- Paramedian: the fold lies slightly to the side of the mid-line and if both are paralysed they are separated posteriorly by a distance of 3.5 mm or 4.0 mm.
- Intermediate (cadaveric): the cord lies in a position which is between paramedian and gentle abduction. The cord is slack and in the same position it assumes in the cadaver, hence the name.
- Gentle abduction: the cord is abducted further than in the cadaveric position, but not fully. This is the position in quiet respiration.
- Full abduction: the cord is abducted to its fullest limit. This position occurs in forced inspiration when the maximal airway is necessary.

The positions assumed by the vocal folds depend upon the damage suffered by the recurrent and superior laryngeal nerves: whether both or either nerves are involved bilaterally or unilaterally as already described. The glottic aperture and degree of flaccidity in the vocal fold determines the degree of breathiness and hoarseness (Casper, Cotton and Brewer, 1986). Aronson (1980) provides a clear account of the flaccid dysphonia problem in vagus nerve lesions. Luchsinger (1965a) analyses the vocal disorders in laryngeal paralysis (paralytic dysphonia) and dysfunction of inidivual muscles.

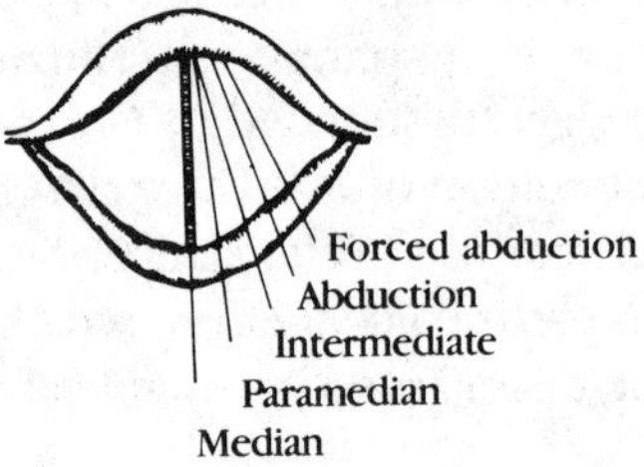

Figure 16.3. Vocal cord palsies: lines of orientation.

Superior RLN lesion

Paralysis of the cricothyroid muscle renders the vocal fold lax since approximation of the cartilages is impossible and the vocal folds cannot be stretched and elongated. At rest and during inspiration the fold may appear normal, but on phonation there is asymmetry of vibration and the paralysed fold is slightly lower than the healthy one. The fold is able to adduct but there is an anterior shift of the fold and the epiglottis to the healthy side presenting a characteristic askew appearance (Tucker, 1980), the 'oblique glottis' (Luchsinger, 1965a). The position of the paretic fold is either paramedian or intermediate, not median (Hirano, Shin and Nozoe, 1977). The voice may be weak and breathy but singing is seriously affected. Aphonia occurs in bilateral paralysis.

Recurrent laryngeal nerve lesion

Paralysis of the RLN affects the whole adductor and abductor phonatory mechanism. The paralysed fold assumes a paramedian position and is flaccid and bowed. The arytenoid cartilage tilts forward without the bracing action of the posterior cricoarytenoid. The interarytenoideus muscle, although having a double innervation, is weak and unable to assist in adduction. The altered voice quality is the result of the loss of mass and stiffness of the paralysed fold as the thyroarytenoid atrophies, in combination with the reduced resistance of the fold to the expiratory air stream and the loss of symmetry (Crumley and Izdebski, 1986). Stroboscopic examination shows an absence of the mucosal wave on the vocal fold which is evidence of a severely damaged fold and indicates poor prognosis (Hirano, Shin and Nozoe, 1977). The voice is hoarse and breathy. The healthy fold can compensate with the affected fold in time and the voice recovers strength considerably if not perfectly.

Bilateral abductor paralysis

If the abductor (posterior cricoarytenoid) is weak the adductors will hold the fold in the mid-line. In this case the voice will not be affected though there will be some inspiratory stridor in forceful breathing and the pitch range will suffer. A bilateral abductor paralysis with both folds in the mid-line is most frequently caused by total thyroidectomy (Singer, Hamaker and Miller, 1985). Bilateral vocal fold palsy is an unusual complication following intubation and is immediately recognisable by the acute onset of respiratory distress and stridor following extubation (Brandwein, Abramson and Shikowitz, 1986).

Although the voice is unimpaired, obstruction of the airway is a hazard in the event of respiratory infections. Lateralisation of one fold will be necessary unless the patient is too frail, in which case a flap-valve cannula can be worn. This 'speaking tube' preserves phonation.

Psychogenic abductor paresis

Occasionally patients may present with symptoms suggesting bilateral abductor vocal fold palsy which are subsequently found to be psychogenic. This condition has been termed 'Munchausen's stridor', 'factitious asthma' and 'emotional wheezing' (Myears *et al.*, 1985) and can be so severe that tracheotomy is performed. Fibreoptic laryngoscopy before and after sedation is proposed by Myears *et al.* (1985) as a method of determining differential diagnosis. They report that in their experience a conversion reaction of this type responds well to psychotherapy, speech therapy and relaxation.

Post-traumatic changes in vocal fold position

Vocal fold paralysis occurring after trauma can recover spontaneously and this must be awaited. Due to atrophy changes in the muscle fibres and partial recovery perhaps of some muscle bundles, the paralysed fold can shift laterallv.

1. The interarytenoideus muscle, being supplied by both right and left RLN, although weakened by unilateral palsy, does retain the possibility of adducting the fold towards the mid-line (from an intermediate to paramedian position). It does not atrophy like the other intrinsic laryngeal muscles and appears healthy and capable (Kirchner, 1983).
2. Atrophy of muscle tissue and fibrosis of the thyroarytenoid muscles shortens the fold and may alter position.
3. Continued tensor action of the cricothyroid muscle, if there is simply a lesion of the RLN, may also assist in medial movement of the fold.
4. The posterior cricoarytenoid is the sole abductor of the vocal fold and is in fact two muscles, the oblique and vertical fibres. Both may not be wholly impaired and the vertical muscle may retain some abductor action (Zemlin, Davis and Gaza, 1984).
5. Besides the propensity in many cases for the paralysed vocal fold to move towards the centre, the healthy fold has a natural tendency when unopposed by its opposite, to pass over the mid-line. This is known as compensation. The arytenoid of the healthy fold passes in front of the prolapsed (tilted) arytenoid of the paralysed vocal fold. The voice can become almost normal (Williams, Farquharson and Anthony, 1975).

Laryngeal Electromyography

Laryngeal electromyography (LEMG) is of great diagnostic value in assessment of the residual functional electrical potential of laryngeal muscles (Hiroto, Hirano and Tomita, 1968). The insertion of needle electrodes into individual muscle fibre bundles and unpredictably placed nerves is difficult and requires much experience. When accurate, the results pinpoint the site of nerve lesions distinguishing myopathy from neuropathy (Parnes and Satya-Murti, 1985) and mechanical fixation from immobility arising from vocal fold paralysis (Hirano, 1981). The degree and extent of paralysis is identifiable and the information provided is useful as a basis for various surgical procedures. To a certain extent prognostic information can be provided for evaluating future function (Hirose, 1985; Parnes and Satya-Murti, 1985). LEMG is also a means of distinguishing between organic and psychogenic disorders. The technique therefore can provide valuable guidelines for remedial speech therapy. The reader is referred to studies by Faaborg-Anderson and Nykobing (1965), Hirano, Shin and Nozoe (1977), and Hirose (1985).

Prognosis

Recovery from paralytic damage to the intrinsic muscles of the larynx is unpredictable as already stated. Recovery from nerve damage frequently takes place and should be given time, from 6 months to a year (Tucker, 1980). Hirano, Shin and Nozoe (1977) in examining the prognostic features of RLN paralysis found none of their group of 167 patients recovered after the 6-month period. Paralysis due to pressure or contusion of the RLN has the best chance of recovery. Intratracheal intubation paralysis has a good prognosis. Neuritis will also resolve and with disappearance of inflammation neuro-electric impulses can travel along the nerve pathway again. Post-influenza laryngeal paralysis can be expected to resolve quickly unless the nucleus has been knocked out, which is quite possible.

The more median the vocal fold position, the greater the action potential of the neuromotor unit and better the chance of spontaneous recovery. If EMG reveals some electrical activity during volitional phonation soon after paralytic trauma this is a favourable sign for recovery. Electrical activity has been registered years after the initial trauma but the vocal fold remains immobile on account of fibrosis and muscle atrophy. In such cases nerve regeneration must have occurred but too late to be functional.

Hirano, Shin and Nozoe (1977) stress the value of indirect laryngoscopy with stroboscopy as an adjunct to EMG. The presence or absence of the mucosal wave over the surface of the paralysed vocal folds is a good diagnostic indicator (Isshiki, 1980). When the mucosal wave is absent the paralysis is severe and chance of recovery slight. Idiopathic paralysis is expected to recover spontaneously before 6 months.

Remedial Surgery

Surgery should not be considered for improvement of glottal closure and voice restoration for at least 6 months, but probably a year to be absolutely sure that no recovery is possible. During the waiting period speech therapy should be given in the hope that exercises will improve mobility of the paretic fold or promote compensatory action in the healthy fold. Moreover, the patient needs psychological support and guidance in how best to manage daily living with impaired voice.

Woodman operation

In bilateral abductor paralysis when there is respiratory distress permanent tracheostomy can be avoided by a Woodman operation (1946) and lateral-isation of one vocal fold. An incision is made along the anterior border of the sternomastoid muscle and the arytenoid cartilage is exposed, disarticulated and all but the vocal process is removed. The vocal process and fibres of the thyroarytenoid muscle are then pulled laterally and sutured to the inferior cornu of the thyroid. The cord is thus fixed in a position of abduction and the vocal fold of the opposite side may be able eventually to pass over the mid-line and approximate with it. The glottic aperture should be 5 mm: if less, the airway is inadequate; if greater the voice will be hoarse or lost (King, 1953). Sometimes the original lateralised position of the vocal fold alters during healing and is shifted by formation of scar tissue. Woodman and Pennington (1976) reported on their mostly successful results using this procedure over a period of 30 years with cases of abductor paralysis.

Laryngofissure and arytenoidectomy

This procedure has been designed to restore the airway following bilateral RLN paralysis with minimal adverse effects on phonation. Following laryngofissure, unilateral arytenoidectomy is performed without lateralisation of the vocal fold (Singer, Hamaker and Miller, 1985). This results in a posterior glottic chink which preserves the airway and competent adduction of the anterior glottis for phonation. Although aware of the possibility of using carbon dioxide laser to perform arytenoidectomy, Singer, Hamaker and Miller (1985) advocate caution. There is danger of glottic scarring reported by some pioneers in this field.

Medialisation laryngoplasty

In unilateral combined paralysis from lesions of the RLN and SLN, the involved fold will be slack and the arytenoid tipped forward and positioned at a lower level than its fellow. In these circumstances Teflon implant may be ineffective and thyroplasty with insertion of a silicon wedge to shift the fold medially is possible (Isshiki, Okamura and Ishikawa, 1975; Isshiki, Tanabe and Sawada, 1978). The operation is performed under local anaesthetic and the patient phonates while the surgeon finds the best position. The cricothyroid muscle is manipulated manually to test whether approximation tenses the fold sufficiently to improve voice. If it does, the cartilages are fixed by surgical suture in the optimum position. Simultaneous vocal ligament tightening in addition to medialisation laryngoplasty is performed in some cases (Koufman, 1986).

Tucker's ansa hypoglossi anastomosis

Tucker (1976, 1978, 1980) advocates nerve and muscle pedicle re-innervation in cases of bilateral abductor paralysis. The procedure involves re-innervating the posterior cricoarytenoid abductor muscle by using a branch of the ansa hypoglossi to the omohyoid muscle. Tucker explains that since the strap muscles are accessory inspiratory muscles they contract on inspiration. The transplanted nerve grows to innervate the abductor muscle and opens the larynx on inspiration. This opens up the airway and remedies breathing difficulties on exertion and the danger of obstruction in respiratory infections. The provision of an adequate airway does not impair the voice. The operation is relatively easy and function returns to the posterior cricoarytenoid after between 6 and 12 weeks. Tucker (1980) reports an 88.6% success rate.

Crumley and Izdebski (1986) have reported results of Tucker's technique for unilateral vocal fold paresis, using ansa hypoglossi–RLN anastomosis. Their study confirmed that this is a simple procedure without serious side effects and is non-invasive in relation to the larynx. Subjective and objective assessment of phonation postoperatively revealed that the resulting voice quality was superior to that obtained by Teflon implant.

Teflon implant

Unilateral RLN paralysis can be treated by implant of Teflon in the affected vocal fold if compensatory action of the healthy fold fails and the voice remains hoarse and weak. Studies of injected Teflon over 20 years agree that it is not carcinogenic and that generally it is well tolerated (Ward, Hanson and Abeymayer, 1985). Teflon injection increases the bulk of the paralytic fold and assists approximation with the healthy fold. Moore *et al.* (1987) suggest that injection into the muscle body stiffens it while leaving the mucosa free as in the normal fold.

Injection of Teflon is most successful when the fold lies in the paramedian or intermediate position. If the glottic aperture is greater it cannot be compensated for by the Teflon implant. If there is doubt about success of the procedure a preliminary trial with injection of Gelfoam is advisable. This disperses after a few days (Tucker, 1980).

Teflon injection takes only a couple of minutes under local anaesthetic and phonation is assessed immediately. Further injections can be given after an interval if further improvement of the voice is required. Oedema sets in almost at once after the injection and the voice deteriorates and becomes hoarse until swelling and inflammation have subsided. This may take a few days or weeks and the larynx may be painful (Nassar, 1977). The patient requires referral to the speech therapist for reassurance that the voice will recover and should be advised to use the voice sparingly until the larynx is comfortable again (Mueller, 1973). After several years a firm rubbery mass is still apparent at the site of the injection (Ward, Hanson and Abeymayer, 1985).

The results of Teflon implant are generally excellent and the success of this treatment is reported in many reviews of patients treated by laryngologists. The principal benefits of Teflon injection are restoration of an efficient cough and increase in vocal intensity. However, the voice is not restored to normal because muscle mass and tension are not the same as those of the normal vocal fold (Crumley and Izdebski, 1986). As a result the voice may be rough or hoarse with pitch breaks and other abnormalities.

Bartelli, Ford and Bless (1986) analysed poor results in 17 adults after Teflon injection. They attributed failure to a number of causes: overfilling supra- and subglottic structures, migration of the Teflon from the vocal folds, granuloma and scar tissue, and stiffness of the injected vocal fold. The condition of the damaged fold was improved by removal of the Teflon and the injection of collagen.

Collagen implant

Injectable collagen is regarded as possibly having certain advantages over Teflon although a cautious approach to its use is advocated (Ford and Bless, 1987;

Spiegel, Sataloff and Gould, 1987). Whereas Teflon is an inert substance, collagen is biologically active (Ford, Gilchrist and Bartelli, 1987). Adverse reactions such as swelling are reported in some cases although it is generally well tolerated. Liquid collagen is more easily and accurately administered than Teflon, which is a thick paste. Collagen has the additional advantage of softening and reducing scar tissue in the treated area.

The implant of collagen into the existing collagen layer of the lamina propria augments normal collagen and stimulates replacement. Ford, Bless and Campbell (1986) reported improvement in vibratory pattern and phonation in 80 patients receiving collagen implant.

Thyrotoxicosis and Thyroidectomy

The most common cause of vocal fold palsies is trauma sustained during thyroidectomy (Holinger, Holinger and Holinger, 1976; Tucker, 1980).

The thyroid gland is situated in the lower neck opposite cervical vertebrae C5–C7 and the first thoracic vertebra. It consists of two lobes formed by an isthmus which crosses the second and third tracheal rings. The lobes are in close relation to the recurrent laryngeal nerves before they enter the larynx via the articulation of the cricoid and thyroid cartilages. These nerves are therefore at risk during thyroidectomy (De Souza, 1980) especially as the course and branching of the nerves vary considerably between individuals and render their identification difficult during surgery.

The thyroid gland controls the metabolism of the body by secretion of the hormone thyroxine. Under-secretion causes myxoedema (p. 199) and excessive secretion causes thyrotoxicosis or hyperthyroidism. Increased metabolic rate disturbs the function of the whole organism and is a true example of systemic disease (Falk and Birken, 1985). The chief symptoms are increased heart beat, sweating, heat tolerance, tremor, weight loss, anxiety and insomnia. There is generalised nervousness and the anxiety symptoms are comparable to those described under anxiety state (p. 198).

Enlargement of the gland may be minimal or visible and palpable. Nodular enlargement may prove to be malignant (Dr Souza, 1980; Allen, 1984; Jiu, Sobol and Grozea, 1985). The popular term for enlarged thyroid gland is 'goitre' and is due to deficiency of iodine in drinking water in many parts of the world beside the deep valley and mountainous districts of the Black Forest, Germany and Switzerland. The addition of iodine salt in the diet prevents occurrence of simple goitre.

Exophthalmic goitre, or Graves' disease, is a more serious form of hyperthyroidism. The most notable symptoms are extreme nervousness, tachycardia and throbbing of the blood vessels, enlargement of the gland and protrusion of the eyeballs due to fatty deposits behind the eyes. Women are more often affected than men in the ratio of 8 : 1. The age of onset is between 16 and 40 years. There is a familial history and the symptoms can be greatly aggravated by shock and stress (Thomson, 1976).

In the early stages of hyperthyroidism it is difficult to distinguish between symptoms associated with thyrotoxicosis and disorders due to hormonal disturbance accompanying the menopause. It is quite probable that the anxiety and apparent hypochondria with complaints of discomfort in the throat or a lump and vocal weakness will be attributed to hysteria. Compression from the gland and systemic disturbance may however be accountable. The speech therapist must be aware of this possibility in assessment of 'functional' cases referred for treatment by the laryngologist.

Sonninen (1960) reported his findings in 131 patients who underwent thyroidectomy. This series included patients without positive evidence of excessive hormone in the blood analysis or enlargement of the gland. Complaints of compression and vocal failure in a shouting test were considered to be diagnostically positive. The tracheal compression symptoms listed by Sonninen are well known to speech pathologists:

- Constant desire to clear the throat – sensations of pressure and pain – paraesthesia.
- Difficulty in swallowing.
- Lowered pitch of speaking voice.
- Lack of volume.
- Difficulty in singing on a high pitch and uncertainty of pitch.

The compression cases may show slight reddening and swelling of the folds, which explains the desire to clear the throat and the discomfort felt.

Antithyroxine medication may control excessive thyroxine in the blood but if unsuccessful, thyroidectomy is performed. All the gland is not removed but a portion is left which it is anticipated will provide normal secretion of thyroxine. If this is underestimated the patient will develop myxoedema and will require thyroxine treatment permanently. The development of myxoedema can be detected a few days after surgery from the characteristic dysphonia – hoarseness and lowered pitch.

Laryngeal Palsy: Adductor Strategies

Eliciting phonation in aphonia

The following exercises are recommended for patients who have undergone the Woodman operation, and those suffering from unilateral vocal fold paralysis. Compensation by the healthy fold may be achieved or a shift in the paralysed fold.

1. Laugh or cough and endeavour to prolong the spasmodic phonation thus achieved into a prolonged vowel.
2. Swallow and phonate /i:/ as recommended by Pollack (1952).
3. Link the fingers, lift the arms to the level of the clavicles and pull against each other while phonating /i:/.
4. Push hands against a table and phonate.

5. Sitting on a chair, push down strongly with hands grasping the seat of the chair on either side.

Froeschels (1948a) who appears to have been the originator of these exercises, stressed that the push must be perfectly synchronised with phonation, voicing being attempted simultaneously with the maximum reflex sphincteric action of the glottis. Moolenaar-Bijl (1956) recommends fast repetition of syllables with /f/ and /s/, but without pushing, as 'a useful laryngeal gymnastic'. Later on, the sustaining of a vowel and vowel glides will increase range and flexibility of phonation. Van Thal (1961) recommended strongly articulated syllables preceded by plosives following production of voice after pushing exercises. The vowel /u:/ is the most propitious and the syllables /bu: bu:/.

These exercises should be practised at frequent intervals throughout the day, but for short periods only. Care must be taken not to strain the laryngeal muscles and produce inflammation and soreness similar to that following vocal strain. In those cases of vocal fold paralysis treated by us, however, it has not generally been found necessary to have recourse to forcing exercises. Voice has developed through use of hard attack and the simple instruction to breathe deeply and voice loudly and firmly. Marland (1952) also reported good results in cases of vocal fold paralysis without forcing exercises. Such exercises are not suitable for induced laryngeal palsy after nerve section.

Vocal prolongation

Difficulty in maintaining voice throughout phrases is encountered initially. A few words may be voiced and then speech deteriorates into a whisper. Voice duration may be increased by the following methods.

1. Singing vowels or humming and feeling the laryngeal vibrations with the finger tips.
2. Phonating a succession of vowels in a staccato string, attempting a glottal plosive on the initiation of each word.
3. Counting or reciting the alphabet starting with one or two numbers or letters and gradually increasing.
4. Speaking phrases of gradually increasing length, e.g. a blue sky; a bright blue sky; a bright blue clear sky etc. aiming to maintain phonation throughout.

Inspiratory phonation

The most common fault after the Woodman operation is the tendency to use inspiratory phonation (Woodman and Pollack, 1950). This must be discouraged since approximation of the folds on inspiration naturally obstructs the airway and reduces the amount of inspired air which, in turn, reduces the amount available for voice. Thus a ruse which temporarily serves to prolong the voicing of a phrase becomes self-defeating.

Persistent glottic chink

When a glottic chink persists despite training in adduction of the folds, the voice remains hoarse but audible. Breath is wasted in phonation and the patient must learn to replenish the breath supply at more frequent intervals than is customary when in possession of a normal larynx. At first there is a tendency to continue speech with very little breath, which produces tension and undermines good breathing patterns, but constant attention to breathing technique will correct this in time.

Chapter 17 Laryngeal Carcinoma: Treatment and Management

Laryngeal carcinoma occurs most frequently in middle-aged or elderly men who smoke. The ratio of men to women is 7 : 1 but there is some evidence that it is increasing among women as their years of smoking increase (Leonard, Holt and Maran, 1972). In the UK approximately 1.5% of new patients with cancer have cancer of the larynx (Berry, 1983) which is the principal reason for the life-saving procedure of laryngectomy.

Although rare under 30 years of age a number of much younger cases is reported in the literature. Recognition of this possibility by professionals is important in relation to early diagnosis and treatment. One of the youngest cases quoted is that of a 20-month-old boy (Peterson, 1973) whose malignant tumour required total laryngectomy. Figi and New (1929) reported on two of their patients, a boy (15 years) and a young woman (24 years) both of whom had squamous cell epithelioma and total laryngectomy was considered to be the only possible procedure because of the extent of the growths. A fibrosarcoma of the larynx in a girl of 15 years described by Garfield Davies (1969) was initially arrested by radiotherapy but necessitated total laryngectomy 15 months later after recurrence. Early cases used to be related to papillomata treated by radiotherapy in childhood (Rabbett, 1965; Vermeuling, 1966) but the danger of this treatment of papillomata is now appreciated.

In rare cases laryngectomy is performed on victims of road traffic accidents when the larynx and trachea are so severely damaged that this surgical procedure is the only method of ensuring a competent airway. Children may also occasionally undergo laryngectomy as the result of laryngeal trauma from ingesting corrosive substances (Jacobs and Abramson, 1980), by penetrating wounds (Gardner, Hill and Carano, 1962) or because of congenital tracheo-oesophageal malformation.

Primary Laryngeal Carcinoma

Laryngeal carcinoma is diagnosed following biopsy of the tumour at direct laryngoscopy.

Tumours can occur at any site in the larynx; they may be glottic, supraglottic or subglottic. Glottic carcinoma is the most common form of intralaryngeal

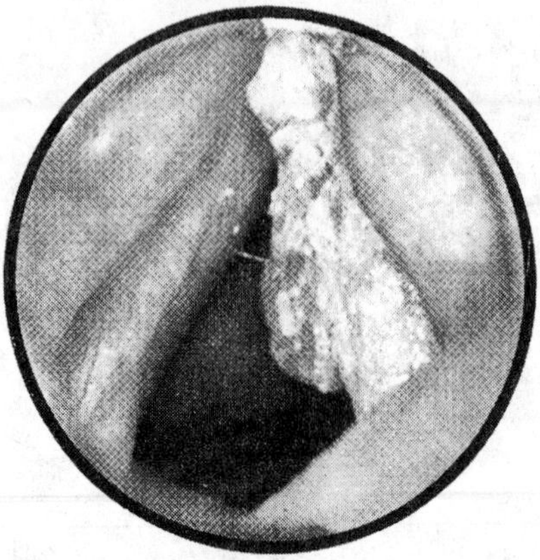

Figure 17.1. Glottic carcinoma (right vocal fold).

growth (Ballantyne and Groves, 1982) and hoarseness is an early symptom. If undiagnosed and untreated the hoarseness will become increasingly severe until stridor occurs as the airway becomes obstructed.

Supraglottic growths may occur in the pyriform fossae, the false vocal folds (ventricular bands), the ventricles and the aryepiglottic region. In the early stages there may be some throat discomfort which is followed by radiating pain to the ear on swallowing. Hoarseness, accompanied by increasing dysphagia, eventually develops as the carcinoma extends.

Symptoms of subglottic carcinoma, which most commonly occurs on the undersurface of the vocal fold, do not arise until a late stage when increasing involvement of the vocal fold produces hoarseness.

Direct extension of a laryngeal tumour in the early stages is confined to the membranes and muscular tissues of the larynx. It is limited by the cartilaginous structures and is therefore of low malignancy. Prognosis for intrinsic laryngeal cancer is better than for any other site in the body.

Any individual's complaints of discomfort or changes of sensation in the throat must not be minimised or disregarded. These symptoms, particularly if they coexist with a dysphonia of 2–3 weeks in the absence of upper respiratory tract infection, require immediate and careful examination by a laryngologist. The majority of laryngeal carcinomata can be cured with radiotherapy and early diagnosis and treatment is vital.

Secondary Carcinoma (Metastasis)

Primary cancer may spread by direct penetration into the surrounding tissue but a more serious risk of secondary growth arises with involvement of the lymphatic glands since cancer may now occur widely throughout the body by lymphatic metastases. As there are practically no lymphatic vessels in the vocal folds, lymphatic metastases will only occur when considerable invasion of the larynx has taken place.

Treatment

The paramount purpose of all treatment of laryngeal carcinoma is to save life. Untreated, the tumour will gradually occlude the airway and result in a distressing death. Preservation of a method of phonation is also considered when making decisions concerning management of the tumour. Radiotherapy and partial laryngectomy are more likely to preserve vocal fold phonation. If total laryngectomy is necessary the preservation or construction of suitable structures for production of pseudo-voice are essential whenever possible.

Radiotherapy

In the UK the treatment of choice is radiotherapy by cobalt unit or megavoltage therapy in order to destroy or arrest active tumour growth and to stimulate fibrous tissue formation. The permanent cure rate is 80–90% and only a small percentage of patients, under 10%, have a recurrence which requires laryngectomy. Ballantyne and Grove (1982) note that there is a slightly higher rate of cure in early cordal growths treated by radiotherapy than by surgery and that there are minimal adverse effects on the voice.

There are considerable differences in attitude among British and American surgeons, the former being usually more conservative (Shaw, 1966; Cheesman, 1983). Some American laryngologists, however, do favour the use of radiation therapy initially when treating certain types of laryngeal carcinoma (Fisher *et al.*, 1986). In the UK it is the convention to perform a total laryngectomy when radiation has failed although in theory it may be possible to carry out a partial laryngectomy. A cordectomy can be carried out if the recurrence involves the same cord to a similar and minimal extent. A simple laryngectomy on the other hand may be considered safer in the long run especially if there is some extension of laryngeal malignancy observable.

On referral for radiotherapy the patient is under the joint care of the radiotherapist and otolaryngologist. Attendance for treatment will be several times each week for several weeks, depending on the size of the irradiation doses being administered. This is a stressful time for the patient who is anxious about the diagnosis of cancer and the possible outcome of treatment. Tissue reaction is usually mild with some reddening of the skin and a dry, sore throat which improves in the early weeks after the end of treatment. Rarely, radiotherapy produces actute oedema and emergency laryngectomy is necessary.

Normal phonation returns on the termination of successful radiotherapy in most cases. Where a degree of dysphonia persists it may be due to permanent changes in the vocal fold or have a psychogenic basis (see Chapter 10). Changes in the vocal fold mucosa not seen on direct laryngoscopy may be established by stroboscopic examination. In some instances persisting dysphonia will be organically and psychogenically based.

Radiotherapy may be used postoperatively if it is found that a tumour has not been completely removed during surgery which has been the first choice of treatment. This pattern of events is more likely in the USA.

The patient is not regarded as having been cured of laryngeal carcinoma until 3 years after completion of radiotherapy without recurrence. Some authorities take a 5-year period. During this time the patient is regularly and frequently reviewed by the otolaryngologist and radiotherapist to ensure that all is well. After this period reviews continue less frequently.

Chemotherapy

In some advanced cases of laryngeal carcinoma, when cancer also involves the lymphatic system, cytotoxic drugs are administered intravenously. There are unpleasant side effects such as severe nausea, vomiting and hair loss.

Surgical procedures

In the UK laryngeal surgery is usually a salvage operation after unsuccessful radiotherapy or tumour recurrence some time after completion of a course of radiotherapy. Total laryngectomy is carried out more frequently than partial laryngectomy. However, for various reasons, in the USA surgery is the preferred treatment and partial laryngectomy is a realistic choice for dealing with early laryngeal carcinoma.

Partial laryngectomy

Partial laryngectomy is far less traumatic than total laryngectomy since the respiratory, phonatory and sphincteric functions of the larynx are retained (Leonard, Holt and Maran, 1972). Recurrence of cancer, of which there is a higher risk than with other procedures, can be treated by radiotherapy or total laryngectomy without any increased hazard to the patient. Postoperative chest infections occur more frequently than after total laryngectomy (Ballantyne and Groves, 1982).

Pressman and Bailey (1968) related surgery to knowledge concerning embryonic development and anatomy of the larynx and the spread of cancer and its escape routes via the submucosal lymphatic compartments. The embryological development of the larynx in two halves and the significance of superficial and deep lymph routes are of prime importance in these surgical techniques. Whereas a superficial tumour in the mucosa of the larynx may freely travel across the anterior commissure and invade the other half of the larynx, the deeper structures and lymph routes do not readily communicate with each other. The interior of the larynx being divided as it were into a number of compartments anatomically segregated from each other, allows a wide variety of surgical procedures. These may be vertical, horizontal and frontolateral procedures, besides supraglottic horizontal procedures combined with radical neck dissection for removal of involved nodes (Shaw, 1966). All methods involve the airway and the voice to a greater or lesser extent. With supraglottic procedures the vocal folds are not involved and the patient's voice will remain unimpaired despite possible difficulties in swallowing.

Lateral partial laryngectomy (laryngofissure with cordectomy)

Cordectomy is performed only in cases of very small, early localised tumour in the anterior part of the vocal fold and on the extreme edge. The interior of the larynx is reached by laryngofissure, also called thyrotomy and thyro-condrotomy, which entails making a vertical medial incision through the anterior angle of the thyroid cartilage. The cord alone is excised in one piece with a surrounding margin of 1 cm of healthy tissue (Jackson and Jackson, 1935).

Hemilaryngectomy (vertico-frontolateral laryngectomy)

In the majority of cases, however, it is considered safer to remove the vocal fold, the ventricular band and the thyroid ala of the affected side. The larynx is left lined with the external perichondrium which heals more readily than if stripped cartilage is left exposed, and the wound heals with the formation of a fibrous band of cicatricial tissue. Thus in the place of the thyroarytenoid muscle a substitute vocal fold conveniently forms. In time the healthy fold may pass over the mid-line to meet the adventitious fold and a serviceable voice be acquired. Teflon injection may be used to improve closure (Dedo, 1976; Biller and Lawson, 1986).

Sessions, Maness and McSwain (1965) reviewed the literature and 40 cases of laryngofissure performed between 1938 and 1963, on 34 males and 6 females. They drew attention to the fact that the resultant voice is dependent on the position of the substitute cicatricial cord. The voice is strong if the healthy fold does not have to pass over the mid-line. The voice depends on the degree of approximation achieved between cicatricial and true cords. Eighteen patients in this series had good voices and 18 only fair voices (four were not followed up).

Kennedy and Krause (1974) reported excellent results in conservative hemilaryngectomy and a 95% 5-year survival rate.

A more recent study by Mohr, Quenelle and Shumrick (1983) also reports good results when patients are carefully selected. They stress the importance of considerable expertise in relation to preoperative and postoperative patient management, endoscopy and surgical skills.

Standard hemilaryngectomy is not appropriate if the subglottic extension of the tumour is 5 mm or more. In such cases extended hemilaryngectomy with cricoid resection can be performed but has a greater complication rate (Biller and Lawson, 1986).

Hemilaryngectomy and skin-graft

Figi (1953) described hemilaryngectomy and skin graft in reconstruction of one vocal fold. Conley (1961, 1962) devised a single-stage operation after partial laryngectomy and removal of both vocal folds, whereby regional flaps are transposed to form imitation vocal folds. Brodnitz and Conley (1967) described the vocal rehabilitation necessary after this procedure. The voice is deep but strong and gentle pushing exercises with great circumspection are advised.

Following the work of Conley (1961) in performing hemilaryngectomy and reconstruction of a substitute vocal cord from a unilateral pedicled skin flap from the neck, Maran, Haast and Leonard (1968) described a vertical hemilaryngectomy operation with cord reconstruction. The sternohyoid and thyrohyoid muscles are cut close to their insertions and a bipedicled muscle transposition is carried out to replace the excised cord. The voice is strong immediately after operation, then deteriorates but improves with healing of the wound. Leonard, Holt and Maran (1972) reported long-term results of this operation on 75 patients operated on during the period 1963–70. They emphasised the need for careful selection of patients; the cancer must be localised and the vocal fold mobile.

Supraglottic laryngectomy

This procedure may be used for treatment of some cases in which carcinoma involves one arytenoid, the medial wall of the pyriform fossa, the aryepiglottic fold or the epiglottis. It allows voice to be unaffected (Burstein and Calcaterra, 1985) but aspiration of fluids may be a complication.

Phonation following laryngofissure

Speech therapy plays an important role in vocal rehabilitation after partial laryngectomy both with and without reconstructive-cord surgery. The substitute cord on the excised side does not project so far towards the mid-line as the normal vocal fold and is also immobile. The healthy fold of the opposite side must be trained to pass over the mid-line and compensate for the deficiency of its fellow in the same way as in a case of total unilateral cord palsy. Forcing exercises (p. 305) are generally recommended but often equally good results may be obtained without the danger of building up laryngeal and pharyngeal tension. The patient is merely encouraged to raise the volume of the voice with good breath support. It may assist to press the wings of the thyroid cartilage between thumb and finger to emphasise tactile and kinaesthetic cues. Relaxation and correct diaphragmatic breathing are vital preliminaries to the vocal exercises since there is considerable air wastage. The practice of strong vowel sounds with hard attack is another useful exercise.

Granulomatous tissue on the healing surfaces may interfere with phonation at first and if it does not disperse spontaneously in the course of 2 or 3 months it may be removed surgically during direct laryngoscopy. The speech pathologist needs to know that this is not a case of local recurrence of tumour, in order to reinforce the reassurances given by the surgeon and to allay the patient's anxiety.

The voice may become comparatively good but it is never quite normal and is generally rather deep and hoarse. Because of the amount of breath wasted in phonation and the precipitate emptying of the lungs, there is always a strong tendency to continue speech in a forced whisper. This involves much tension in an attempt to achieve the previous length of phrase despite inadequate breath pressure. The patient must be taught first to increase usual breath capacity and then to obtain better control over expiration. When approximation of adventitious cord and the vocal fold is poor, there is sometimes a tendency to attempt vocalisation on inspiration. The patient must be taught to inspire more frequently and to use shorter phrases. A pocket amplifier can be used very successfully to boost vocal volume.

Some improvement in tone can be obtained by the usual vocal exercises. Increased range may also be achieved by practising scales, attempting to sing and speaking phrases with various intonation patterns. Many patients thus acquire surprisingly serviceable voices in a very short time. On the whole the vocal results with the elderly are disappointing. Levin (1962b) makes the following observations based on wide experience.

> Following healing, repeated observation of these patients indicates that there is a partial or complete replacement of the removed fold by a scar tissue band. Since approximation is only partial or non-existent, the voice is very harsh and seriously impaired. The outgoing air cannot be interrupted properly. There are extraneous harsh noises as a result of the more or less continuous flow of air.

The exceptional case of a reasonably pleasing voice can occur, however.

Total laryngectomy

Carcinoma which is not cured by radiotherapy or partial laryngectomy necessitates total laryngectomy.

If the tumour is causing dyspnoea a tracheotomy may be performed before the main operation but generally this is done at the same time, although preceding laryngectomy. The new airway ensures freedom from breathing complications as far as possible and gives the surgeon freedom of action in the laryngeal field above.

A U-shaped flap is raised to expose the larynx which is removed in its entirety and the resulting defect in the pharyngeal wall is carefully closed. The hyoid bone is usually excised with the larynx (Cheesman, 1983); this is particularly important when the anterior commissure is involved in the carcinoma and there is danger of the pre-epiglottic space being invaded (Ballantyne and Groves, 1982). However, preservation of the hyoid bone has been advocated, and Vrticka and Svoboda (1961) report that an intact hyoid bone was found much more frequently in their good speakers. They point out that preservation of the hyoid often signifies preservation of the strap muscles whose importance for facilitating aspiration of air into the oesophagus for production of pseudo-voice was emphasised as early as 1922 by Seeman. Of course, removal of all malignant cells must have priority.

The trachea and oesophagus are now entirely separate with respiration and expectoration taking place via the permanent tracheal stoma. The patient wears a tracheostomy tube in the early stages of recovery until there is no danger of the stoma stenosing. In normal recovery the nasogastric feeding tube, which is inserted during surgery, remains *in situ* for approximately 10–14 days.

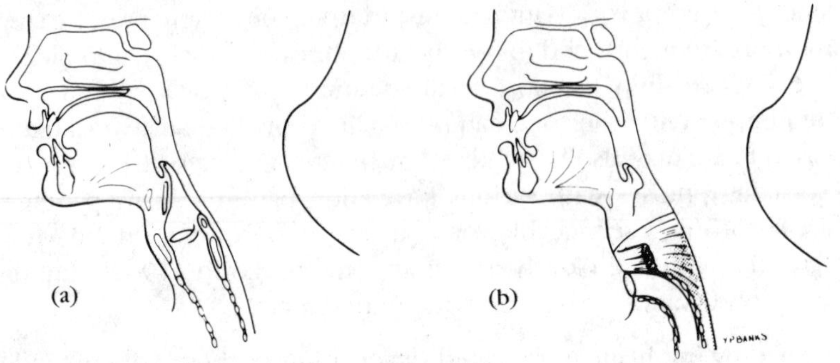

Figure 17.2. Vocal tract: (a) prelaryngectomy; (b) postlaryngectomy.

Radical neck dissection (block dissection)

Metastases of malignant cells in the lymph glands of the neck necessitates radical surgery if the patient has previously had radiotherapy. The throat will be flatter and tighter than after simple laryngectomy because additional tissue has been removed. An uncomfortable consequence of the unavoidable removal of the spinal accessory nerve in this procedure results in a 'dropped' shoulder. In addition to experiencing discomfort the patient's arm movements on the affected side become restricted so that the hand and arm cannot easily be raised above shoulder level. Carrying any weight on the affected side, e.g. shopping, is only possible for short periods. A course of physiotherapy may be helpful.

Pharyngolaryngectomy

Radiotherapy has a low success rate in cases of carcinoma in the hypopharynx and the postcricoid and cervical oesophagus. Consequently, surgical removal of the larynx, pharynx and variable amounts of the oesophagus is necessary. In addition, most cases will need a unilateral or bilateral block dissection. Repair presents many problems and sacrifice of the cricopharyngeal sphincter means that voice production will be difficult.

Oesophageal reconstruction

In repair of the cervical oesophagus a single-stage operation and Thiersch graft round a Portex tube may be used in reconstruction and was first described by Negus. This procedure is fraught with difficulties (Harrison, 1964). Stenosis of the pharynx and oesophagus resulting in dysphagia may occur, the patient having to be admitted to hospital for bougienage and stretching of the reconstructed tube under general anaesthetic. Plastic surgery for reconstruction of the pharynx and oesophagus is possible from thoracic flaps but this multiple-stage operation necessitates long hospitalisation. In view of the fact that recurrence is anticipated within 2–3 years it is not generally considered worth while. Greene examined a Canadian patient who had had this treatment and not only did her throat appear normal externally but she had an excellent and fluent voice.

Stuart (1966), because of the difficulties of reconstruction and hazards of operation, and of the short life expectancy, advocated insertion of a plastic tube prosthesis. These patients obtain characteristically hollow and sometimes quite strong voices with great ease and without speech instruction.

Stomach and colon transplants

Lewis (1965) drew attention to the formidable procedures in bringing up stomach or colon through the thorax to the neck. A major abdominal operation is added to extensive neck surgery. He advocated reconstruction of the pharynx by local cervical skin flaps or tubed pedicle flaps migrated from the chest wall. Pectoralis major myocutaneous flaps (Murakami *et al.*, 1982) and quilted, skin-grafted pectoralis major flaps (Robertson and Robinson, 1984) continue to be used and researched in relation to reconstructing the cervical oesophagus following pharyngolaryngectomy.

A good pseudo-voice develops after repair by skin flaps. This operation however is not suitable after irradiation therapy, so the numbers who can benefit are few in the UK.

Experimentation

Studies have also been carried out using a posteriorly based tongue flap for reconstructing the hypopharynx following total laryngectomy with subtotal pharyngectomy (Calcaterra, 1983). Rehabilitation was rapid and articulation unaffected.

All these procedures of reconstruction, whether partial or total, are vulnerable to fistula, stricture and the death of the patient (Fee, 1984). The survival rate in total reconstruction is poor. The priority of surgery in these cases is to use the most straightforward procedure in order to achieve acceptable swallowing without subjecting the patient to endless surgery in the last months of life (Fee, 1984).

Pharyngolaryngo-oesophagectomy

Extensive involvement of the oesophagus besides larynx and pharynx presents even greater difficulties than those already described in connection with laryngectomy. Stomach pull-up and colon transplant are used in reconstruction of the oesophagus.

Ranger (1964, 1983) and Le Quesne (1964) carried out immediate repair after pharyngolaryngectomy and oesophagectomy by creating a pharyngogastric anastomosis. Stomach and duodenum are mobilised and transplanted into the neck to form a continuous tract between pharynx and stomach. There is no difficulty in swallowing postoperatively and this surgical procedure is suitable in irradiated cases. Pseudo-voice can be as satisfactory as oesophageal speech.

The operation is hazardous and even if the patient survives the prognosis is not good. The balance of prolonging life and the quality of that life has to be considered by the surgeon. Harrison (1964) remarked that the surgeon has both 'moral and technical responsibilities' and quoted Gardham: 'How often by prolonging life do we really add to its sum of happiness and how often do we prolong the quantity of life at the expense of its quality?' Although these decisions are not made by the speech pathologist an awareness of them helps to maintain perspective and to plan the rehabilitation programme. As Ranger (1983) realistically points out, even those patients who die of the disease before the 3-year stage of survival can be helped by alleviating their swallowing problems and prevented from dying of dysphagia.

The voice will be weak but some patients do develop good voice. Voice results are similar with stomach and colon transplants. Lall and Evison (1966) reported on the performance of four patients: one developed excellent speech and another a reasonable voice. X-ray showed narrowing of the transplant while the diaphragm obtained air fluctuation. The patient who showed no narrowing of the reconstructed oesophagus had only a strong whisper as did the last patient who was unable to shift air in the tube transplant. We have had patients who produced satisfactory functional voice.

The pharyngo-oesophageal segment

The acquisition of an acceptable voice is a secondary aim of laryngectomy surgery. If survival is a realistic goal the subsequent quality of life is a major consideration and satisfactory communication must be considered in making surgical decisions. Oesophageal and tracheo-oesophageal voice are dependent on the pharyngo-oesophageal segment (called P-E segment because of initial introduction of the term in the USA) which is vibrated by air introduced into the oesophagus by the alaryngeal speaker and acts as a substitute vibrator or pseudo-glottis.

The P-E segment is the upper oesophageal sphincter at the level of cervical vertebrae 5 to 7 (C5–C7) and is composed of fibres of the inferior pharyngeal constrictor muscle, the cricopharyngeus muscle and the upper fibres of the oesophagus. At rest, the sphincter is in a tonic state and only relaxes on swallowing to allow entry of the bolus into the oesophagus.

The sectioning of the constrictor muscles during laryngectomy reduces the tonicity of the P-E segment and thus its effectiveness for pseudo-voice (Singer, Blom and Hamaker, 1986). Repair of the sphincteric muscles may also affect acquisition of pseudo-voice if it results in a hypertronic segment. The appropriate tonicity of the P-E segment and its site, width and length are important factors affecting the acquisition of oesphageal voice.

Bentzen, Guld and Rasmussen (1976) made a distinction between high and

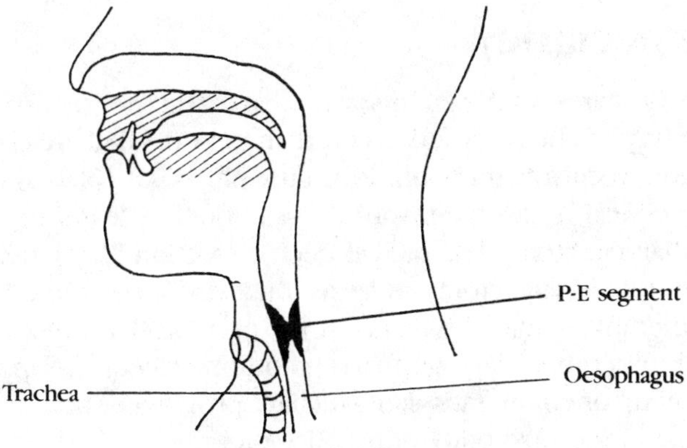

Figure 17.3. P-E segment.

low positioned pseudo-glottis in a video-radiographic study of 41 patients. The high situation was at the level of C4–C5 and the low situation at C6–C7. The high pseudo-glottis, especially with posterior muscular rigidity, produced the best voice. These findings can be related to Simpson's surgical techniques which aim to provide an optimally functioning P-E segment (Simpson, Smith and Gordon, 1972).

Although it may vary widely there are certain irregularities of the P-E segment which operate against good functional control over the vicarious lung, glottis and resonator (Singer and Blom, 1980; Perry and Edels, 1985). Inability to produce voice because of an inadequate P-E segment is discussed in the next chapter.

Postlaryngectomy Complications

Uncomplicated recovery from total laryngectomy allows removal of the nasogastric feeding tube within 10–14 days of surgery and the early stages of acquiring voice can be initiated. A number of complications may prolong this stage of recovery, however. The incidence of problems increases when more radical and extensive surgery is necessary and if the patient has had radiotherapy preoperatively. The irradiated tissue is ischaemic and this results in slower and less satisfactory healing.

A fistula will occur if the surgical repair fails to heal or breaks down at a later stage. It may heal spontaneously if it is small. Following block dissection or procedures such as laryngopharyngo-oesophagectomy a large fistula may require plastic surgery. In this case a well-vascularised pedicle of non-irradiated skin is brought up to make the repair.

Other problems include postoperative bleeding and wound infection. Removal of the thyroid and parathyroid glands with disruption of the endocrine system will require adjustment with appropriate supplements of thyroxine and calcium.

Life Expectancy

Berry (1983) states that patients who have had no recurrence 3 years postoperatively can be regarded as cured. In tumours that are confined to the larynx without vocal fold immobility the cure rate is 90–100% by radiotherapy. When the cervical nodes are involved the outlook is less sanguine.

Pharyngolaryngectomy and radical neck dissection may have just as good results as simple laryngectomy as far as longevity is concerned if combined with radiotherapy. Ranger (1983) is of the opinion that 20–25% of patients who have undergone laryngopharyngo-oesophagectomy and immediate stomach pull-up or colon transplant will have prolonged survival, with normal swallowing and the possibility of pseudo-voice.

Some individuals in the laryngofissure and laryngectomy categories live to normal old age and eventually die from other causes. Guthrie (1966) reported the case of a man who underwent laryngectomy when 35 years of age and was still alive 42 years later. Usually the outlook is more optimistic for the aged than for the young because carcinoma tends to be more ebullient in youth than in old age when the rate of cell replacement is slowed down.

Surgical Speech Rehabilitation

In addition to improving techniques for prolonging life and facilitating oesophageal speech, surgeons have sought to develop surgical procedures which provide the patient with voice. By diverting expired lung air through a surgically constructed tube or fistula into the vocal tract, air is vibrated as it passes into the pharyngeal cavity and phonation is generated. Fistula voice is similar to oesophageal but is much less arduous to acquire if surgery is successful. It is of higher pitch and greater fluency. The pitch is more acceptable to women laryngectomees (Snidecor, 1968; Edwards, 1976). Edwards (1983) and Singer, Blom and Hamaker (1983) have given succinct accounts of the history of surgical speech rehabilitation.

External fistula speech (prosthesis and air shunt; reed-fistula speech)

The first artificial larynges consisted of a membrane or reed vibrator activated by lung air from a tube fitted into the tracheal stoma. The 'voice' thus created was piped into the mouth and shaped by articulation into intelligible speech (Hunt, 1964; Holinger, 1975). The reed type of vibrator is still in use in Holland, Spain and Japan. A further development in fistula speech is the adaptation of the reed vibrator for use in conjunction with a constructed skin tube in the neck. This pipes vibrated air into the pharynx thus producing more natural speech and a less conspicuous speech aid.

Taub's Voicebak

Stanley Taub (1975) devised this valved prosthesis which fits into a fistula opening into the trachea above the tracheostoma. It is activated by air shunted upwards from the usual tracheal opening. The superior fistula can be created at any time after laryngectomy. The voice created is claimed to be good and the patient can laugh, shout, whisper and even sing. Healing difficulties make this an unsuitable procedure for patients who have had radiotherapy, in addition to which the equipment is expensive and awkward and requires regular maintenance.

Weinberg and Shedd – reed-fistula speech

Weinberg, Shedd and Horii (1978) used a modified form of the Tokyo external pneumatic artificial larynx and a surgically created pharyngeal fistula. These researchers reported promising progress with four patients but noted that the procedure does not merit consideration as a routine method in pharyngo-laryngectomy. They also mention the need for a speech therapist to help the patient with management of the prosthesis and fistula speech after the operation.

Internal fistula speech

This category includes procedures where a fistula is constructed so that pulmonary air is directed into the vocal tract at some point. Various techniques have been used but the success achieved by the originator is often not duplicated by others.

The Asai technique

In 1959 Ryozo Asai of the University of Kobe, Japan, first reported his now famous three-stage operation which constructs a dermal tube from the tracheostoma to a pharyngeal fistula at about the level of the hyoid bone. The first stage is performed at the time of the laryngectomy and the next two follow at intervals of a month later. Digital closure of the stoma while speaking enables a moving column of air from the lungs to be directed through the tube into the pharynx. Miller (1967, 1968) performed operations of this type in the USA and found that only 20% of patients achieved good voice and that there was a high proportion of patients in whom saliva entered the trachea. Asai (1972) reported good speech results of surgery in 72 patients. This operation has not been adopted universally because good surgical and speech results are difficult to achieve. Some patients have to exert digital pressure on the neck at the level of the internal pharyngeal exit, others have difficulty in swallowing. Healing can present difficulties and strictures commonly develop in the dermal tube. It is not a viable procedure after radiotherapy which precludes further surgical interference of this type after laryngectomy.

Serafini operation

Arslan and Serafini (1972) reported success with an operation which involves raising the trachea and suturing it to the hyoid so that it is continuous with the hypopharynx. This maintains respiration through mouth and nose in addition to phonation. The editor of *The Laryngoscope*, in which this report was published, commented upon the problems arising from this operation. Pulling up the trachea created swallowing difficulties and two-thirds of the patients had breathing difficulties and required tracheostomy tubes *in situ*.

Staffieri technique

Staffieri's operation designed in the early 1970s to construct a neoglottis did produce some good voice results and has been adopted by many surgeons. This procedure has also been bedevilled by aspiration and stenosis (Singer, Blom and Hamaker, 1983).

Tanabe, Honjo and Isshiki neoglottic construction

A new technique for neoglottic construction has been evolved by Tanabe, Honjo and Isshiki (1985) using the upper tracheal rings in an attempt to overcome the complications of postoperative stenosis and aspiration. Following tracheotomy and laryngectomy, the upper three tracheal rings are used to create a neoglottis with the first ring being sutured to the oesophageal wall. Seven of the eight patients in the study are reported to use voice which is superior to oesophageal voice when judged on the basis of duration and intelligibility. The neoglottis in the eighth patient was closed due to aspiration.

Tracheo-oesophageal flap

Experimentation continues in the search for a satisfactory method of internal fistula speech. A new technique performed on 19 patients in China is reported (Li, 1985). A tongue-like tracheo-oesophageal flap is transposed into the oesophageal lumen in a downwards direction through the tracheo-oesophageal fistula. Li reports that voice is produced effortlessly when the stoma is occluded with the finger and that speech therapy is not required. During swallowing, food and liquids are prevented from entering the trachea by the flap covering the fistula.

Blom–Singer tracheo-oesophageal puncture (T-E puncture) and prosthesis

In 1980 Singer and Blom first reported on their prosthesis which is introduced into the oesophagus via the tracheostoma through a fistula in the posterior tracheal wall. Pulmonary air enters the prosthesis and is directed by the duckbill valve into the oesophagus where it vibrates the P-E segment for production of pseudo-voice. When first developed the T-E puncture was performed some time after laryngectomy (secondary voice restoration). Primary restoration may also be undertaken now at the time of the laryngectomy (Hamaker *et al.*, 1985; Trudeau, Hirsch and Schuller, 1986). The procedure is easily reversible as the fistula closes spontaneously if the valve is not inserted. Originally it was necessary for the patient to use finger occlusion of the tracheostoma but a suitable tracheostoma valve was developed to eliminate manual occlusion (Blom, Singer and Hamaker, 1982). Constant improvements of prosthesis and valve continue.

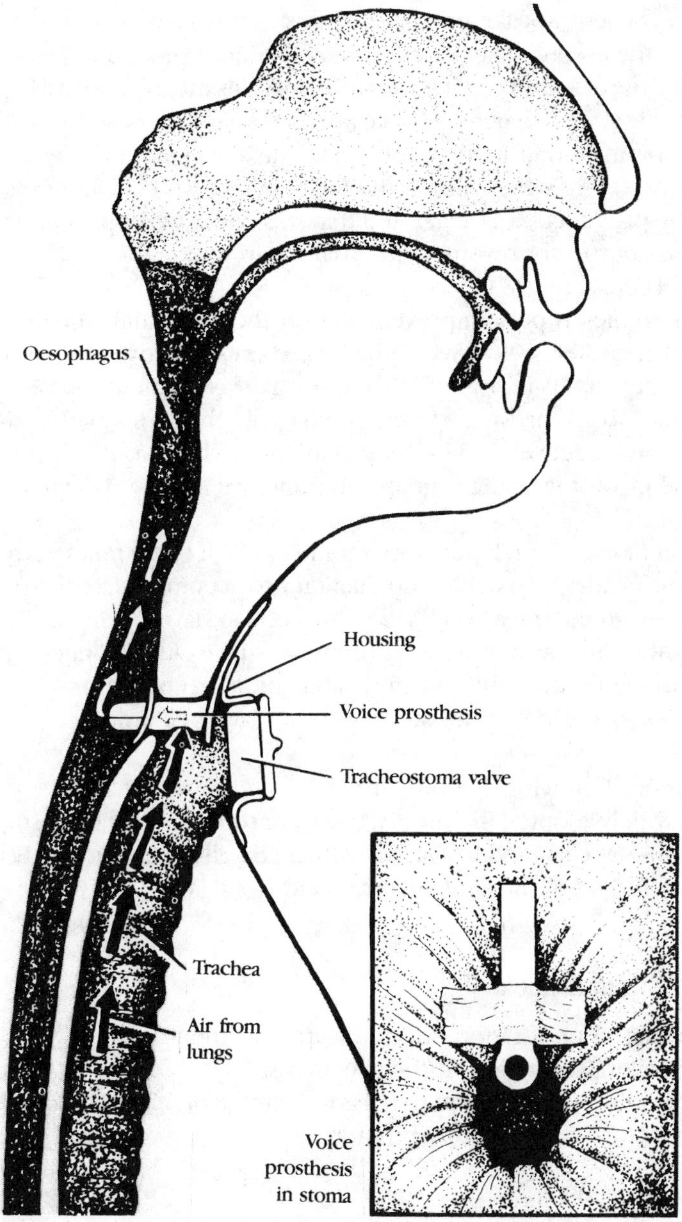

Figure 17.4. Blom–Singer valve in use. (Reproduced by permission of the American Hospital Supply Corporation.)

Patient selection for T-E puncture

Suitable patients are carefully selected. Of paramount importance in the criteria for patient selection is a suitable P-E segment. This is investigated by an air insufflation test (Taub test). A catheter is introduced into the oesophagus through the nose to just below the P-E segment, approximately to the level of the tracheostoma. The patient is at rest as air is insufflated and air subsequently leaving the oesophagus vibrates the P-E segment producing oesophageal voice. The patient speaks on the egressive air stream so that quality and duration of the pseudo-voice can be assessed (Singer and Blom, 1980). If there is no oesophageal sound or if it is unsatisfactory this may be due to a hypertonic or hypotonic P-E segment or because of pharyngo-oesophageal spasm. Reflexive spasm is confirmed by the effectiveness of a parapharyngeal injection of local anaesthetic which allows the P-E segment to relax and oesophageal voice to be produced. It is suggested that this patient group should undergo pharyngeal constrictor myotomy in order to overcome the problem (Singer, Blom and Hamaker, 1983).

Various studies report improvements on the air insufflation test (Blom, Singer and Hamaker, 1985) which has relied on subjective evaluation of the sound produced. It is argued that objective assessment of oesophageal insufflation, which provides intraoesophageal pressure measurements, is essential for effectively identifying patients who would benefit from pharyngeal myotomy at the time of P-E puncture (Baugh, Lewin and Baker, 1987).

Good candidates for T-E puncture should have adequate pulmonary reserve and a stoma of adequate depth and diameter to accommodate the prosthesis without obstructing the airway. They also need to have the manual dexterity and motivation to clean and insert the valve successfully (Singer and Blom, 1980). Although successful speech rehabilitation is reported to be as high as 80–90% this procedure is not suitable for all laryngectomees.

Complications following T-E puncture

Although widely adopted in America there are reports of major postoperative complications at early and late stages which give rise to caution in use of this procedure in the UK (Silver, Gluckman and Donegan, 1985; Andrews *et al.*, 1987).

Early complications include:

- Oesophageal perforation during creation of the fistula.
- Severe allergic reaction to the prosthesis.
- Severe cellulitis in the peristomal area; leakage of saliva and food through the puncture resulting in aspiration.

Later complications include:

- Enlargement of the T-E fistula.
- Pneumonia as a result of recurring aspiration.
- Aspiration of the prosthesis.
- Fistula migration.
- Tracheal stoma stenosis.
- Oesophageal stenosis.

The incidence of problems has been found to be similar whether or not the patient has had radiotherapy but when complications occur in the irradiated patient they are more severe. The surgeons reporting these problems consider that when benefits are weighed against the risks it is worth while continuing with the procedure (Silver, Gluckman and Donegan, 1985). Some patients prefer to remain voiceless following complications rather than risk encountering further difficulties.

Avoidable problems also occur with the prosthesis if it is not kept scrupulously clean. The oesophageal end of the valve is vulnerable to the accumulation of food deposits. Colonisation by fungi must be constantly removed if health and voice quality and efficiency are to be maintained (Izdebski, Ross and Lee, 1987).

Tracheo-oesophageal speech

Singer and Blom (1980) reported fluent voices in 90% of their first 60 patients who underwent T-E puncture. There are reports that the percentage of patients continuing to use T-E fistula voice in the long term is less than this (Wetmore *et al.*, 1985). It appears that careful patient selection and a well-trained team whose members are well integrated will maintain a high long-term percentage of successful users. The speech pathologist has a key role in the assessment and treatment of these patients (Perry, 1983).

Studies of the effectiveness of tracheo-oesophageal voice are generally favourable. An important feature is the relative preservation of speech rate and voice duration, and normal prosody as a result of using the pulmonic air stream. This is unlike many oesophageal speakers where the rate is markedly slower than in laryngeal speakers and where pauses for air injection may disturb prosody (Robbins *et al.*, 1984). For this reason, when acoustic speech parameters are evaluated, T-E puncture speech bears more similarity to laryngeal speech than traditional oesophageal speech (Robbins *et al.*, 1984; Williams and Watson, 1987). However, both types of speech have been rated as comparable in studies of intelligibility and overall communicative effectiveness (Tardy-Mitzell, Andrews and Bowman, 1985; Williams and Watson, 1985). Merwin, Goldstein and Rothman (1985) maintain that the quality of voice in both methods of alaryngeal phonation is similar.

The low intensity of oesophageal speech, 6–10 dB below laryngeal voice, is a common problem for the laryngectomee. T-E puncture speech is approximately 10 dB louder than normal voice and the fundamental frequency of connected speech is similar to that of laryngeal speech (Robbins *et al.*, 1984).

Other advantages of the procedure include the speed with which most speakers attain pseudo-voice with minimal speech therapy. In many instances voice is regarded as superior to that achieved by oesophageal speakers (Williams and Watson, 1985, 1987). Perhaps most important of all when successful, it may be a method of giving voice to a laryngectomee who has been unable to acquire traditional oesophageal voice.

The development of the Blom–Singer valve has been a major contribution to the process of providing voice for the laryngectomee which has wide acceptance throughout North America. The role of the speech pathologist includes involvement in a team approach for the evaluation of suitable candidates and postoperatively in applying appropriate therapeutic skills. It must be remembered that although voice may be excellent in appropriately selected patients in whom there are no surgical complications, the procedure is not without its problems even when performed by the most competent surgeons.

Panjé Voice Button

This small prosthesis devised by Panjé (1981) also allows pulmonic air to be shunted into the oesophagus. Creation of the fistula is an out-patient procedure and the prosthesis is placed in position with an inserter.

Life after Laryngectomy

Respiration

Immediately following surgery the radical change in the anatomy of the breathing mechanism no longer allows air to be warmed and filtered before entering the lungs. A humidifer is used in the early days postoperatively in order to avoid crusting around the tracheostoma and the accumulation of 'tacky' mucus.

Respiratory complications

The most common and troublesome postoperative complication is bronchitis induced by the aspiration of secretions into the bronchi during surgery. The patient is distressed by the difficulty in breathing and becomes exhausted by the effort to expectorate mucus. A cannula is inserted into the tracheal opening at first; this cannula consists of two tubes fitting one within the other. The outer tube is left in position until the wound is healed, but the inner tube can be removed, cleaned and sterilised frequently by a nurse. Suction apparatus is also used to extract mucus via the tracheostoma. This provides temporary relief for the patient and prevents the formation of bronchial plugs of mucus which can cause asphyxia. In most patients these problems resolve in the early days and weeks of recovery and suction apparatus will not be necessary for long. If patients have had chronic respiratory problems preoperatively, however, or if they are asthmatic their management will present a greater problem.

Persistent postlaryngectomy bronchial mucus may hold up the patient's recovery and discharge from hospital for several weeks. Breathing exercises may be prescribed by the surgeon, also postural drainage of the lungs, which is undertaken by the physiotherapist. If this is the case and the speech therapist wishes to give instruction in breathing for speech, contact should be made with the physiotherapist in order to avoid possible conflict of exercises and instructions. If the breathing technique taught by the physiotherapist is different from that of the speech therapist, and it may be, then the latter must explain that her instructions relate exclusively to the breathing patterns necessary for speech and not the chest condition.

Management

It is important that the patient should be rid of bronchial infection as soon as possible for, quite apart from the considerations of health, it renders the acquisition of oesophageal voice difficult on account of the interference with breathing for speech. Patients with bronchial congestion cannot produce voice easily. Unfortunately, congestion cannot be cured in heavy smokers who develop emphysema and the mucus may be too viscid to remove from the upper trachea by coughing. Some patients always carry a pair of tweezers or forceps in order to extract particularly 'stringy' mucus near the tracheostoma; a small mirror completes the equipment required and they are able to ensure a patent airway. Patients should be advised not to use a paper tissue to clear mucus around the rim of the stoma or just inside because this can result in irritation which triggers the cough reflex. Rapid inspiration of air can suck the tissue into the trachea and result in asphyxiation. One of our patients almost succumbed to this fate. Fortunately, an exceptionally forceful cough finally removed the obstruction three miles after he had left home on the way to the nearest hospital.

Tracheostoma protection

Even when the laryngectomee has recovered from the immediate effects of surgery and has been discharged home, inspired air should be warmed and moistened so that tracheal and lung secretions are easily removed. The trachea should not be exposed to sudden temperature changes. Stoma protectors of various types are available.

Laryngectomy bibs (Buchanan laryngectomy protector; Mediquip laryngectomy bib)

These are made of a light-weight material which absorbs mucus and so protects clothing. The bib is either tied round the neck or has Velcro tabs; it is washable.

Foam squares (Laryngofoam)

These disposable foam filters are held in place over the stoma by a hypoallergenic adhesive strip. They are not suitable for patients with a very forceful or productive cough unless worn with a laryngectomy bib. Patients who need the square only for warming, filtering and moisturising air wear them under normal clothing.

Romet filters

This protector is worn inside the open neck of a blouse or shirt and looks like the neck of a light-weight sweater. It is bib-shaped with a ribbed neck band with Velcro fasteners and comes in several colours. It can be worn without additional stoma protection although many patients prefer to have either a foam square or bib as additional protection. These filters are washable.

Loss of nasal breathing

The laryngectomee cannot nose-blow and is therefore unable to clear the nose of mucus. Although this is no longer the airway, patients report that this is particularly unpleasant during a head cold.

Olfaction

Loss of smell is often noticed, due to inability to inhale through the nose and stimulate the olfactory nerve endings. The sense of taste is also impaired since we scent flavours and taste salt, sweet, sour and bitter. The laryngectomee will complain that food no longer tastes so good and that appetite is lost. Inhalation of air into the oesophagus as for oesophageal voice production by change in thoracic pressure, when mastered, can be used to inhale air in through the nose. Explanation of cause and effect and practise in sniffing will help in restoration of olfaction. Movements of the back of the tongue making contact with the soft palate can agitate nasal air.

Expectoration

Without closure of the vocal folds the patient is unable to build up subglottic air pressure in the normal way in order to clear obstructions from the airway. Although the glottis is usually considered a necessary part of the mechanism of coughing, the laryngectomee is able to cough efficiently using the abdominal muscles and diaphragm for increasing intrathoracic pressure.

The most difficult and unacceptable aspect for the patient to tolerate, if a normally sensitive individual, is the tracheal opening and airway. In some patients this takes precedence in importance over loss of voice. It is particularly difficult to cope with coughed-up mucus discreetly and excessive coughing may be an affliction for many weeks after leaving hospital.

Whereas blowing the nose and wiping the mouth with a handkerchief are socially permissible, wiping mucus from the stoma and attacking the problem under blouse, shirt or 'bib' is another thing altogether. Embarrassment may at first prevent a patient from leaving the house and this may contribute substantially to depression.

Violent coughing can render a patient incontinent. One patient with a persistent irritating cough could not go back to work for 18 months for this reason despite acquiring excellent speech early. In these cases physio-therapists can help with enuresis procedures.

Swallowing

The majority of patients are aware of changes in the efficiency of their swallow mechanism even when there are no marked problems. Food and liquid usually need to be taken rather more slowly than preoperatively if accumulation of solids in the pharynx and nasal regurgitation of fluids are to be avoided. The patient can be encouraged to perceive the pharynx as a funnel which empties rather more slowly than preoperatively. The practice of taking slightly smaller mouthfuls of food, chewing it carefully and not taking another mouthful until the previous bolus is swallowed soon becomes established.

Dysphagia

Dysphagia will occur in some patients as a result of the surgery required. Although there is no danger of food being aspirated (except following surgical speech restoration procedures), the pharyngeal phase of swallowing may present problems for a number of reasons.

In some patients a band of scar tissue at the base of the tongue occurs as a result of the surgical closure of the defect in the pharyngeal wall. During swallowing this scar tissue band is pulled posteriorly so that a pouch develops at the base of the tongue in which food collects, simultaneously occluding the pharynx so that the bolus cannot enter the oesophagus (Logemann, 1983a).

Stenosing of the hypopharynx and oesophagus may result from a necessarily tight closure when pharyngolaryngectomy has been carried out. Swallowing will be slow and restricted because of the narrow lumen and loss of pharyngeal peristalsis. The narrowing may be corrected by dilatation or further surgery. Careful consideration and experimentation will be necessary to determine which foods can be eaten most easily. Apparently obvious substances such as mashed potatoes and minced meat are often far from ideal because of the way in which they accumulate and clog the pharynx. The dietitian will give advice to ensure that nutrition is balanced when a diet of suitable texture has been decided upon.

When the cricopharyngeal muscle has been removed in extensive surgery together with the cardiac sphincter, regurgitation may occur if the patient has eaten a particularly large meal or bends over too soon after eating. Ranger (1983) also notes that in some of these patients food drains into the duodenum from the stomach too rapidly. This gives the patient a feeling of fullness, faintness, tachycardia and nausea accompanied by sweating for an hour or two after a heavy meal. This condition is known as 'dumping'.

It is interesting to consider the study conducted by Mendelsohn and McConnel (1987) which demonstrated the importance of laryngeal elevation as a major factor in controlling sphincter function in the P-E segment, in addition to the cricopharyngeal muscle. As described elsewhere, the cricopharyngeus muscle acts as a sphincter which relaxes to allow the bolus to pass into the oesophagus. Using manofluoroscopy, a technique combining manometry and videofluoroscopy, it can be seen that rapid elevation of the larynx produces the drop in pressure and transient negative pressure observed in the P-E segment as the bolus passes through. Mendelsohn and McConnel also established that if laryngeal elevation is impaired, the pressure drop during deglutition is slower and the fleeting negative pressure does not occur. It can be concluded, therefore, that if the larynx is so crucial to the function of the P-E segment during deglutition, all laryngectomees will almost certainly have less efficient patterns of swallowing than preoperatively even if more obvious problems are not apparent.

The inability to speak and eat at the same time presents obvious social difficulties. Many patients will eat only with members of the family and avoid eating in restaurants.

Defaecation

It is important that the laryngectomee maintains a diet that reduces the possibility of constipation. The loss of the glottis which closes during exertion may make effortful defaecation a problem.

Smoking

Patients are advised to stop smoking but some continue to do so being of the opinion that there is little point in closing the stable door after the horse has bolted. It is possible to use the buccinator muscles for suction and aspiration of air through the nose as with smelling.

Baths and showers

Care has to be taken not to inhale water into the tracheostoma when taking a bath or shower or hair washing. A plastic stoma apron should be worn tied round the neck for protection.

Lifting

The maintenance of thoracic pressure is difficult for prolonged fixation of the thorax to meet the demands of manual work, but even so, many patients are able to continue employment in jobs such as porters or dockers. Their previously well-developed muscles in the back, shoulders, arms and elsewhere appear able to compensate for the loss of the glottis in this respect. If the patient has a dropped shoulder, of course, lifting weights will not be possible and even turning the steering wheel of a heavy goods vehicle will be difficult.

Swimming

Swimming is not normally possible unless special apparatus is worn and instruction given by an experienced instructor. Laryngectomee associations (see p. 372) can provide information.

(a)

(b)

(c)

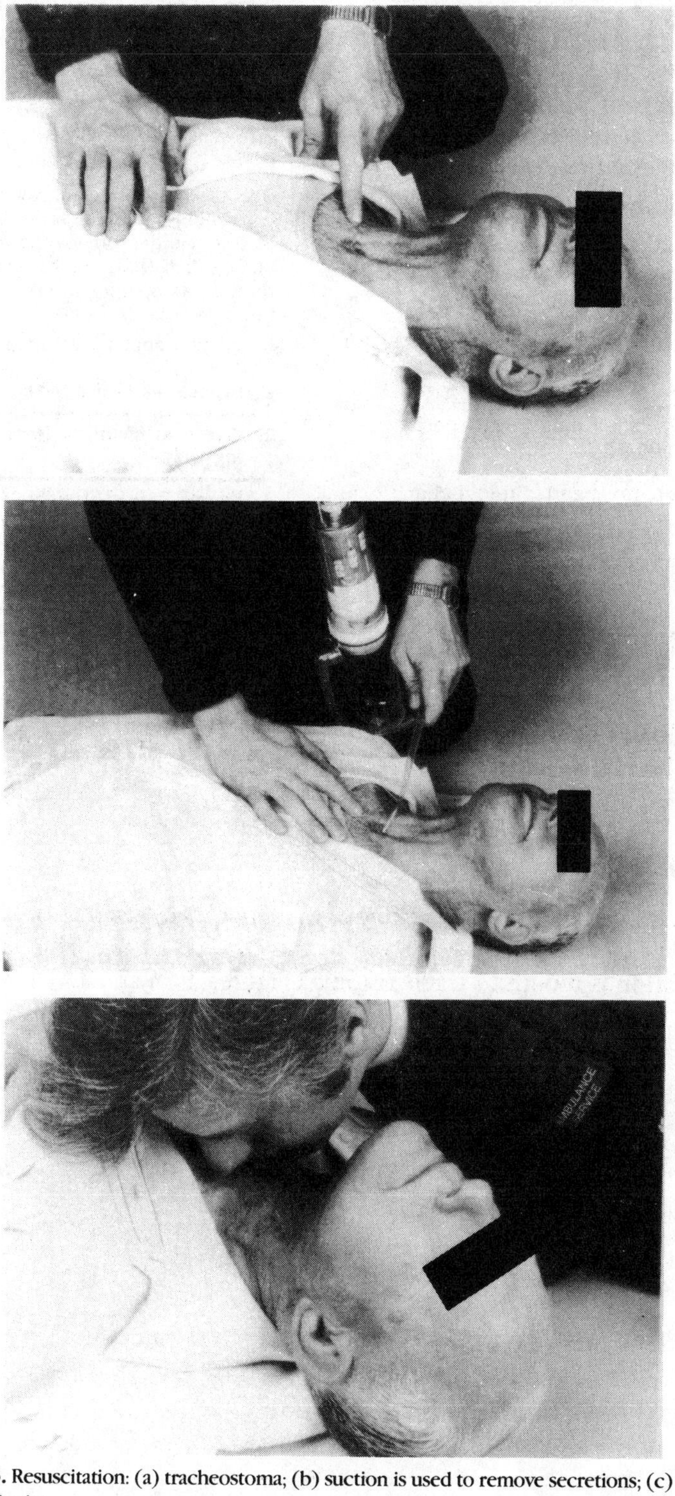

Figure 17.5. Resuscitation: (a) tracheostoma; (b) suction is used to remove secretions; (c) mouth-to-neck resuscitation.

EMERGENCY!

I am a
Partial Neck Breather
(LARYNGECTOMEE)

I breathe MAINLY through an opening in my neck, very little through my nose or mouth.

If I have stopped breathing:

1. Expose my entire neck. Pinch my nose between the middle two fingers of your hand, and cover my lips with the palm of same hand. Press thumb on upper neck under chin.

2. Give me **mouth to neck breathing only.**

3. Keep my head straight-chin up.

4. Keep neck opening clear with clean CLOTH (not tissue)

5. Use oxygen supply to neck opening, ONLY, when I start to breathe again.

BE PROMPT-SECONDS COUNT
I NEED AIR NOW!

EMERGENCY!

One or more occupants of this car is a Total Neck Breather. He (or she) is a Laryngectomee and has **NO VOCAL CHORDS!** He breathes only through an opening in his neck. Not through nose or mouth.

If he has stopped breathing:

1. **Expose the Entire Neck.**
2. **Give Him Mouth to Neck Breathing Only.**
3. **Keep His Head Straight - Chin Up.**
4. **Keep Neck Opening Clear With Clean Cloth (Not Tissue).**
5. **Use Oxygen Supply To Neck Opening, Only, When He Starts to Breathe Again.**

BE PROMPT — SECONDS COUNT
HE NEEDS AIR NOW!

Figure 17.6. Emergency card and car sticker.

Resuscitation

It is essential that everyone working in the emergency services or involved in first aid is aware of neck breathing in the laryngectomee. This means that resuscitation is mouth to tracheostoma (Figures 17.5 and 17.6).

Chapter 18 Total Laryngectomy: Acquisition of Pseudo-voice

The subject of laryngectomy is an area of speech pathology which has been exceptionally well documented and researched. Many articles tracing the historical developments in surgery since Bilroth performed his first laryngectomy on 31 December 1973 are available in journals of otolaryngology. Outstanding books on the acquisition of pseudo-voice and the management of the laryngectomee are those by Damsté (1958), Snidecor (1968), Boone (1977), Diedrich and Youngstrom (1977), and Gardener (1978). A clear and comprehensive account of laryngectomy from diagnosis to rehabilitation can be found in Edels (1983).

The Pharyngo-oesophageal (P-E) Sphincter

The importance of the P-E segment of suitable tonicity for oesophageal speech has been discussed in the previous chapter. As early as 1937 Stetson published the first X-ray study of laryngectomee speech. He discovered that the pseudoglottis is formed by the oesophageal sphincter and that the valvular lips are separated as air bursts through them and then recoil and close automatically as the air pressure below them drops. This mechanism is much the same in fact as for laryngeal phonation. The sphincter in normal individuals is tightly closed in order to prevent this happening and the entry of air into the stomach during the respiratory cycle (Bateman and Negus, 1954). After laryngectomy the muscles may be relaxed to take advantage of this normal physiological process.

Pseudo-voice requires a moving column of air to pass through the segment causing it to vibrate. This air must first be introduced into the oesophagus. The segment is composed of striated muscle innervated by the recurrent laryngeal nerve, and voluntary relaxation and tension of the sphincter can be acquired for oesophageal voice production (Levin, 1962b).

Seeman (1959) claimed to have been the first to determine by lateral radiography that the oesophagus acts as a vicarious or substitute 'lung' and the oesophageal sphincter as a pseudoglottis. As cited in Kallen's (1934) review of research, Seeman drew attention to the fact that:

(a) (b)

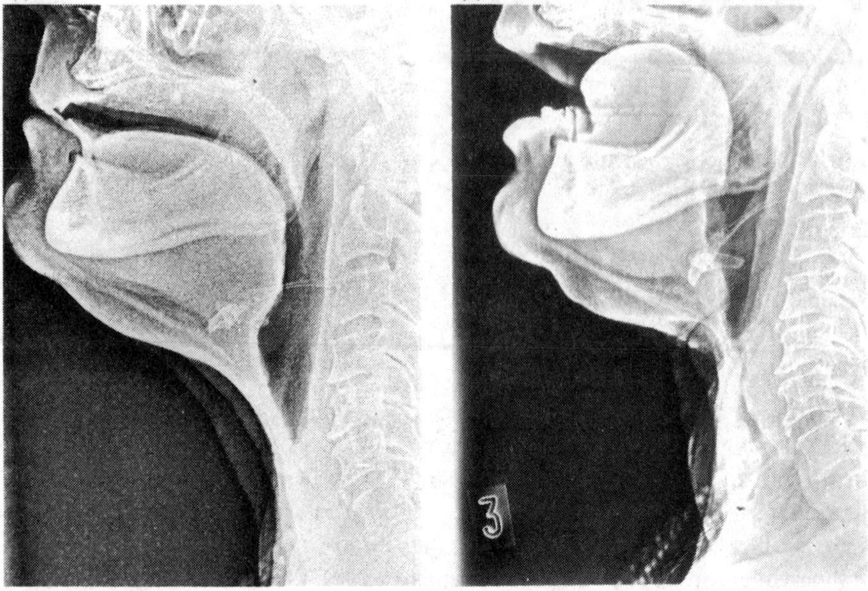

Figure 18.1. Postlaryngectomy xeroradiographs. (a,b) Patient 1: total laryngectomy, fluent speaker (male). (a) At rest – the P-E segment is at the level of the junction of C5 and C6; the posterior wall of the pharynx bulges forwards. (b) Producing /i:/ – the P-E segment is vibrating as air returns from the capacious 'vicarious lung' (oesophagus).

> The cervical and upper portions of the oesophagus contain transverse striated muscle fibres, the muscles of the lower part are smooth. As the recurrent laryngeal nerve gives off branches some of which (the so-called rami oesophagei nervi recurrentis) are distributed to the oesophagus, the phenomenon associated with phonation is probably the result of an irradiation to the musculature of the oesophagus of the nerve impulses attending phonation.

Seeman sought to prove that phonatory contractions in the cervical and upper portions of the thoracic oesophagus were genuinely active and not dependent upon respiratory movements. Only in the middle and lower thoracic oesophageal sections did he observe changes in the lumen effected by thoracic movement. In skilful laryngectomised speakers it seems possible that there is extension to the oesophageal sphincter of the nerve impulses for normal laryngeal phonation, though this is naturally difficult to prove. In one of our most proficient speakers the cricopharyngeal bands on either side were seen in the laryngoscopic mirror to approximate in the mid-line exactly like bulky vocal folds as he phonated, and to relax and separate on inhaling.

The adaptation of the upper oesophagus to function as a vicarious lung can be seen clearly in xeroradiographs. It is obvious that the volume of air available for voice production is far less than when a pulmonic air supply is available. Stetson (1937) thought that the oesophageal air reservoir consisted of only 2.5 cm^3. Snidecor and Isshiki (1965) discovered, however, that airflow is

(c) (d)

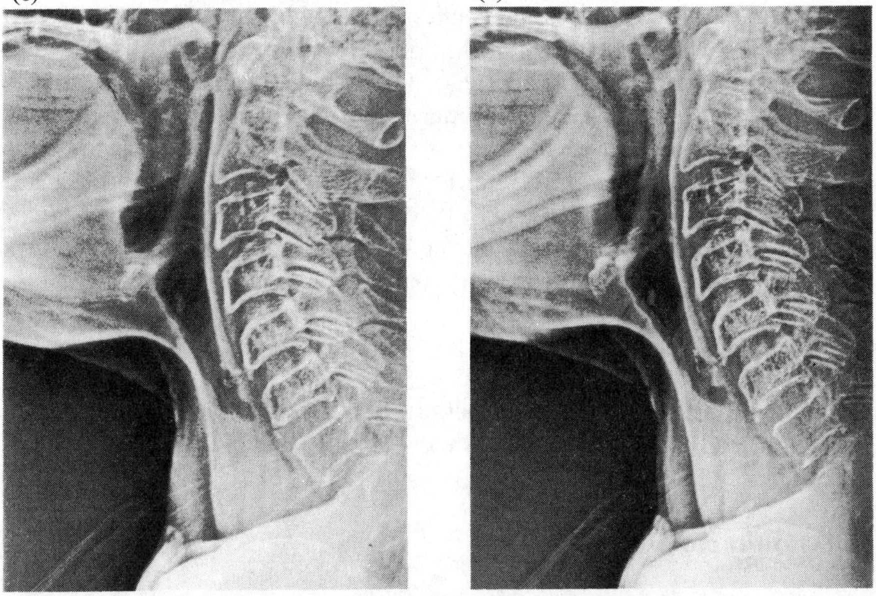

Figure 18.1. (contd). (c,d) Patient 2: total laryngectomy; fluent speaker (female). (c) At rest – the P-E segment is at the level of the junction C6 and C7; the anterior wall of the pharynx bulges to meet the posterior. (d) Producing /i:/ – the shallow P-E segment vibrates on returning air. Note the small air reservoir in comparison with patient 1; although a fluent speaker, patient 2 needs to charge the oesophagus with air frequently in order to maintain fluent speech.

(a) (b)

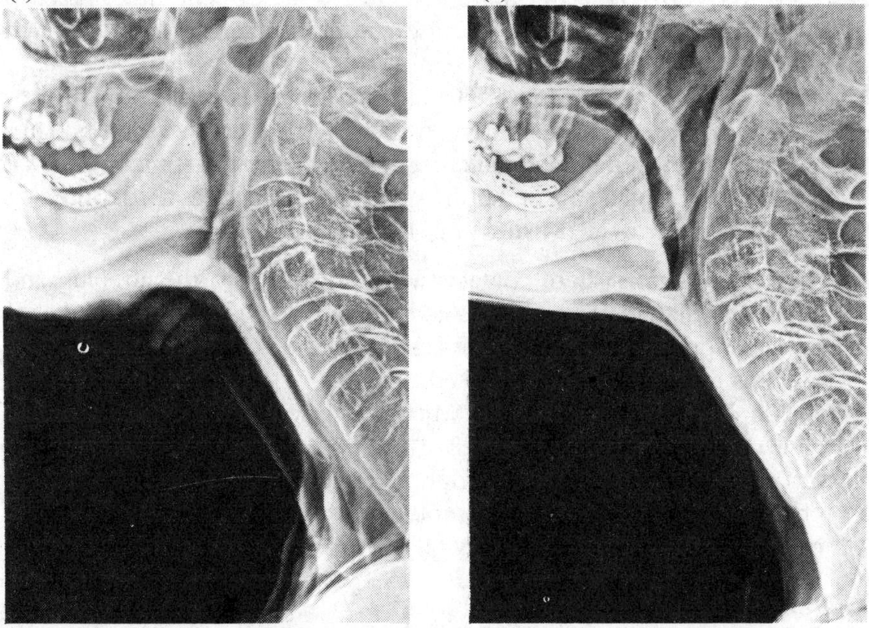

Figure 18.2. Patient 3: pharyngolaryngectomy (male). (a) At rest – there is no P-E segment. (b) Attempting to produce /i:/. Oesophageal voice can only be produced in single syllables with great effort. There are swallowing difficulties. Patient 3 uses an electronic larynx very successfully.

(Figures 18.1 and 18.2 reproduced by permission of Dr Frances MacCurtain, National College of Speech Sciences, London.)

considerably higher than this and volume per syllable ranged from 5 cm^3/s to 16 cm^3/s and 27 cm^3/s to 72 cm^3/s in good speakers.

All research workers and experienced speech clinicians who have to rely upon their powers of observation are agreed that fluent oesophageal speech is perfectly synchronised with the normal respiratory cycle. Bateman and Negus (1954), Di Carlo, Amster and Herer (1955), Robe *et al.* (1956), Vrticka and Svoboda (1961, 1963) and Isshiki (1965, 1968) are unanimous that fluent oesophageal speech occurs only during lung expiration and that it is always prefaced by lung inspiration as in normal speech.

Methods of Air Intake

There are three main methods of charging the oesophagus with air: injection, inhalation and swallowing. The latter is not suitable for oesophageal speech.

Injection method

Standard injection

Standard injection consists of compressing air in the oral cavity by sealing the lips, closing the palatopharyngeal sphincter and compressing the cheeks while the tongue pumps the air posteriorly into the pharynx. As the compressed air descends to the hypopharynx the fibres of the P-E segment either relax to allow air into the oesophagus or the air pressure is sufficient to pass through the sphincter.

Diedrich and Youngstrom (1966), by means of lateral X-ray studies, examined tongue movements during air intake in 20 laryngectomees. They noted that these movements are different from a swallow movement, also that the quicker the air intake the better the speech as long pauses reduce fluency. Standard injection revealed two types of tongue movement:

1. Glossal press consists of contact by the tongue with the alveolus, and frequently middle of the tongue contact with the hard palate, while the posterior portion moves backwards but fails to touch the pharyngeal wall. The lips may be opened or closed.
2. Glossopharyngeal press occurs when the tip and middle of the tongue contact the alveolus and hard palate, and posterior tongue moves back to make contact with the posterior pharyngeal wall, whilst the hypopharyngeal cavity may be completely obliterated. There is palatopharyngeal closure and lips may be open or closed.

Consonant injection

This term is used to describe the method whereby air injection occurs simultaneously with articulation of consonants, particularly voiceless plosives. This technique always involves closure of the palatopharyngeal sphincter but approximation of lips, and the tongue tip with the alveolar ridge, or posterior tongue with the velum will vary according to the consonant being produced. Articulation assists injection.

Inhalation method (insufflation or aspiration)

At rest the oesophagus below the P-E segment is closed. On inspiration the drop in thoracic pressure also results in a fall in pressure in the oesophagus. Air then flows into the oesophagus from the pharynx in order to equalise pressure. (This transfer of air may not occur if the P-E segment is tense or hypertonic.) The air is then held in the oesophagus by closure of the P-E segment once the air pressure is equalised, and will subsequently be used for oesphageal voice. During 'inhalation' the tongue never occludes the oral cavity (Diedrich and Youngstrom, 1966) and there is little or no movement of the dorsum of the tongue. The lips are open, there is no velopharyngeal closure and the airway from lips to pharyngo-oesophageal junction is open.

Air swallowing

This is not a viable method of air intake for speech because of the time delay between air intake and return which disrupts fluency. It may also result in discomfort as air accumulates in the stomach. Nevertheless, occasional instances of air swallowing in the early stages of treatment may help the patient to identify the sound and sensation of air passing through the P-E segment as air from the stomach is released.

Importance of insufflation

The various methods used by oesophageal speakers were highlighted by Isshiki (1965, 1968). Six speakers of variable proficiency were assessed. It was found that air intake and use, in conjunction with respiration and vocalisation, vary greatly with individual speakers. Some speakers injected air while speaking and as they exhaled, which is what other researchers have found. All speakers apparently 'inhaled' air into the oesophagus synchronously with lung inspiration. Some speakers relied more on injection than inhalation. Negative pressure in the oesophagus during lung inhalation assists injection of the air by the injection method. The more effective and larger the air intake, the better the speech. Lung expiration and speech are synchronised. A slow and normal deep breathing movement itself did not insufflate air into the oesophagus. This is important and confirms the observation that a quick diaphragmatic pant is necessary for sucking air into the oesophagus and needs to be developed by the patient.

Diaphragmatic action

Samuel and Adams (1976) examined the role of oesophageal and diaphragmatic movements in successful speakers. The neoglottis relaxes as the diaphragm descends and near the end of the diaphragm's descent the oesophagus suddenly dilates like an inflated sausage-shaped balloon. As the diaphragm ascends, the lower end of the oesophagus collapses and the upper segment increases slightly in diameter with increased air pressure. The neoglottis opens and the neck of the balloon undergoes controlled release until emptied as the diaphragm reaches maximum ascent. There is good co-ordination between movements of neoglottis and diaphragm. The quality of speech is related to the length of the oesophageal dilatation. (These authors note that emphysema (see p. 10) will interfere with lung flow and control.)

Lateral thinking in therapy

Traditionally, various advocates of either injection or inhalation have stressed the advantages of their preferred approaches to air intake and these are discussed on p. 351. It is advisable for the therapist to be flexible, however, and to use the approach which appears to be easiest for the patient. In the early stages an exploratory and empirical approach is appropriate. The rigidity of one fixed approach may exclude potentially successful routes to achieving oesophageal voice. It is obviously unwise to confine speech therapy to teaching one method but advisable to introduce a combination of methods, since this is actually what takes place when fluent speech is mastered.

Air-shunt after Loss of P-E Segment

In pharyngolaryngectomy, since the upper portion of the oesophagus and the hypopharyngeal muscular tissue have been excised, the P-E segment is lost. Without the pseudoglottis, fluent speech is much more difficult to acquire but voice is possible and injection and inhalation can be used in the same way. If there is sufficient narrowing of the reconstructed tube vibration may be obtained for weak voice as the air is expelled. The air charge is under very little control during speech, of course, and is quickly lost, generally after one or two syllables. Air intake has to be accomplished very frequently and voice is tiring for the individual to maintain. At first, too, the throat muscles may ache with fatigue rather readily. The voice may be deeper than oesophageal voice after simple laryngectomy. Air has to be aspirated rather than injected and overbreathing and dizziness can develop.

Very rarely, the reconstructed oesophagus, without causing difficulty in swallowing, presents sufficient narrowing at some point to offer resistance to the outgoing air. Then the voice is produced as loudly and as fluently as that obtained by the patient who has undergone simple laryngectomy. Only one of our patients has obtained speech of such high standard, but Dornhurst and Negus (1954) stated that the difficulty in producing the necessary narrowing of the oesophagus should not be insuperable. Where no such narrowing exists, digital pressure on the front of the neck or a specially designed band, or even just a collar worn moderately tightly, may be sufficient to create an adequate pseudoglottis.

We have had three patients who developed the knack of vibrating air in the reconstructed pharynx on both ingoing and outgoing air. Air was moved by means of rapid lung inspiration and expiration. No air injection took place. This method of voice production was a great advantage because it doubled the number of syllables for each air charge and speech was fluent and rapid as a result, though the voice was weak. In these patients the method was not taught but developed naturally and spontaneously and was encouraged because of its effectiveness. It is not an appropriate method for acquiring oesophageal voice after simple laryngectomy.

Colon transplant cases may obtain a whisper or audible voice with little trouble and more easily than in the case of simple laryngectomy, with the anastomosis of colon and hypopharynx providing a narrowing which acts as a pseudoglottis. Lall and Evison (1966) described four cases of colon transplant subjected to cineradiographic examination during speech:

Case 1
Case 1 had a good voice and a reservoir of air which rose, with the help of the diaphragm, through an upper narrowed segment of the transplant.

Case 2
Case 2 had no narrowing, air was shunted up by the diaphragm; a soft whisper was possible.

Case 3
Case 3 did not retain air in the tube and failed to coordinate diaphragmatic movement with voice.

Case 4
Case 4 had an excellent colonic voice; the cervical portion of the tube from the level of C7 to the first thoracic vertebra was noted to be collapsed at rest and the segment vibrated in phonation.

Patients who can only obtain a soft voice may be helped by an amplifier.

Success and Failure Rates in achieving Oesophageal Voice

There is general recognition that a substantial number of laryngectomees do not achieve successful oesophageal voice.

The incidence of failure is difficult to establish because of the variability in standards of what constitutes good, bad and indifferent. The basis for selection of cases varies between assessors and the standards of assessment. Diedrich and Youngstrom (1966) estimate that a third fail and Edwards (1976) agrees. Goode (1975) at the Stanford Medical Centre places failure rate as high as 50% and makes the point that it takes 12 months of arduous endeavour to attain real proficiency. Blom, Singer and Hamaker (1986) also state that although traditionally considered to be the method of choice, oesophageal voice cannot be achieved by more than half those patients who try to acquire it. They also qualify this statement by adding that the standard of oesophageal speech when acquired is very variable. Schaeffer and Johns (1982) note reports of success ranging from 98% to 25% and conclude that it is reasonable to assume that at least one-third of laryngectomees fail to achieve satisfactory oesophageal communication.

Reasons for failure

Inadequate P-E segment

Recent work has clarified the various insufficiencies of the P-E segment which occur as a direct result of the type and extent of surgery. Perry and Edels (1985) conducted a videofluoroscopic study of 8 oesophageal speakers and 42 'failed' oesophageal speakers. They concluded that the latter could be divided into four groups, each with a clearly identifiable inadequacy of the P-E segment:

Hypotonic (group 1)
In the hypotonic group the P-E segment does not close and is functionally ineffective, resulting in a weak voice which may be improved by exerting digital pressure (Logemann, 1983b).

Hypertonic (group 2) and spasmodic (group 3)
The tight P-E segment of the hypertonic and spasmodic groups can affect both air intake and expulsion and it is these groups which might benefit from pharyngo-oesophageal myotomy (Henley and Souliere, 1986) or pharyngeal plexus neurectomy (Singer, Blom and Hamaker, 1986).

Stricture (group 4)
This was defined as fibrous tissue which did not dilate during swallowing and some of these patients exhibited the pouch at the base of the tongue described by Logemann (1983a) and discussed in Chapter 17.

It is significant that all the patients in this study who failed to develop oesphageal speech had anatomical or physiological problems to account for their failure. In the past, failure to achieve voice has frequently been attributed to lack of motivation. The importance of motivation cannot be undervalued but this study highlights appropriate assessment of the P-E segment when voice is not developing satisfactorily. Referral to a specialist centre with viseofluoroscopy is necessary.

Neurological damage

Damage to the pharyngeal and lingual nerve supply produces muscular weakness, especially of the tongue, which impedes air injection and articulation. Swallowing difficulties may also occur as a result of neurological damage.

The other reasons for failure can be listed as follows:

- Amount and timing of radiotherapy.
- Old age and frailty accompanied by lack of drive to learn.
- Deafness and inability to monitor speech.
- Low intelligence and inability to master the new muscular condition.
- Rejection of oesophageal speech on aesthetic and social grounds. These patients may prefer to use 'whispered' speech or an electronic larynx rather than what they or their fellows regard as 'belching'.
- Previously inadequate speech.
- Unsympathetic spouse or a partner who is deaf.
- Depression.
- Insufficient and/or inadequate speech therapy.

Superior Oesophageal Voice

The oesophageal speaker can become so fluent that strangers do not realise the true nature of the disability and may ask whether the speaker has a cold or laryngitis. This is a tribute indeed to the naturalness of the voice which up to this time no artificial larynx has been able to emulate.

Pitch and quality

Studies indicate that pitch and quality in oesophageal speech appear to be interdependent (Williams and Watson, 1985) as are pitch and intensity (Snidecor and Curry, 1959). Gimson (1962) states that variations of intensity on the same frequency may induce impression of pitch change. In order to raise the pitch, greater volume has to be employed necessitating replenishment of the oesophageal reservoir. For a drop in pitch, less intensity must be used. The accomplished speaker may have a range of an octave but the fundamental pitch is an octave lower than normal voice. Damsté (1958) in a study of 20 male patients found a median pitch of 67.5 Hz and Snidecor and Curry (1959), 63.3 Hz. Kallen (1934) noted that movements of the head and neck could contribute to pitch change and this aspect might be utilised for emphasis and expressiveness in speech. Understandably, oesophageal speakers with pitch levels and inflection variations approximating those of a laryngeal speaker are considered most acceptable (Hyman, 1979).

The quality of oesophageal voice is rough by reason of the crude vibration and cricopharyngeal muscle recoil. Harmonic analysis by sonograph shows the two vowel formants of oesophageal voice to be 'fuzzy'. Although quality of the vowels may be improved by carefully adjusted articulation and the raising of resonance pitch, much improvement of the partials is not feasible on account of the poor quality of the fundamental note (Snidecor, 1968).

Duration and rate

Length of phrase varies considerably. Snidecor and Curry (1960) measured the number of syllables per breath intake of superior laryngeal speakers. They found that the mean lowest consecutive sequence consisted of 3.8 syllables and the highest 8.7, with an overall average of 4.98 syllables. The extreme range in these subjects was 22 syllables in one speaker, and Snidecor (1968) is of the opinion that 11–12 syllables is a very satisfactory number for superior speakers.

Snidecor and Isshiki (1965) expressed the opinion that the number of syllables per air charge is not of crucial importance and that the speed of utterance is a preferable indicator of similarity to normal speech. A good average rate is between 80 and 120 words per minute (words/min) although a very superior speaker was found to achieve 153 words/min. (Laryngeal speakers have a rate of 166 words/min.) Speech rate entirely depends on the efficiency of the air charge. The latency period – from the start of injection or inhalation of air into the oesophagus until pseudo-voice is produced – is approximately 0.5 second in superior oesophageal speakers. Snidecor concluded:

> There is no magic in a long phrase. Clearness, ease of speech and reasonable rate of words per minute should take precedence over any struggle to break records in regard to words per air charge.

Volume

The chief handicap, even in the most excellent speakers, is the lack of volume and this is especially felt when speaking against background noise such as at a party, in the street, in an office or restaurant. Clarke and Hoops (1970) found that laryngectomees' speech deteriorated with increased speech-type background noise, not in intelligibility but in general speech proficiency, with a decrease in phrase length, and increase in lung airflow. An amplifier counteracts this problem.

Articulation

Superior oesophageal speech is not attainable without excellent articulation, however good the oesophageal voice itself. Hyman (1979) noted that oesophageal speakers considered to be intelligible have articulation that is correctly identified 90% of the time.

Studies analysing the acoustic features and differences in speaking proficiences of laryngeal, oesophageal, electronic larynx and tracheo-oesophageal speakers may be of interest to the reader (Robbins *et al.*, 1984; Merwin, Goldstein and Rothman, 1985; Williams and Watson, 1985, 1987).

Management and Treatment

The patient who is about to undergo laryngectomy does not usually see the speech therapist until the traumatic period of diagnosis and failure of radiotherapy is over and surgery is essential. As a member of a team consisting of laryngologist, radiotherapist, nursing sister, physiotherapist, medical social worker and other professionals, the speech therapist's involvement begins at a relatively late stage. The patient and family are contending with distress resulting from unsuccessful intervention and the anticipation of surgery.

The speech therapist's goals throughout can be broadly divided into those related to the acquisition of an acceptable and efficient method of communication, and those concerned with the patient's adjustment to the consequences of laryngectomy.

Preoperative contact

In ideal circumstances the speech therapist should visit the patient and, if possible, the spouse during the days prior to laryngectomy. The interview must be tailored to the needs of each patient and for this reason may be brief or, in some cases, very lengthy indeed. It will be relaxed and unhurried and will take place where there is privacy and little chance of interruption.

Although it is carried out in a conversational setting the therapist will incorporate specific goals into what should be dialogue, not an out-pouring of factual information. These goals include:

1. Establishing patient/therapist relationship and understanding.
2. Informal evaluation of communication skills.
3. Observing the patient's emotional status.
4. Providing reassurance and information about postoperative communication.

Throughout the interview the therapist will provide information but this should be simple and straightforward and should not overwhelm. Patients vary enormously in what they want to know and in what they have understood and remembered of the explanations given to them by other team members. The speech therapist is only one member of a team where the ward sister is usually the chief source of information and reassurance. Medical social workers will also be providing advice. In addition to keeping each other informed, all professionals involved should know what the surgeon has told the patient so that conflicting information and terminology relating to the disease is avoided. In the USA surgeons discuss cancer openly with their patients but in the UK 'growth' and 'tumour' are used in an attempt to soften the blow. Patients tend to be told that they have cancer only if they ask the question directly. It is not the speech therapist's task to inform the patient that the condition is cancer (Greene, 1980b).

Many patients are reassured by the explanation that it is the voice alone which will be lost. As the terms 'speech', 'language' and 'articulation' are used interchangeably in general conversation some patients are surprised and heartened to learn that they will not be like the stroke victim who has lost his 'voice', but that it will be possible to mouth words clearly in structured sentences. A demonstration of clear speech without voice by the therapist can be reassuring.

It is helpful to see patient and spouse together so that the family is involved in treatment from an early stage and domestic relationships can be observed. The spouse can provide essential support for the laryngectomee after hospitalisation but will also need considerable support to deal with a potentially frightening and distressing situation from the early stages. For this reason the therapist may also arrange an interview with the spouse alone at some time so that the family's fears and concerns may be discussed freely.

By the end of preoperative contact with the speech therapist, whether on one or more occasions, the patient should be confident that treatment will be with a clinician who will ensure a satisfactory means of communication postoperatively.

Preoperative visit by a laryngectomee

The patient will find it reassuring and encouraging to be visited by a laryngectomee with good speech and tact. Tremendous harm can be done to a vulnerable patient by an unsuitable visitor, however efficient the pseudo-voice, and the effects may be long lasting and militate against successful therapy.

If possible, a good oesophageal speaker of the same sex and similar age should visit – someone who is able to empathise with the patient rather than embark on a detailed and horrendous account of his or her own operation. In general patient and spouse do not react adversely to a less than ideal voice regarding quality and loudness, but they are dismayed by a speaker with noisy stoma blast which highlights for them the permanent tracheostoma.

Consideration must be given to the comparability of the necessary surgery in each case. It is cruel and pointless to introduce a visitor who has had 'simple' laryngectomy to the prospective laryngopharyngo-oesophagectomy patient when the task of acquiring pseudo-voice may be very different. In these cases we do not arrange for a laryngectomised visitor to demonstrate but we assure the patient that a loud whisper will be achieved quite easily and mention the various artificial larynxes and amplifiers available (see p. 367).

The speech therapist should mention the prospective visitor to the patient and respect the wishes of the individual who does not want to meet the laryngectomee at this stage. The majority of patients welcome the opportunity. Others, understandably, feel that they cannot cope with yet another person and new experience when there can be no choice as to whether or not they undergo surgery. A visit may be more valuable postoperatively.

The visiting oesophageal speaker should be accompanied by the speech therapist initially. If visitor and patient establish a good relationship the therapist can leave them to talk freely.

Psychological Effects of Laryngectomy

However excellent the surgical result and speech therapy, progress will not be made if the patient's emotional reaction to the situation is not considered. The speech therapist, by keeping in touch with the patient before and after operation, pays out a lifeline onto which he can hold and the strength of which even the therapist may not fully realise. The operation of laryngectomy is one of the most traumatic and mutilating procedures and emotional trauma is unavoidable but can be alleviated by good management.

Acute depression often interferes with speech progress. Fontaine and Mitchell (1960) stressed the emotional and sexual difficulties which may arise after laryngectomy. They emphasise the need for cooperation between medical social worker and speech therapist in the alleviation of anxiety, and of obtaining adjustment of interpersonal relationships within the patient's family before voice can be expected to develop. Heaver and Arnold (1962) emphasise the same point and write as psychiatrist and laryngologist 'coordinately' as follows:

> A pathologic reactive depression is the usual sequel to the doctor's dictum that the larynx is cancerous, that it must be removed at once, and that natural speech no longer will be possible. Fright, anxiety, insomnia, confusion, self-pity, fear of death, and suicidal impulses pervade and devitalise the patient's psychic energy. It also should be remembered that a depression occasionally masquerades as euphoria.

This last sentence is often true in our experience when the patient is in hospital, depression overcoming him when he returns home. It is also our experience that with increasing information being provided by health education agencies and the media, patients generally have greater understanding of anatomy, physiology and medical conditions. As a result, fewer individuals appear to experience panic and despair to the same extent that patients exhibited 25 years ago.

Laryngologist's role

The laryngologist's ability to establish rapport with the patient and family preoperatively is vital. If the patient has complete confidence in the surgeon anxiety can be markedly reduced. Barton (1965) examined the adjustment of 50 patients to total laryngectomy (among whom there were five suicides) and of 50 patients to partial laryngectomy. He concluded that the individual's adjustment to the disease and operation should be of primary concern to the surgeon. Many patients are ill before the operation and are overwhelmed by the catastrophe. Instability in a patient in the past is an indication for extra care and vigilance in rehabilitation, and psychotherapy may be advisable. Inability to speak and express fears causes acute anxiety. Lack of motivation in learning to speak is a danger signal.

Marital relations

Of major importance is the understanding and forbearance of spouse and family. Sleeping together, Barton says, is a haunting experience; coughing of the patient may alarm the partner who becomes tired and over-wrought. We have had many spouses describe the hours they spend awake at night, particularly in the early stages, as they listen for their partner's breathing and periodically check that blankets are not covering the stoma. Even when the patient has fully recovered from surgery, the spouse can be so repulsed by the tracheostoma that the couple's sexual relationship is seriously affected. This, in combination with the communication difficulties, can have a devastating effect on the marriage and referral to appropriate counselling services will be necessary.

Warning signs

Murphy, Bosna and Ogura (1964) reviewed 24 laryngectomised patients, four of whom were judged to be suffering from depression, and three of whom had not returned to work. These researchers were not interested in the technicalities of diagnosis by experts and whether the depression was reactive, endogenous, psychotic or neurotic. Whether depression antedates surgery they think is fortuitous. Whether depression is a reaction to surgery is not germane since they believe the general symptoms, course, treatment and final outcome are the same. Depression in the absence of other psychiatric illness is readily treatable with gratifying results. These authors describe depression as a sustained mood of dejection, sadness and joylessness. Other symptoms are:

- Insomnia.
- Undue fatigue.
- Anorexia.
- Disinterest.
- Social withdrawal.
- Crying spells.
- Feelings of helplessness.
- Impaired concentration.
- Indecisiveness.
- Neglect of personal cleanliness or grooming.
- Either a passive wish for death or thoughts of suicide.

Many of these symptoms are normal in the circumstances after laryngectomy and resolve themselves spontaneously. Real depression is characterised by the persistence for months of a cluster of these symptoms, Murphy, Bosna and Ogura (1964) emphasise. This needs psychotherapy, discussion and support, combined with antidepressant drug therapy. These authors noted significant details related to their group of patients: age, education, employment history, marital relations, alcohol abuse, psychiatric history and the estimated importance of speech in the patient's usual employment. None of these factors or group of factors was predictive of the patient's final adjustment, mastery of oesophageal speech or return to work.

Fear of cancer

The laryngectomee has to deal with the fears experienced normally by anyone suffering from cancer in addition to the specific anxieties of disfigurement, communication problems and eating and breathing difficulties (Harris, Vogtsberger and Mattox, 1985). When cancer is diagnosed the victim feels helpless to control the course of the illness and may withdraw emotionally from others while experiencing anger, isolation and loneliness. There will also be considerable fear of various treatments such as surgery, radiation and medication. The severity of these reactions may be reduced by the doctor's and surgeon's sympathetic discussion preoperatively. The psychosocial implications of laryngectomy are frequently not discussed (Berkowitz and Lucente, 1985).

Effect on self-image

The operation is an amputation and many patients will go through a long period of grieving for the loss of this part of themselves and its significance. Some men mourn the lost laryngeal voice which was part of their masculinity while women may find the deeper oesophageal voice unfeminine and regret the loss of a beautiful voice. Even when oesophageal voice is excellent the subtle paralinguistic features previously possible can no longer be produced (see Chapter 1).

Emotional expression

Without the larynx the normal routes of catharsis for emotional relief are also curtailed. The inability to shout or sob is frequently mentioned by patients as an added frustration at times of stress. Similarly, enjoyment of humour is reduced with the inability to laugh out aloud.

Our society is highly verbal and good communication skills, rightly or wrongly, are equated with intelligence. The opposite is also true and many laryngectomees feel socially devalued. They may have to contend with the 'Does he take sugar?' syndrome, when enquiries are directed to companions of the laryngectomee, in addition to other social indignities. Rehabilitation must take into account all these distressing features. Surgeons who are sensitive to the distress of their patients are driven to seek alternatives in partial laryngectomy and fistula speech as described earlier. There is no doubt that laryngectomy is psychologically far more traumatic than the operation itself. There is a need for weeks and often months to reassure patient and family and to ward off depression and despair in which loss of speech is the focal factor. The misery of being unable to communicate must be recognised and, from the beginning, the patient must be helped to communicate as effectively as possible by the most efficient means.

Postoperative Management

To maintain contact the speech therapist should visit the patient as soon after the operation as is allowed even if this visit is fleeting. Ideally, during the period of 10 days to a fortnight while the nasogastric tube remains *in situ*, daily visits should continue. In the first few days of recovery swelling and stiffness around the neck and mandible will restrict movement. Strenuous attempts at speech may damage the wound so the patient is encouraged to articulate clearly but gently. This relaxed 'whisper' is intelligible and some voiceless consonants can be heard so that the patient is encouraged. An intraoral speech aid, such as the Cooper-Rand oral vibrator, can be used effectively at this stage. This will be rendered easier if the patient has experimented with it before the operation in the course of reassurance strategies.

We discourage written communication as far as possible when clearly articulated speech is much less tedious and frustrating. Other benefits of this approach include maintaining the mobility of articulatory muscles, especially the tongue, which may be paretic or stiff following surgery. Encouraging relaxed and accurate articulation is also an ideal basis for pseudo-voice. A realistic approach must be employed and some patients may prefer written communication. Their frustration should not be compounded by the feeling that the speech therapist has 'forbidden' them to use writing.

In cases where healing is delayed and the nasogastric tube is retained for some weeks because of a fistula, the surgeon should be consulted concerning the advisability of whispering and the possible danger of exaggerated articulatory movements of the tongue pulling at the wound. Much depends upon the height of the fistula in the pharyngeal wall and also the manner of speech - some patients put far too much effort into whispering.

Similarly, even when recovery has been straightforward and the nasogastric tube removed, therapy directed at achieving voice should not begin without the surgeon's agreement. In practice it is usually possible after the patient has successfully taken two 'meals' by mouth. To inject air into the oesophagus before healing is complete may result in rupturing the sutures.

Eliciting Pseudo-voice

The speech pathologist knows that this is likely to be a tense and anxious time for the laryngectomee; voice is desperately desired and yet thoughts of failure intrude. With some patients the therapist's task is made easy if relaxed, firm patterns of clear articulation have been established while the nasogastric tube is in place. Also if there is an ideal P-E segment, vibration of the segment will occur spontaneously with the articulation of certain plosive consonants. Therapeutic intervention is directed at maintaining relaxed speech, slightly slower than normal, so that maximum benefit may be derived from injection of air into the oesophagus. These patients progress rapidly with appropriate support. The laryngectomee whom we treated and who was speaking with fluent oesophageal voice 2 weeks after removal of the nasogastric tube is an exception, unfortunately. Such patients owe their success to the surgeon's skill and their own determination rather than to the attentions of the speech therapist.

It is important that any attempts at producing voice are not introduced in a pass/fail setting. The patient and therapist should perceive this as an exploratory situation in which the therapist is experimenting with various strategies in order to ascertain the most promising route for treatment. The first aim is production of a sound; it does not matter how this is achieved, but achieved it must be at the earliest possible moment after the removal of the larynx. This is for purely psychological reasons because the thing the patient fears most is remaining silent. Failure to achieve voice after laryngectomy has the most depressing and disastrous effect upon the patient and may delay speech for many months even when it is physically possible. Some patients find the analogy of learning to swim is an everyday example which puts the task ahead of them into perspective. Once the 'knack' of keeping afloat for one or two strokes has been acquired it is only a matter of time and practice before longer distances can be swum in style. Once a sound has been produced, by whatever method, accidentally or intentionally, the rest is practice and refinement.

Exploration of the patient's voice potential is based on the three ways in which the oesophagus may be charged with air.

Injection

Experimentation should be tried using consonant/vowel (CV) combinations with voiceless plosives, e.g. /p t k st sk sp skr/ followed by vowels, preferably those requiring marked mouth opening, e.g. /pɑː/ /tɑː/ /kɑː/. The patient should be relaxed, especially in shoulder, neck and jaw muscles. No more effort should be put into articulation than for the normal articulation of these consonants. If the therapist can produce these sounds with pseudo-voice and demonstrate what is desired this is helpful. It gives the patient something to imitate and also does much to remove embarrassment at what the patient may regard as 'belching'. However, if the therapist is unable to produce oesophageal voice a passable imitation can be achieved by using excessively creaky voice.

Many patients will use spontaneously a combination of standard injection and consonant injection even at this early stage. Most find it helpful if the therapist acts as a visual model so that the degree of pressure and timing of articulation can be seen. This is a technique for ensuring that excessive effort is not used. Our experience is that it is equally, if not more, important for the laryngectomee to see what has to be done and how to do it, as it is to hear pseudo-voice. Practice before a mirror and with another laryngectomee is helpful.

The image of having a bubble of air in the mouth (Diedrich and Youngstrom, 1977) which is firmly compressed and squeezed into the pharynx and then released on saying /pɑː/ is frequently successful. From the beginning it is important that on all CV combinations voicing is encouraged without delay after injection of air. Patients frequently equate effort with probable success but forceful injection will drive air down to the stomach or the P-E segment will tighten and prevent injection.

Although it would appear logical to instruct the patient in breathing, drawing attention to the fact that quick, brief inspiration should preface speech may possibly cause confusion. Some say it provides too many things to concentrate upon at once. By the time the patient has mastered easy injection in successive syllables it is generally found that chest expansion takes place prior to speech unconsciously as it did preoperatively. This is one reason why the naturally good speaker before laryngectomy is often the naturally good speaker afterwards. The possession of good kinaesthetic sense and naturally good habits of breathing and articulation appear to be important factors influencing the speech progress of the laryngectomee. Tongue exercises may be necessary to improve speech clarity, especially with a lingual paresis following block dissection with laryngectomy.

Inhalation

The patient may be able to produce voice easily by 'inhaling' air through open lips, with tongue relaxed, and then phonating on prolonged vowels as the air returns in conjunction with expiration. If not, and this is more probable, various methods can be experimented with:

1. Simulate a long relaxed yawn in which air may enter the oesophagus and then be expelled.
2. Sniff air in through the nose, lips closed, tongue flat with slight forward thrust of the mandible which enlarges the pharyngeal cavity and is a method often used by laryngectomees for recharging of air. Placing the hand on the throat under the chin checks excessive jaw thrust.
3. A four-step procedure for trapping air in the oesophagus may be used (Gately, 1971):
   (a) open mouth wide, flatten tongue;
   (b) close lips with little or no elevation of the mandible; puckering lips;
   (c) bring teeth together;
   (d) hold nose.
4. Blow bubbles through a straw into water.

When an individual is tense and breathing is shallow, and preoperative speech patterns were poor, proper instruction in relaxation and central breathing is essential. The slightly exaggerated and rapid descent of the diaphragm is an obvious feature of every proficient oesophageal speaker. If a patient is unable to achieve coordination of respiratory and articulatory muscles, speech will lack fluency, and injection and inhalation of air into the oesophagus will not be synchronised.

It is advisable to instruct the patient in relaxation and correct breathing technique as soon as possible and this should form part of every treatment session. Initially exercises need not be linked to phonation. The patient may learn to produce voice by the injection method independently as previously described and, if the oesophageal voice is effortless, then attention may only be drawn to the connection between voice and respiration at a later stage. Some patients never work on relaxation and breathing and produce excellent results but the majority need help in these areas early in treatment in order to increase the air reservoir and so obtain greater duration and volume of voice.

Di Carlo, Amster and Herer (1955) found that abdominal expansion in breathing occurred in their poor speakers and thoracic expansion in their better speakers. Abdominal breathing is to be discouraged and the intercostal diaphragmatic method emphasised. The quick, pant-like intake essential for drawing air into the oesophagus (Isshiki, 1968) can be encouraged by panting exercises for toning up the muscles and by sitting upright, abdominal muscles firm, not sagging.

Injection and inhalation

The danger of confusing the patient with 'breathing exercises' and encouraging increased blowing from the stoma is not so great as the antagonists of the inhalation method believe. The patient has nothing to learn, inspiration and expiration coincide with the preparatory and active phases of speech in exactly the same way as they did preoperatively. There is, on the other hand, a real danger in concentrating exclusively upon air injection. This is an unnatural process quite foreign to the reflex habit patterns of the individual, and as difficult to acquire as any other new skill demanding muscular coordination invariably is in adult life. It is quite common to find patients concentrating upon injection to the complete cessation of respiration. The breath is held while injection and ejection of air take place and the abdomen and thorax are held rigid. Attention must be paid to the necessity of relaxing and coordinating respiration with inhalation of air into the oesophagus and production of voice. As stated earlier, negative pressure in the thorax aids inhalation of air into the oesophagus, hence the need to synchronise exactly inhalation with the quick inspiration of lung air. In fluent speakers consonant injection plays an important role in recharge of air and voice duration.

Pharyngeal voice

The injection method alone may encourage the undesirable pharyngeal voice with its Donald Duck quality. The P-E segment tends to be tightly closed when this method of air charging is used, air is trapped in the hypopharynx and is vibrated at a site between the base of the tongue and the posterior pharyngeal wall of the oropharynx. Patients with a tense, hypertonic or spasmodic P-E segment are particularly liable to develop pharyngeal voice.

Pharyngeal voice must never be allowed to become established because it is extremely difficult to unlearn and unpleasant to listen to. Relaxation and a firm but gentle approach to articulation and air charging while learning the injection method reduces possible development of this distinctive and unpleasant form of voicing. The inhalation method counteracts pharyngeal voice. If in doubt as to whether the initial sounds made by the patient are pharyngeal or oesophageal, patient and therapist can verify vibration of the P-E segment (rather than a higher and unsuitable pseudoglottis) by placing the finger tips on the front of the neck at the level of the previous site of the larynx. Vibrations will be felt here if the P-E segment is acting as the pseudo-glottis.

Buccal speech

When the P-E segment is tight and does not allow inhalation, turbulent air can be used in the mouth to produce a quasi whisper. Tense articulation while attempting to achieve oesophageal speech may also give rise to buccal whisper. Air is vibrated orally by vigorous movements of the tongue and is also pushed between the constricted cheek muscles and the lateral dental arch. If buccal whisper develops it must be discouraged immediately and speech therapy must concentrate on relaxed articulation.

Air swallowing

Although not viable as a method of air intake for oesophageal speech, swallowing air and vibration of the P-E segment as the air is expelled may be a useful start to therapy. If the patient has not lost the facility for 'burping' it may be possible for air to be eructated from the oesophagus immediately. The necessary kinaesthetic and tactile sensations will be familiar and control can be readily obtained over relaxation and dilatation of the cricopharyngeal sphincter.

Many patients, however, find it difficult to overcome their dislike of oesophageal speech because of its similarity to belching against which there are strong taboos in Western society. This is, of course, a strong argument against advocating air swallowing and belching as the first method of instruction. Another objection is the long latency period between air intake and sound production. This technique, aided by aerated drinks, may serve a temporary purpose if other methods do not produce results but since it has to be unlearned at some stage, it is wasteful of effort if another method can be readily mastered. No proficient oesophageal speaker uses air swallowing for charging the vicarious lung.

Establishing Oesophageal Voice

Voluntary control

Once oesophageal voice has been obtained the next task is to bring CV production under voluntary control so that there is consistency of performance. Relaxed and effortless repetition of syllables reinforces kinaesthetic feedback. Progress from this level should not be made until syllables are consistently being produced successfully. Edels (1983) recommends a 90% success rate before a more ambitious step is taken.

It is essential that from the earliest stages of therapy, bad habits of voice production, discussed on p. 362, are not allowed to develop. The temptation to progress in the face of these faults may be great but will be disastrous eventually. It is extremely difficult to unlean them and they detract from, or delay, the acquisition of good oesophageal voice. The faults may arise purely as a result of the patient's poor technique. More significantly, the P-E segment may be hyper- or hypotonic and as a result the patient is forced to use inappropriate manoeuvres in an attempt to produce voice.

Monosyllables

Different syllables beginning and ending with voiced and voiceless plosives and containing different vowels can now be practised. It is generally found that some consonant combinations are more helpful than others with individual patients. These assist in the acquisition of the knack of flattening the tongue to the roof of the mouth, forcing compressed air from the oral cavity into the pharynx and so into the oesophagus. Consonant combinations such as /sk/, /tʃ/, /skr/ may be found helpful, and words beginning with these sounds can be practised. Treatment should be adapted to individual needs. Gradually all consonants and vowels are worked on obtaining clear and effortless phonation.

In most cases it is advisable to leave the nasals /m/ and /n/ till late because they allow the escape of air through the nose and render air compression difficult. The speaker learns, however, to overcome the difficulty by using insufflated air only or by putting an unreleased plosive equivalent before the nasal in order to silently compress the air, e.g. (b)man; (d)no.

The consonant /h/ is very difficult as its normal mode of articulation by laryngeal whisper is, of course, no longer possible, and should be taught last, if at all. A good imitation can be produced by lifting the back of the tongue as for the voiceless palatal fricative in 'loch' as suggested by Paget (1930) and Oswald (Hodson and Oswald, 1958). A slight pause before the following vowel is also an effective substitute for /h/ (Greene, 1980b).

The aim of a short latency period (Edels, 1983) is added to the goal of consistency in voice production in these exercises. The latency period is the time between injection of air into the oesophagus and sound being introduced at the P-E segment. It is fundamental to fluent oesophageal speech that this should be as short as possible. As in other aspects, this is enhanced by a relaxed and effortless technique.

Monosyllabic and polysyllabic words leading to phrases

These build on the early achievements of phoneme production. All tasks are directed at duration of the sound for continuous fluent speech. Breathing technique can now be positively linked with speech as the length of phrases is extended. For example:

Part - party - part-time
Don't - don't go - don't go back
Scratch - scratch it - scratch it off
Try - try to - try to go
Pack - pack it - pack it up

In this way the laryngectomee also learns to use the consonant at the end of a word to air charge for a subsequent word beginning with a vowel.

Easy mechanical exercises such as saying 'chapter 1, chapter 2, chapter 3' etc. are helpful as are counting, days of the week etc. Duration of voice is also encouraged by practising strings of CVC syllables where the consonants are plosives, e.g. /kæp - kæp - kæp; tʌt – tʌt – tʌt/.

The next stage is to use short sentences, omitting 'difficult' consonants, for example:

bake a cake	cup of coffee
kick the cat	pint of bitter
take it back	go to bed

Volume

Direct work on increased volume is not appropriate in the early stages of treatment. Effort is counterproductive and causes tightening of the P-E segment and reduction in volume. An amplifier enables the patient to relax and volume frequently increases spontaneously, continuing when the amplifier is switched off.

When pseudo-voice is well established, increase in volume of oesophageal voice can be achieved by stronger inspiration and expiration and slightly exaggerated articulation which increases the air reservoir and assists in more forceful ejection. Care must be taken to avoid forcing the voice and the development of tension and stoma blast. As the voice improves, volume improves spontaneously in many patients and, in all cases, it is related to relaxation.

Increase of range and flexibility of the vocal note

This is important if oesophageal voice is to emulate laryngeal intonation.

1. Syllables with rising and falling intonation are practised.
2. Short phrases and sentences said by the therapist with varying intonation and stress patterns are imitated by the patient.
3. The patient places the forefinger and thumb on either side of the throat at the level of the pseudoglottis and experiment with varying pressures and changing note and pitch. This is repeated without external pressure while endeavouring to reproduce the necessary muscular adjustment by ear alone (Stetson, 1937).
4. As the patient becomes more accomplished singing familiar tunes can be attempted. Although the whole melody will not be possible the mental

concept of melody results in pitch changes. The attempt at singing also develops breathing technique and inhalation.

5. Rhymes with emphasised rhythm can be used to encourage the normal rhythms of speech and these give an impression of improved intonation in connected utterance.

Development of intelligibility

The truly proficient speaker can be understood without being seen. This is essential if the telephone is to be used. A hierarchy of tasks helps to minimise failure.

1. Ten easily produced words are listed which the patient reads aloud clearly while the therapist watches. The therapist looks away from the patient who says the words at random for repetition by the therapist. A score of identifiable words is kept for future comparison. This is repeated with different lists of words and phrases until there is a consistently high achievement level, with the therapist identifying and helping to correct behaviours which reduce intelligibility.
2. The patient lists words and phrases which are unknown to the therapist. It is advisable to confine the list to five words initially until reasonable success is assured. Gradually the lists and length of phrases can be increased until the patient reads from text with the therapist repeating each phrase.
3. Finally, telephone practice should be preceded by demonstrating the importance of holding the mouthpiece to the mouth so that the sound of air from the stoma is not picked up. Increased effort will reduce effectiveness. Ideally, the patient should have telephone practice from an adjacent room so that problems can be immediately analysed and discussed.

Assessment of Progress

Assessment of the laryngectomee's progress can be divided into evaluation of pseudo-voice, communication skills and general rehabilitation (Perry, 1983). The perceptual and instrumental evaluations described in Chapters 6 and 7 are relevant. Rating scales are useful in providing objective measurements of progress and motivate therapist and patient to raise their aims and achieve more ambitious targets. Some scales are qualitative, as for example, the seven-point scale devised by Wepman *et al.* (1953). Others, like Berlin's four-skills measurement (1963) are quantitative.

Wepman's oesophageal speech rating scale

This scale is based on the fact that when developing oesophageal voice, most laryngectomees pass through recognised stages of development in a natural progression.

The levels of the scale can be briefly described as follows.

Level Description

7 No oesphageal sound production, no speech. There is neither involuntary nor voluntary audible air movement through the P-E segment. At this level the patient may not attempt to speak or is only mouthing words.

6 Involuntary oesophageal sound production, no speech. Involuntary oesophageal sound occurs during speech and/or at rest. It indicates that although as yet uncontrolled the patient has the potential for oesophageal voice.

5 Voluntary sound production part of the time, no speech. The patient is able to produce some oesophageal sound at will but in the early stages this is infrequent. Wepman *et al.* (1953) stress the importance of this level which demonstrates that voluntary control is possible in addition to confirming the suitability of the P-E segment for oesophageal sound production.

4 Voluntary sound production most of the time, vowel sounds differentiated, monosyllabic speech.

3 Oesophageal sound produced at will, single word speech. Although there is no continuity, single words are produced with pseudo-voice.

2 Oesophageal sound produced at will with continuity; word grouping. Oesophageal speech is not automatic and the patient is conscious of careful production of pseudo-voice. Short phrases are voiced but oesophageal sound fails if the patient hurries in an attempt to increase phrase length.

1 Automatic oesophageal speech which is rapid, continuous, automatic and effortless.

Table 18.1 A rating scale for oesophageal speech

Level	*Oesophageal sound production*	*Speech proficiency*
7	None	No speech
6	Involuntary only	No speech
5	Voluntary part of the time	No speech
4	Voluntary most of the time	Vowel sounds differentiated Monosyllabic speech
3	At will	Single word speech
2	At will with continuity	Word grouping
1	Automatic	Oesophageal speech

From Wepman *et al.* (1953).

Berlin's measurement of four skills

Berlin (1963, 1965; Berlin and ZoBell, 1963) stresses that this scale is designed to chart progress in acquiring pseudo-voice in the early stages. It is not adequate for assessing the overall efficiency of communication using oesophageal voice. Berlin's patients were seen for half-hour treatments, two or three times daily. The four skills are:

1. Ability to phonate reliably on demand: the patient is asked to inflate the oesophagus and to phonate /ɑ/. Twenty attempts are made. Only vocalisations lasting longer than 0.4 second are considered successful. A success rate of almost 100% after 10–14 days occurred in Berlin's patients who developed into good speakers.
2. Short latency between inflation of the oesophagus and vocalisation. Potentially good speakers can have an average latency of 0.5 second by day 18.
3. Adequate duration of phonation: the patient produces /ɑ/for as long as possible following one inflation. This can be sustained for approximately 3 seconds by day 24 in good speakers.
4. Ability to sustain phonation during articulation: 8–10 CV syllables on one inflation can be expected from a potentially good speaker by day 25.

Extensive reviews of oesophageal and laryngectomee assessment procedures can be found in the laryngectomy texts named at the beginning of this chapter. Relevant research papers have been collected by Weinberg (1980).

Electronic Larynx

We believe that every laryngectomee should be allowed to try out instruments, be shown how to use them to best advantage and decide whether or not to use one. The majority of patients prefer oesophageal voice and dislike the sound of the electrolarynx, and also the inconvenience and constant reminder it provides of disability. On the other hand there is no doubt that a vibrator is often a necessary aid in the early stages of treatment and to some it makes life worth while. Various models of artificial larynx are available and are described on p. 367.

In the past vibrators were only presented to patients as a consolation prize when attempts at producing oesophageal voice had failed. This philosophy is still adhered to by some surgeons who refuse to allow the speech therapist to introduce such equipment to the laryngectomee. It then becomes a mark of failure with the attendant negative feelings that this engenders.

It is now realised that use of an artificial larynx does not necessarily mean that the patient will give up trying to speak with oesophageal voice. On the contrary, most patients dislike the gadgets and want to learn to speak without them, but it can save the frustration and misery of not being able to talk freely at home, and in fact help a patient to relax and learn oesophageal voice more easily. Use of a vibrator requires slow clear speech and encourages practice in phrasing. Diedrich and Youngstrom (1966), Gardener (1978) and Salmon (1978) and Greene (1980b) strongly advocate use of a vibrator from the outset. Lauder (1968), himself a laryngectomee and qualified speech pathologist, stressed that a laryngectomee can be in dire straits without an artifical larynx. Moreover, there is no proof that use of a vibrator excludes the ultimate mastery of oesophageal voice. He very sensibly points out that the use of one mode of communication at any one time does not exclude the other.

Both natural and artificial voice may be used to meet different contingencies. We can cite examples of patients who speak naturally and adequately at home but need a vibrator in the noisy surroundings of work or when using the telephone. If deprivation of a vibrator means staying off work longer than is necessary once the patient is physically fit, then the aid is essential. The speechless patient who lives alone or is alone at home for long periods is reassured that a telephone can be used if a vibrator is available.

Further advantage is that a vibrator placed on the area of the neck near the cricopharyngeal muscle, innervated as it is by branches of the recurrent laryngeal nerve, is positively conducive to facilitation of voluntary control in oesophageal speech. The feedback and monitoring of one's own speech is so important that it seems likely that sound heard and strong vibrations felt from a vibrator in the dead space left after laryngectomy, helps in the establishment of a link between neuromuscular and auditory pathways consistent with the principle of biofeedback.

Quite apart from the physical impossibility of a patient being unable to produce audible voice, some patients have a personal preference for using an artificial larynx and dislike oesophageal voice intensely. This preference should be respected. The therapist should not adopt an attitude of disapproval or entertain any secret feeling that the patient should have persevered with oesophageal voice (Greene, Atkinson amd Watson, 1974). Sometimes, moreover, the therapist is under the impression that the patient's speech is perfectly adequate when it is not, sincerely believing it to be better when produced naturally than when using an artificial sound source. Professional training and skill in interpreting mediocre speech production may unwittingly influence judgement. McCroskey and Mulligan (1963), in rating the relative intelligibility of oesophageal and artificial larynx speech, discovered that naive listeners rate the artificial larynx as having higher intelligibility, while students and therapists rated oesophageal speech higher.

Williams and Watson (1985) found that naive judges did not rate oesophageal speakers as being significantly more intelligible than electrolarynx speakers in their study comparing oesophageal, tracheo-oesophageal and electrolarynx speakers. This study also produced the surprising result that the three laryngectomee groups were not rated differently on pitch and quality by naive or expert listeners. In fact oesophageal and electrolarynx speakers were not rated significantly different in overall communication effectiveness.

Training in use of electronic larynx

The patient needs training in how to use the vibrator. It is not enough, as often happens, for the instrument to be thrust into the patient's hand with the exhortaton to 'Try that'. The following factors should be considered when supplying and using the artificial larynx:

1. It must be explained that the vibrator only provides the sound source for speech and that the clarity and rate of utterance are provided by the speaker.
2. A demonstration of the way in which the instrument is used is helpful and

enables the patient to start to become accustomed to the mechanical sound. Patients are frequently surprised and disconcerted by the loudness of the artificial larynx when they use it themselves. Any steps that can be taken to desensitise a patient to the volume, prior to placing the instrument on the neck, are necessary in order to reduce the possibility of rejection.

3. The patient can be given the opportunity to become familiar with the vibrator by handling it, getting used to the amount of pressure required on the button and trying it out on the palm of the hand. In this way the importance of placing the whole of the vibrating diaphragm at the head of the vibrator onto the skin surface becomes clear. If complete contact is not maintained unpleasant ambient noise occurs.
4. In some patients the area of the neck to be used for placement of the head of the artifical larynx is obvious. A flat area, near the original site of the larynx, which can be reached without changing head posture unnaturally is ideal. Where surgery has been extensive finding a suitable area may take some time. It is helpful to experiment with different artificial larynges with varying head sizes. Occasionally, if considerable tissue has been removed a patient will experience nausea if the vibrator is positioned too anteriorly. Some patients are able to use the vibrator on the cheek successfully. The optimal position for use is obvious when the patient is asked to articulate vowels, words, phrases and eventually connected speech.
5. Having found the ideal position it may be necessary to mark the patient's skin in some way, for example with a marker pen, until the movement of correct placement is automatic. The neck often lacks normal sensation and as a result it is difficult to find the right spot quickly which is essential for conversation. We find it helpful for certain patients to sit in front of a mirror and just practise placing the vibrator correctly. When this movement is established the same task is carried out without visual monitoring.
6. Practice is required in timing the onset and cut-off of 'voice' with articulation. Routine drills may be used initially such as counting, days of the week etc. until conversational standard is reached.
7. Some patients frequently need reminding that they only have to articulate, not attempt to produce voice. Other problems include the tendency to articulate quite silently and a demonstration of the sound of articulation without voice is useful. Patients also try to separate syllables so that normal prosody is disrupted. Work on articulation and the preservation of normal prosody are essential elements of learning how to use a vibrator successfully.

Reasons for failure to use an artificial larynx

1. Inadequate pharyngeal air-filled space for picking up vibrations from the vibrator.
2. Lack of sensation in the skin of the neck and 'neck hardness'.
3. Hearing impairment and inability to monitor artificial voice produced.

Hearing should be tested and a hearing aid provided although this may not help patients to monitor speech any better when using a vibrator.

4. Nervousness with a noisy gadget and, in the elderly, reactions too slow to manipulate an on-off switch between phrases.
5. Poor articulation and inability to adjust the degree and speed of oral movements to obtain maximum benefit from the vibrator.
6. A reluctance to speak audibly by any method, for various reasons ranging from a reluctance or need to achieve maximum rehabilitation, to a preference for a 'whisper' which is sufficient for the patient's lifestyle.

Attempts to introduce a vibrator should not be abandoned if they are unsuccessful initially. A patient may be able to use a vibrator efficiently, as neck anaesthesia resolves or attitude changes, even if there has been earlier failure. With patience and determination even the most inept patient can frequently be taught to use an artificial larynx (Verdolini *et al.*, 1985).

Laryngectomee Teachers

In the USA laryngectomee teachers are employed in many centres to teach laryngectomees. Lauder (1965) reported on the questionnaire he carried out to obtain the views of distinguished American speech pathologists on this controversial question. Although this is not the practice in Europe, speech results with a laryngectomee teacher can be excellent. The laryngectomee teachers observed by Greene (1980b) were far more exacting in the practice of exercises than the average speech therapist. There seems to be no reason why laryngectomees who have successfully completed an appropriate course should not be used as an adjunct in the normal clinical team, working under qualified speech therapists, especially where there is a shortage of speech therapists (Lauder, 1965, 1968).

General Principles of Therapy

Frequency and duration of therapy

Ideally, in the early stages of treatment patients should be seen daily. If this is not possible a minimum of two or three treatments per week is essential. The length of each treatment should be governed by the patient's recovery from the operation, the amount of direct work that can be tolerated, and the amount of counselling and supportive discussion which are deemed necessary.

Some oesophageal sound should be achieved as early as possible and by 3 months postoperatively a substantial amount of oesophageal voice should be in use. A patient who is progressing satisfactorily can often be discharged or placed on less frequent appointments at this stage. If there is no functionally useful voice by 3 months, further investigation of the P-E segment should be considered if all other aspects of the treatment situation are satisfactory (Perry and Edels, 1985). Frequently, patients are still without voice at this stage but subsequently develop satisfactory voice while perservering with therapy without any other intervention. It seems probable that these patients have a less than ideal P-E segment postoperatively, although not grossly abnormal, and that necessary adaptations of the hypopharynx occur which enable voice to be produced as the cut muscles recover function.

Less frequent visits may continue for approximately a year. In many instances the oesophageal voice continues to improve during the 2 or 3 years after completion of formal therapy before finally stabilising.

Practice

Regular practice of exercises achieved successfully in the clinic are essential reinforcement of the new behaviour patterns. We recommend that patients practise for 5 minutes each hour in the early stages of treatment. Longer than this is inadvisable because muscle fatigue may cause deterioration in performance which leads to discouragement and excessive effort in compensation. The therapist should clearly indicate the material to be practised. It is unwise for the patient to attempt tasks which have been unsuccessful in the clinical situation and where faulty technique may develop without guidance.

Group treatment

Most patients require individual attention from the speech therapist during treatment but group therapy is a valuable supplement, although not always possible because of the small number of laryngectomees in many clinics. The great difficulty, once voice is achieved, is in overcoming self-consciousness. The beginner feels oesophageal voice is conspicuous and socially unacceptable. Women especially may dislike the deep voice, which is harder to accept in the female than in the male patient. Working in a group in a sympathetic atmosphere where everyone is in the same predicament breeds confidence, and gives the patient the courage eventually to speak freely at home and in the outside world. The congratulations and obvious pleasure of more experienced members of the group when a newer member achieves and uses voice, is valuable encouragement and reinforcment.

Common Faults in Oesophageal Speech

The faults and difficulties which commonly arise in learning oesophageal speech are frequently due to generalised tension which interferes with the rhythmic coordination of articulation and respiration. It arises out of the excessive effort which the individual uses in the attempt to vocalise. The therapist must be able to recognise these faults as soon as they show signs of developing so that they are not allowed to become established.

Air swallowing

An excessive amount of air may be directed into the oesophagus and then enter the stomach, causing distension of the gas cap. This will cause considerable discomfort and the accidental eructation of air interrupts speech, to the embarrassment of the speaker, or causes uncontrolled voicing. Patients complain of indigestion and need explanation. This difficulty arises in patients who have been allowed to develop air swallowing or very forceful injection. Both faults must be eliminated as methods of air intake. The individual generally manages to make this adjustment after a few weeks and so prevent air from entering the stomach. It will be necessary to inspire less forcibly before speaking and also to reduce the over-forceful movements of the back of the tongue which are nearly always found to accompany the intake of air in these patients.

Accumulation of air in the stomach may also be due to poor diaphragmatic intercostal breathing. It is possible to hold the abdominal wall rigid and use upper thoracic breathing so that in a fluent speaker air enters the stomach inadvertently. Concentration on using the abdominal muscles to expel air during speech using the normal intercostal diaphragmatic method will correct this fault.

Stoma blast

Noisy exhalation of air from the stoma can be troublesome and the noise of exhaled air so loud that it masks the voice. This is generally the result of excessive effort in an attempt to eject air from the oesophagus and acquire a louder voice. Tension in the throat and upper thorax are evident, and as muscular tonicity increases the voice fades. Relaxation, central breathing, lack of effort and further drills in the easy injection and expulsion of air from the oesophagus must be practised. Practice with an amplifier is generally successful as the patient no longer strives to increase volume and, as a result, relaxes.

Bubbling in the trachea is of course difficult to avoid when mucus is present and occurs in heavy smokers. The treatment of the chest condition is the only remedy. Patients who have learned to speak well often lose their voices with a respiratory infection as a result of excessive mucus. This can be readily understood in relation to the importance of breathing in the production of oesophageal voice. When speech deterioration in these circumstances takes place the patient should be reassured by an explanation of its cause and assured of its temporary nature.

Noisy air intake ('klunk')

A gulping sound, rather like a noisy swallow, often precedes voice in the initial stages of voice acquisition. It is caused by air being forced under pressure through a tense P-E segment on air intake. The gulp occurs if over-forceful injection is employed. Air charging will also be noisy in patients using the inhalation method when there is excessive glossopharyngeal tension. If 'klunk' becomes part of the kinaesthetic pattern of air charging and is not corrected immediately it is extremely difficult to unlearn.

At the first signs of this problem it is advisable to go back to the initial stages of the treatment programme with general relaxation and diaphragmatic breathing. Emphasis should be placed on the importance of a relaxed technique and less pharyngeal tension. Air intake with mouth shut and tongue tip pressed behind front teeth will help correction of the exaggerated posterior movement of the tongue when 'klunk' occurs with glossopharyngeal press.

Perseverence in improving the method of air intake is worth a temporary set-back in speech performance. This problem highlights the importance of ensuring maximum performance with minimal faults at each stage of treatment before progressing with the therapeutic plan. Use of an amplifier is recommended.

Double pump

This problem occurs in patients using the injection method. Instead of making one firm contact for air intake, a double or multiple 'munching' action is used. This inevitably impairs normal speech rhythms and is visually intrusive and confusing for the listener. It arises in the early stages when the laryngectomee lacks confidence in the newly learned skill of charging the oesophagus with air; the 'insurance policy' of double pump is employed. If it appears as an emergent fault at the beginning of treatment, higher stages of the treatment plan should not be attempted until the patient is consistently achieving voice easily on syllables without the fault. If the behaviour pattern is established a return to earlier stages of treatment is necessary.

Grimacing and 'button-holing'

Grimacing due to over-exaggerated articulation is a minor problem which develops through the anxiety to be understood when the voice is weak. An inclination to 'button-hole' the listener and to stand too close for comfort may also develop for the same reasons. It is sufficient just to draw the individual's attention to these quite unconscious speech habits for them to be corrected. Videorecording will be useful at this stage with these patients.

Lack of fluency

Proficiency in the ability to obtain and maintain a sufficient air reservoir for phrases of more than a few words is mainly a matter of time. Poor coordination and poor breathing are the prime causes of limited phrase length, unless there is an inadequate P-E segment. The inveterate talker is the one who finds the limits imposed by laryngectomy the most frustrating; tense, rapid speech accompanied by gesticulation overrides the newly acquired technique of oesophageal voice. Insistence upon slower speech, the need for patience and the reassurance that the correct technique voice duration will gradually be extended will improve the situation.

Even a slight and transient pharyngeal tension will render a proficient speaker speechless. The cricopharyngeal sphincter is as vulnerable to emotional changes in the laryngectomee as it is in the laryngeal speaker and patients will lose their voices if embarassed, angry or in a state of emotional upheaval. The voice may also be lost if attempts are made to shout in emotion, to call someone or to overcome background noise. Any increase in tension, however caused, will reduce the potential phrase length.

Common Problems arising during Rehabilitation

By the very nature of the major surgery that the laryngectomee has undergone there will be various problems in most cases. The speech pathologist must be alert to the fact that the difficulties described by the patient may signal a serious underlying aetiology and that the otolaryngologist's opinion is necessary. Reassurance and advice outlining the appropriate strategies for dealing with the problem are generally sufficient.

Regurgitation of food

In the early stages of recovery the patient may need to adjust the rate at which food and drink are taken. If there is narrowing of the pharynx/oesophagus a build-up of food may accumulate. Similarly, very rapid drinking, particularly of gassy drinks, may cause nasal regurgitation. It is usually sufficient to eat and drink more slowly. If the problem is severe and shows no sign of improving, further investigation will be necessary (see 'Swallowing and dysphagia', p. 229).

Throat tightening 4–6 weeks postoperatively

Some patients are very perturbed that the throat gets tighter and swallowing may become more difficult in the early postoperative weeks. This appears to be related to healing processes and in most cases this sensation resolves in subsequent weeks but will need attention if it persists.

Swallowing problems are common after extensive surgery and the dietitian's advice will be sought.

Debris from the stoma

Debris is sometimes expelled from the tracheostoma following surgery and patients may be frightened by scabs which they expectorate. Examination by the otolaryngologist is advised.

Neck hardness

Following radiotherapy and surgery the neck and surrounding area may be extremely hard as a result of postradiotherapy fibrosis and oedema. Although it does not entirely resolve the stiffness becomes less obvious.

Adverse listener reaction

People do not intend to hurt but are often unintentionally tactless through simple embarrassment in the face of a misfortune they little understand. Instead of treating the patient normally they may be over-sympathetic or on the other hand apparently callous. It helps the patient to discuss and laugh over listener reactions.

> Case note
>
> A transport driver who was excellently adjusted and spoke well before going back to work was infinitely depressed by his reception when he resumed his duties. He did not know, he said, which was the harder to bear; the men ragging him over his oesophageal voice, or the tender sympathy of the girl in the canteen whose eyes filled with tears whenever he asked for a cup of tea.

Laryngectomees frequently complain of the following reactions:

- The tendency to shout at the laryngectomee 'as if I were deaf and daft'.
- Whispering at the patient as if in a conspiracy of quiet voices.
- Not looking at the patient. Some listeners cannot make eye contact because of their embarrassment, while others turn their ear to the laryngectomee in an attempt to hear more successfully, when 'lip-reading' is more effective.
- Cutting conversations short. This is perhaps understandable on the part of the listener who is having difficulty in understanding an inexperienced speaker, but it is still hurtful.
- The 'Does he take sugar?' syndrome of speaking to the laryngectomee through a companion.
- The listener who pretends to understand what is being said, when asking for clarification would be the less complicated and kinder course.
- The listener writing down the response to the laryngectomee when the patient is using written communication.
- Adverse reactions on the telephone. These occur when the patient is telephoning a stranger and fall into two broad categories. The listener may think that the laryngectomee is joking and putting on a funny voice, in which case they laugh or become angry. Alternatively they think that they are answering an obscene call so they subject the caller to abuse or slam down the receiver. These reactions on the telephone can be reduced if the laryngectomees state immediately that they have had a throat operation which has affected the voice. If a laryngectomee is anxious about using the telephone, voice may be slow in starting or frail when the call is answered so that the patient puts down the receiver. Some people find it helpful to have an introductory sentence pre-recorded which clarifies the situation and allows the patient to relax before speaking. A telephone with an integral amplifier is useful for the patient with quiet oesophageal voice (see p. 115).

Frustration with reactions such as these are frequently at their height in the home. The family can be advised not to expect too much at first, to watch the patient's lips and to listen without interruption and to make every endeavour to understand. The spouse must be cautioned not to pursue everyday tasks when being addressed but to encourage speech in every way possible. The use of a self-erasing pad is better than the patient suffering the exasperation of not being understood in the early stages of acquiring voice.

Stoma management

Practical management of the tracheostoma is discussed on p. 326. Adverse reactions to the patient can be reduced by careful management of the stoma. Laryngectomy protectors fulfil a practical and aesthetic function of which some patients will need to be made aware if they are to be successfully rehabilitated. It is not socially acceptable for the laryngectomee to leave the stoma unprotected and the majority of patients take care to dress suitably. Some patients do not appear to be sensitive about their appearance or perhaps wish to obtain sympathy by drawing attention to their disability, leaving the stoma uncovered. A man can wear a collar and tie if he wishes, or a cravat. The Romet filter is popular with men and women because it looks like a sweater but the stoma remains accessible after coughing for wiping away mucus. If a shirt or blouse is buttoned up to the neck the second button can be removed from the shirt edge and sewn to the site of the button hole so that the shirt looks properly buttoned but the opening provides access for cleaning the stoma. Blouses with high necklines or bows look attractive, and scarves and jewellery can also be used without impairing breathing.

Laryngectomy Clubs

Counselling and emotional support from the speech therapist is an integral part of vocal rehabilitation but membership of a laryngectomy club is invaluable as a source of additional support and information for laryngectomees and their famlies. No-one can give more sincere and realistic help in adjustment to all the physical changes which are to have widespread repercussions in everyday life than another laryngectomee. This fact is clearly illustrated in the book *Larynectomy is not a Tragedy* by Norgate (1984) himself a laryngectomee and founder of the Cancer Laryngectomy Trust. Lauder's (1968) book *Self-help for the Laryngectomee* gives a similar perspective.

Speech therapists generally believe they can provide all the answers but this is a fallacy, hence the need for laryngectomy clubs. Anxieties and questions concerning breathing, speaking, coughing, nose-blowing and other aspects of changes which may be embarrassing or infuriating can be discussed. Horror may be felt at the prospect of permanently breathing through a hole in the neck and fears concerning loss of sexual attractiveness torment both men and women. These things can be explained by professional staff but relaxing with other laryngectomees, sharing the same problems, visiting a club where spouses can meet, makes the stressful early days easier for both patient and family (Parkes, 1975).

In the UK, the National Association of Laryngectomee Clubs (NALC), affiliated to the International Association founded by Warren Gardener in the USA, promotes rehabilitation through clubs run by laryngectomees, usually with the support of a speech therapist. These associations provide up-to-date information concerning speech aids for laryngectomees, emergency cards and stickers identifying their condition in case of accident, and regular news letters. The Cancer Laryngectomy Trust provides similar services besides helping patients in financial straits.

Many clubs also seek to publicise the existence of this patient group and its problems by arranging meetings with members of police, fire, ambulance and medical services. In particular, the importance of mouth-to-neck resuscitation and the necessity for emergency services to be on the alert for neck-breathers is emphasised.

The traditional objection to laryngectomee clubs is that deaths are depressing for the remaining members. Our experience is that patients in these groups are generally realistic about their situation. When a member is ill the support the group gives is encouraging for all concerned and if death occurs the spouse derives comfort from being able to talk to club members who have become understanding friends. Inevitably, a death causes grief but, on balance, the benefits of a club outweigh the potential disadvantages.

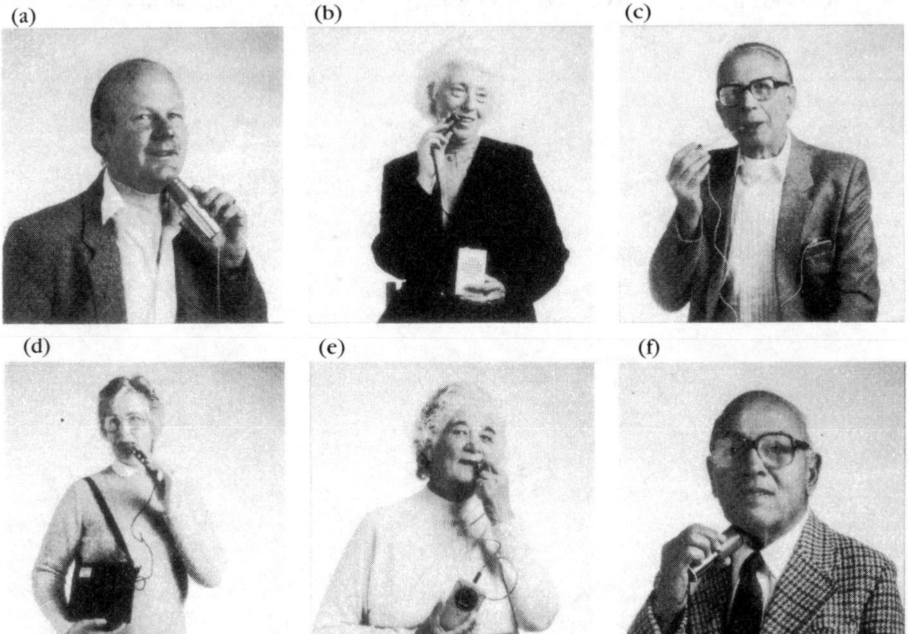

Figure 18.3. Artificial larynges and amplifiers. (a) Servox Electronic Speech Aid; (b) Mediquip Amplifier; (c) Cooper-Rand Electronic Speech Aid; (d) Voicette Amplifier; (e) Cooper-Rand Amplifier; (f) Jedcom MK3 Larynx. (Courtesy of Thackraycare, Leeds.)

Communication Aids for Laryngectomees

Portable amplifiers which can be used by laryngectomees during therapy and on a day-to-day basis if the voice is weak are described in Chapter 7.

Artificial larynges

Most models consist of a hand-held sound generator with a vibrating diaphragm at one end which is held to the neck (or cheek in some cases) during speech. There are controls for adjusting volume, pitch and quality. Recent developments provide the possibility of intonation in some models (e.g. Servox Intone).

An intraoral speech aid, such as the Cooper-Rand, delivers sound through a plastic tube, the tip of which is positioned in the mouth. Some of the 'neck' vibrators also have an oral adaptor. This enables the patient to use an artificial larynx immediately after surgery or when the neck is unsuitable for conventional artificial larynges.

Current artificial larynges include (see Appendix I for addresses):

- Servox Electronic Speech Aid (Thackraycare).
- Servox Intone (Thackraycare).
- Cooper-Rand Electronic Intra-oral Speech Aid (Thackraycare).
- Bart's Artificial Larynx Mark II (Jedcom Medical Ltd).
- Companion Intra Oral Larynx (Jedcom Medical Ltd).
- Jedcom MK3 Electronic Artificial Larynx (Jedcom Medical Ltd).

Appendices

Appendix I: Manufacturer's addresses

Brüel and Kjaer
18 Naerum Hovedgade,
DK-2850 Naerum,
Denmark
Telephone: (45) 02 80 05 00

Brüel and Kjaer (UK) Ltd
Harrow Weald Lodge,
92 Uxbridge Road,
Harrow,
Middlesex HA3 6BZ,
UK
Telephone: 01-954-2366

Entomed AB
Box 16015,
S-200 25 Malmo,
Sweden
Telephone: (0)40-18 40 61
(UK suppliers of glottal frequency analyser:
Millgrant Wells,
Rugby
Telephone: 0788-61185)

Jedcom Medical Ltd
Rue Fondon,
St Peter
Jersey, Channel Islands
Telephone: Jersey (0534) 46494

Kay Elemetrics Corporation
12 Maple Avenue,
Pine Brook,
NJ 07058-9798,
USA
Telephone: (201) 227-2000

Laryngograph Ltd
1 Foundry Mews,
Tolmers Square,
London NW1 2PE,
UK
Telephone: 01-387-7793

Mediquip Surgical Supplies Ltd
Unit 10, Oakwood Industrial Park,
Gatwick Road,
Crawley,
W. Sussex RH10 2AX,
UK
Telephone: 0293-546144/5

Mercury Electronics (Scotland) Ltd
Pollok Castle Estate,
Newton Mearns,
Glasgow G77 6NU,
UK
Telephone: 041-639-4944

Thackraycare
45–47 Great George Street,
Leeds LS1 3BB,
UK
Telephone: 0532-430028

Winslow Press
Telford Road
Bicester, Oxon OX6 0TS,
UK

Appendix II: Vocal Profile Analysis Protocol

Speaker: ______________________ Sex: ____________ Age: ____________

I VOCAL QUALITY FEATURES

	FIRST PASS			SECOND PASS						
CATEGORY	Neutral	Non-neutral		SETTING	Scalar Degrees					
					1	2	3	4	5	6
Vocal Tract										
1. Labia				Lip Rounding/Protrusion						
				Lip Spreading						
				Labiodentalization						
				Extensive Range						
				Minimised Range						
2. Mandibular				Close Jaw						
				Open Jaw						
				Protruded Jaw						
				Extensive Range						
				Minimised Range						
3. Lingual Tip/Blade				Advanced						
				Retracted						
4. Lingual Body				Fronted Body						
				Backed Body						
				Raised Body						
				Lowered Body						
				Extensive Range						
				Minimised Range						
5. Velopharyngeal				Nasal						
				Audible Nasal Escape						
				Denasal						
6. Pharyngeal				Constriction						
7. Larynx Position				Raised						
				Lowered						
Phonation Type										
				Harshness						
				Whisper(y)						
				Creak(y)						
				Falsetto						
				Modal Voice						
Tension										
8. Supralaryngeal				Tense						
				Lax						
9. Laryngeal				Tense						
				Lax						

"VOCAL PROFILES OF SPEECH DISORDERS" Research Project. (M.R.C. Grant No. G978/1192)
Phonetics Laboratory, Department of Linguistics, University of Edinburgh.

Date of Analysis: ______________ Tape: ______________ Judge: ______________

II PROSODIC FEATURES

CATEGORY	Neutral	SETTING	MILD	MOD	EXTREME
1. Pitch		High Mean			
		Low Mean			
		Wide Range			
		Narrow Range			
		High Variability			
		Low Variabaility			
2. Loudness		High Mean			
		Low Mean			
		Wide Range			
		Narrow Range			
		High Variability			
		Low Variability			
3. Tremor		Present			

III COMMENTS

CATEGORY	FIRST PASS		SECOND PASS Scalar Degree Inappropriate		
	Appropriate	Inappropriate	1	2	3
1. Breath Support					
2. Continuity		Interrupted			
3. Rate		Fast			
		Slow			
4. Rhythmicality					

5. Other (including posture, diplophonia, etc.)

Reproduced by permission of Professor John Laver, Dr S. Wirz, Dr J. Mackenzie-Beck and Dr S.M. Hiller.

Appendix III: Addresses of Societies and Communication Aids Centres

Societies

Association for all Speech Impaired Children (AFASIC), 347 Central Markets, Smithfield, London EC1A 9NH
Tel: 01-236-3632/6487

Association to Combat Huntington's Chorea, 34a Station Road, Hinckley, Leicestershire LE10 1AP
Tel: 0455-615-558

The British Association of Bobath Trained Therapists (BABITT), Bobath Centre, 5 Netherhall Gardens, London NW3 5RR

Cancer Laryngectomy Trust, Enderleigh, Brant Avenue, Illingworth, Halifax HX8 8DL
Tel: 0422-244165

Cleft Lip and Palate Association (CLAPA), Dental Department, Hospital for Sick Children, Great Ormond Street, London W1CN 3JH
Tel: 01-405-9200, ext. 286

International Association of Laryngectomees (IAL), 777 Third Avenue, New York. NY 10017, USA
Tel: 212-371-2900

International Society for Augmentative and Alternative Communication, ISAAC UK, 25 Mortimer Street, London WC1N 8AB
Tel: 01-637-5400

Motor Neurone Disease Association, 58 Hazelwood Road, Northampton NN1 1LN
Tel: 0604-22269/2239

The Multiple Sclerosis Society, 25 Effie Road, London SW6 1YZ

The National Association for Deafened People (NADP), 8 Maybush Walk, Olney, Bucks MK46 5NA

The National Association of Layngectomee CLubs (NALC), 39 Eccleston Square, London SW1 1PB
Tel: 01-834-2857

Parkinson's Disease Society, 36 Portland Place, London W1N 3DG
Tel: 01-323-1174

Royal National Institute for the Deaf (RNID), 105 Gower Street, London WC1E 6AH
Tel: 01-387-8033

VOCAL (Voluntary Organisations Communication and Language), South Western Hospital, St Peter's Office, Landor Road, London SW9 7AA

Communication Aids Centres (England and Wales)

Boulton Road, West Bromwich, Birmingham
Tel: 021-553-0908

Castle Farm Road, Newcastle-upon-Tyne
Tel: 091-284-0480

Charing Cross Hospital, Fulham Palace Road, London W6
Tel: 01-748-2040

Frenchay Hospital, Bristol BS16 1LE
Tel: 0272-565656

Roakswood Hospital, Fairwater Road, Llandaff, Cardiff
Tel: 0222-566281

The Wolfson Centre, Mecklenburgh Sqaure, London WC1N 2AP
Tel: 01-837-7618

Bibliography

ABBERTON, E. (1987). An introduction to voice research within phonetics departments within the U.K. *Voice Research Society Newsletter* **2**, 3.

ABBERTON, E. and FOURCIN, A. (1984). Electrolaryngography. In C. Code and M. Ball (Eds) *Clinical Phonetics*. London: Croom Helm.

ABERCROMBIE, D. (1967). *Elements of General Phonetics*. Edinburgh: Edinburgh University Press.

ABRAMSON, A.L., STEINBERG, B.M. and WINKLER, B. (1987). Laryngeal papillomatosis: clinical, histopathologic and molecular studies. *Laryngoscope* **97**, 678.

ADDINGTON, D.W. (1968). The relationship of selected vocal characteristics to personality perception. *Speech Monogr.* **35**, 429.

AGGER, W.A. and SEAGER, G.M. (1985). Granulomas of the vocal cords caused by *Sporothrix schenkii. Laryngoscope* **95**, 595.

AGOSTINI, E. and SANT'AMBROGIO, G. (1970). In E.J.M. Campbell, E. Agostini and J. Newsom Davis (Eds) *The Respiratory Muscles: Mechanics and Neural Control*, 2nd edn. London: Lloyd-Luke.

ALLAN, C.M. (1970). Treatment of non-fluent speech resulting from neurological disease - treatment of dysarthria. *Br. J. Dis. Commun.* **5**, 1.

ALLEN, G.W. (1984). Neoplasms of the thyroid gland. In G.M. English (Ed.) *Otolaryngology*, Vol. 5. London: Harper & Row.

ALVIN, J. (1961). Music therapy and the cerebral palsied child. *Cerebral Palsy Bull.* **3**, 255.

AMADO, J.H. (1953). Tableau général des problèmes posés par l'action des hormones sur le dévelopment du larynx. *Ann. Otolaryngol (Paris)* **70**, 117.

ANDREWS, J.C., MICKEL, R.A., HANSON, D.G., MONAHAN, G.P. and WARD, P.H. (1987). Major complications following tracheoesophageal puncture for voice rehabilitation. *Laryngoscope* **97**, 562.

ANDREWS, A.H. and MOSS, H.W. (1974). Experience with carbon dioxide laser in the larynx. *Ann. Otol.* **83**, 462.

ANDREWS, S., WARNER, J. and STEWART, R. (1986). EMG biofeedback and relaxation in the treatment of hyperfunctional dysphonia. *Br. J. Dis. Commun.* **21**, 353.

ARGYLE, M. (1970). *The Psychology of Interpersonal Behaviour*. Harmondsworth: Penguin.

ARNOLD, G.E. (1957). Vocal rehabilitation of paralytic dysphonia 111. Present concepts of laryngeal paralysis. *Arch. Otolaryngol.* **65**, 317.

ARNOLD, G.E. (1958). Dysplastic dysphonia. *Laryngoscope* **68**, 142.

ARNOLD, G.E. (1962). Vocal nodules and polyps: Laryngeal tissue reaction to habitual hyperkinetic dysphonia. *J. Speech Dis.* **27**, 205.

ARNOLD, G.E. and HEAVER, L. (1959). Spastic dysphonia. *Logos* **2**, 3.

ARONSON, A.E. (1971). Early motor neurone disease masquerading as psychogenic breathy dysphonia - a clinical case presentation. *J. Speech Hear. Dis.* **36**, 115.

ARONSON, A.E. (1973). *Audio Seminars in Speech Pathology: Psychogenic voice disorders*. Philadelphia: W.B. Saunders.

ARONSON, A.E. (1980). *Clinical Voice Disorders*. New York: Thième Stratton.

ARONSON, A.E. and DE SANTO, L.W. (1983). Adductor spastic dysphonia: three years after recurrent laryngeal nerve re-section. *Laryngoscope* **93**, 1.

ARONSON, A.E. and HARTMAN, D.E. (1981). Adductor spastic dysphonia: a sign of essential (voice) tremor. *J. Speech Hear. Dis.* **46**, 52.

ARONSON, A.E., BROWN, J.R., LITIN, E.M. and PEARSON, J.S. (1968a). Spastic dysphonia 1. Voice, neurologic and psychiatric aspects. *J. Speech Dis.* **33**, 203.

ARONSON, A.E., BROWN, J.E., LITIN, E.M. and PEARSON, J.S. (1968b). Spastic dysphonia 2. Comparison with essential (voice) tremor and other neurologic and psychogenic disorders. *J. Speech Dis.* **33**, 219.

ARSLAN, M. and SERAFINI, I. (1972). Restoration of laryngeal functions after total laryngectomy in the first 25 cases. *Laryngoscope* **82**, 1319.

ASAI, R. (1972). Laryngoplasty after total laryngectomy. *Arch. Otolaryngol.* **95**, 114.

ATEN, J.L., McDONALD, A., SIMPSON, M. and GUTTIERREZ, R. (1984). In M.R. McNeil, J.C. Rosenbek and A.E. Aronson (Eds) *The Dysarthrias: Physiology, acoustics, perception, management*. San Diego: College-Hill Press.

BAKEN, R.J. (1977). Estimation of lung volume change from torso hemicircumference. *J. Speech Hear. Res.* **20**, 808.

BAKEN, R.J. (1987). *Clinical Measurement of Speech and Voice*. London: Taylor & Francis.

BAKER, D.C. and SAVETSKY, L. (1966). Congenital partial atresia of the larynx. *Laryngoscope* **77**, 616.

BALLANTYNE, J.C. and GROVES, J. (1982). *A Synopsis of Otolaryngology*, 3rd edn. Bristol: John Wright and Sons.

BALLANTYNE, J. and MARTIN, J.A.M. (1984). *Deafness*, 4th edn. Edinburgh: Churchill Livingstone.

BARIMO, J.P., HUBAL, M.B., SCHEUERLE, J. and RITTERMAN, S.J. (1987). Postnatal palatoplasty: implications for normal speech articulation. *Scand. J. Plast. Recontr. Surg.* **21**, 139.

BARLOW, W. (1955). In D.O. O'Neill (Ed.) *Modern Trends in Psychosomatic Medicine*, Chap. 17. London: Butterworths.

BARLOW, W. (1959). Anxiety and muscle tension pain. *Br. J. Clin. Prac.* **13**, 339.

BARTELLI, T.E., FORD, C.N. and BLESS, D.M. (1986). Teflon injection of vocal folds: an analysis of poor results. *I.A.L.P. 20th Congress Report*, Vol. 2. Abstract 17, 283.

BARTON, R.T. (1965). Life after laryngectomy. *Laryngoscope* **75**, 1408.

BASSICH, C.J. and LUDLOW, C. (1986). The use of perceptual methods by new clinicians for assessing voice quality. *J. Speech Hear. Dis.* **51**, 125.

BATEMAN, G.H. and NEGUS, V.E. (1954). *Speech after laryngectomy. British Surgical Progress*. London: Butterworths.

BAUGH, R.F., LEWIN, J.S. and BAKER, S.R. (1987). Preoperative assessment of tracheoesophageal speech. *Laryngoscope* **97**, 461.

BAYNES, R.A. (1966). An incidence study of chronic hoarseness in children. *J. Speech Dis.* **21**, 172.

BENNETT, S., BISHOP, S. and LUMPKIN, S.M.M. (1987). Phonatory characteristics associated with bilateral diffuse polypoid degeneration. *Laryngoscope* **97**, 446.

BENTZEN, N., GULD, A. and RASMUSSEN, H. (1976). X-ray videotape studies of laryngectomised patients. *J. Laryngol.* **90**, 655.

BERKOWITZ, J.F. and LUCENTE, F.E. (1985). Counselling before laryngectomy. *Laryngoscope* **95**, 1332.

BERLIN, C.I. (1963). Clinical measurement of oesophageal speech: I. Methodology and curves of skill acquisition. *J. Speech Hear. Dis.* **28**, 42.

BERLIN, C.I. (1965). Clinical measurement of oesophageal speech: III. Performance of non-biased groups. *J. Speech Hear. Dis.* **30**, 174.

BERLIN, C.I. and ZO BELL, D.H. (1963). Clinical measurement during the acquisition of oesophageal speech: II. An unexpected dividend. *J. Speech Hear. Dis.* **28**, 389.

BERNSTEIN, L. (1979). Cleft lip and palate. In G.M. English (Ed.) *Otolaryngology*, Vol. 4. (1987) New York: Harper & Row.

BERRY, R.J. (1983). Radiotherapy and chemotherapy. In Y. Edels (Ed.) *Laryngectomy: Diagnosis to rehabilitation*. London: Croom Helm.

BERRY, R., EPSTEIN, R., FOURCIN, A., FREEMAN, M., MacCURTAIN, F. and NOSCOE, N. (1982). An objective analysis of voice disorders (Part 1 and 2) *Br. J. Dis. Commun.* **17**, 67.

BILLER, H.F. and LAWSON, W. (1986). Partial laryngectomy for vocal cord cancer with marked limitation or fixation of the vocal cord. *Laryngoscope* **96**, 61.

BLESS, D.M. and ABBS, J.H. (Eds) (1983). *Vocal Fold Physiology*. San Diego: College-Hill.

BLOM, E.D., SINGER, M.I. and HAMAKER, R.C. (1982). Tracheostoma valve for post-laryngectomy voice rehabilitation. *Ann. Otol.* **91**, 576.

BLOM, E.D., SINGER, M.I. and HAMAKER, R.C. (1985). An improved oesophageal insufflation test. *Arch. Otolaryngol.* **3**, 211.

BLOM, E.D., SINGER, M.I. and HAMAKER, R.C. (1986). A prospective study of tracheo-esophageal speech. *Arch. Otolaryngol.* **112**, 440.

BOLLIER, B. and DABUL, B. (1976). Therapeutic approaches to apraxia. *J. Speech Hear. Dis.* **41**, 268.

BONCHARD RYAN, E. and GILES, H. (Eds) (1982). *Attitudes towards Language Variation*. London: Edward Arnold.

BONE, R.C. (1986). Laryngeal papillomatosis. In G.M. English (Ed.) *Otolaryngology*, Vol. 3 (1987). New York: Harper & Row.

BONE, R.C., FEREN, A.P. and NAHUM, A.M. (1976). Laryngeal papillomatosis: immunologic and viral basis of therapy. *Laryngoscope* **86**, 341.

BOONE, D.R. (1977). *The Voice and Voice Therapy*, 2nd edn. London: Prentice Hall.

BORNHOLT, A. (1983). Interferon therapy for laryngeal papillomatosis in adults. *Arch. Otol.* **109**, 550.

BOSMA, J.F. (1953). Studies of disabilities of the pharynx resultant from poliomyelitis. *Ann. Otol.* **62**, 529.

BOURHIS, R.Y. (1985). The sequential nature of language choice in cross-cultural communication. In R.L. Street and J.N. Cappella (Eds) *Sequence and Pattern in Communication Behaviour*. London: Edward Arnold.

BOWDEN, R.E.M. (1972). Innervation of intrinsic laryngeal muscles. In B. Wyke (Ed.) *Ventilatory and Phonatory Control Systems*. Oxford: Oxford University Press.

BRADLEY, P.J. and NARULA, A. (1987). Clinical aspects of pseudodysphagia. *J. Laryngol. Otol.* **101**, 689.

BRAIN, W.R. (1985). In R. Bannister (Ed.) *Brain's Clinical Neurology*, 6th edn. Oxford: Oxford University Press.

BRALLEY, R.C., BULL, G.L., GORE, C.H. and EDGERTON, M.T. (1978). Evaluation of vocal pitch in male transsexuals. *J. Commun. Dis.* **2**, 443.

BRANDWEIN, M., ABRAMSON, A.L. and SHIKOWITZ, M.J. (1986). Bilateral vocal cord paralysis following endotracheal intubation. *Arch. Otolaryngol. Head Neck Surg.* **112**, 877.

BRENNAN, H.G. (1979). Treatment of the aging face. In G.M. English (Ed.) *Otolaryngology*, Vol. 4 (1987). New York: Harper & Row.

BRIDGEMAN, E. and SNOWLING, M. (1988). The perception of phonemic sequence: a comparison of dyspraxic and normal children. *Br. J. Dis. Commun.* **23**, 245.

BRODNITZ, F.S. (1988). *Keep your Voice Healthy* New York: Taylor & Francis.

BRODNITZ, F.S. (1959). *Vocal Rehabilitation*. Rochester, Minn: American Academy of Ophthalmology and Otolaryngology.

BRODNITZ, F.S. (1961). Contact ulcer of the larynx. *Ann. Otol.* **74**, 90.

BRODNITZ, F.S. and CONLEY, J.J. (1967). Vocal rehabilitation after reconstructive surgery for laryngeal cancer. *Folia Phoniatr.* **19**, 89.

BRONDBO, K., ALBERTI, P.W. and CROWSON, N. (1983). Adult recurrent multiple laryngeal papilloma. *Acta Otolaryngol.* **95**, 431.

BROWN, R.G., MacCARTHY, B., GOTHAM, A.M., DER, G.J. and MARSDEN, C.D. (1988). Depression and disability in Parkinson's disease: a follow-up study of 132 cases. *Psychol. Med.* **18**, 49.

BUCKINGHAM, H. (1979). Explanation in apraxia with consequences for the concept of apraxia of speech. *Brain Language* **8**, 202.

BUMSTEAD, R.M. (1982). Velopharyngeal incompetence. In G.M. English (Ed.) *Otolaryngology*, Vol. 4 (1988). New York: Harper & Row.

BUNCH, M.A. (1976). A cephalometric study of structures of the head and neck during sustained phonation of covered and open qualities. *Folia Phoniatr.* **28**, 321.

BUNCH, M.A. (1982). *Dynamics of the Singing Voice*. Vienna: Springer-Verlag.

BURKOWSKY, M.R. (1968). Vocal ulcers in a seventy-one year old male. *J. Speech Dis.* **33**, 268.

BURNS, P. (1986). Acoustical analysis of the underlying voice differences between two groups of professional singers: opera and country and western. *Laryngoscope* **96**, 549.

BURSTEIN, F.D. and CALCATERRA, T.C. (1985). Supraglottic laryngectomy: series report and analysis of results. *Laryngoscope* **95**, 833.

BZOCH, K. (1964). The effects of a specific pharyngeal flap operation upon the speech of 40 cleft palate persons. *J. Speech Dis.* **29**, 264.

BZOCH, K.R. (1979). Rationale, methods and techniques of cleft palate speech therapy. In K.R. Bzoch (Ed.) *Communication Disorders relating to Cleft Lip and Palate*. Boston: Little, Brown and Co.

CALCATERRA, T.C. (1983). Tongue flap reconstruction of the hypopharynx. *Arch. Otolaryngol.* **109**, 750.

CALNAN, J. (1953). Movements of the soft palate. *Br. J. Plas. Reconstr. Surg.* **13**, 275.

CALNAN, J. (1955). Diagnosis, prognosis and treatment of palato-pharyngeal incompetence with special reference to radiographic investigations. *Br. J. Plas. Reconstr. Surg.* **16**, 352.

CAMPBELL, E.J.M. (1974). Muscular activity in normal and abnormal ventilation. In B. Wyke (Ed.) *Ventilatory and Phonatory Control Systems*. Oxford: Oxford University Press.

CAMPBELL, E.J.M., AGOSTINI, E. and DAVIS, J.N. (1970). *The Respiratory Muscles: Mechanics and neurol control*, 2nd edn. London: Lloyd-Luke.

CANTRELL, R.W. (1983). Laryngeal trauma reviewed. *Arch. Otolaryngol.* **109**, 112.

CAPPELLA, J.N. and STREET, R.L. (1985). Introduction: a functional approach to the structure of communicative behaviour. In R.L. Street Jr and J.N. Cappella (Eds) *Sequence and Pattern in Communicative Behaviour*. London: Edward Arnold.

CAPPS, F.C.W. (1958). The Semon Lecture: Abductor paralysis in theory and practice since Semon. *J. Laryngol. Otol.* **72**, 1.

CASE, J.L. (1984). *Clinical Management of Voice Disorders*. Rockville, MD: Aspen.

CASPER, J., COTTON, R. and BREWER, D. (1986). Selected therapy techniques and laryngeal physiological changes in patients with vocal fold immobility. *Folia Phoniatr.* **38**. XXth Congress of IALP.

CAVANAGH, F. (1955). Vocal palsies in children. *J. Laryngol.* **69**, 399.

CAVO, J.W. (1985). True vocal cord paralysis following intubation. *Laryngoscope* **95**, 1352.

CHEESMAN, A.D. (1983). Surgical management of the patient. In Y. Edels (Ed.) *Laryngectomy: Diagnosis to rehabilitation*. London: Croom Helm.

CHERRY, J. and DELAHUNTY, J.E. (1968). Experimentally produced vocal cord granulomas. *Laryngoscope* **78**, 1941.

CHERRY, J. and MARGULIES, S.I. (1968). Contact ulcer of the larynx. *Laryngoscope* **78**, 1937.

CLARKE, W.M. and HOOPS, H.R. (1970). The effect of speech-type background noise on oesophageal speech production. *Ann. Otol.* **79**, 653.

CLIFFORD, E. (1979). Psychological aspects of cleft lip and palate. In K.R. Bzoch (Ed.) *Communicative Disorders relating to Cleft Lip and Palate*, 2nd edn. Boston: Little and Brown.

COHN, A.M. and PEPPARD, S.B. (1979). Laryngeal trauma. In G.M. English (Ed.) *Otolaryngology* (1987). New York: Harper & Row.

COLTON, R.H. and STEINSCHNEIDER, A. (1980). Acoustic relationships of infant cries to the Sudden Infant Death Syndrome. In T. Murry and J. Murry (Eds) *Infant Communication: Cry and early speech*. Houston, Texas: College-Hill Press.

CONLEY, J.J. (1961). Glottic reconstruction and wound rehabilitation. *Arch. Otol.* **74**, 21.

CONLEY, J.J. (1962). Rehabilitation of the airway system by neck flaps. *Ann. Otol.* **71**, 924.

COOK, T.A., BRUNSCHING, J.P., BUTEL, J.S., COHN, A.M., GOEPFERT, H. and ROWS, W.E. (1973). Laryngeal papilloma: etiologic and therapeutic considerations. *Ann. Otol.* **82**, 649.

COOPER, M. (1971). Papilloma of the vocal folds: a review. *J. Speech Dis.* **36**, 51.

COOPER, M. (1974). Spectrographic analysis of fundamental frequency and hoarseness before and after therapy. *J. Speech Hear. Dis.* **39**, 286.

COOPER, M. and NAHUM, A.M. (1967). Vocal rehabilitation for contact ulcer of the larynx. *Arch. Otolaryngol.* **85**, 41.

COTES, J.E. (1979). *Lung Function*, 4th edn. Oxford: Blackwell Scientific.

COTTAM, P. J. and SUTTON, A. (1986). *Conductive Education: A system for overcoming motor disorder*. London: Croom Helm.

COTTON, E. (1965). The institute for movement therapy and school for 'conductors', Budapest, Hungary. A report on a study visit. *Develop. Med. Child Neurol.* **7**, 437.

COWIE, R., DOUGLAS-COWIE, B.A. and KERR, A.G. (1982). A study of speech deterioration in post-lingually deafened adults. *J. Laryngol. Otol.* **96**, 101.

CRITCHLEY, M. (1939a). Spastic dysphonia: inspiratory speech. *Brain* **62**, 96.

CRITCHLEY, M. (1939b). *The Language of Gesture*. London: Edward Arnold.

CRITCHLEY, M. (1949). Observations on essential voice tremor. *Brain.* **72**, 113.

CRUMLEY, R.L. and IZDEBSKI, K. (1986). Voice quality following laryngeal reinnervation by ansa hypoglossi transfer. *Laryngoscope* **96**, 611.

CRYSTAL, D. (1976). *Child Language, Learning and Linguistics: An overview for the teaching and therapeutic professions.* London: Edward Arnold.

CRYSTAL, D. (1980). *Introduction to Language Pathology.* London: Edward Arnold.

CRYSTAL, D. (1981). *Clinical Linguistics*. London: Edward Arnold.

CRYSTAL, D. (1982). *Profiling Linguistic Disability*. London: Edward Arnold.

CURLE, R.J. (1979). Therapeutic methods for the incompetent soft palate. In R.R. Ellis and F.C. Flack (Eds) *Diagnosis and Treatment of Palato-glossal Malfunction*. London: College of Speech Therapists.

CURRY, E.T. (1949). Hoarseness and voice change in male adolescents. *J. Speech Dis.* **14**, 23.

DABUL, B. and BOLLIER, B. (1976). Therapeutic approaches to apraxia. *J. Speech Hear. Dis.* **41**, 268.

DAMSTE, P.H. (1958). *Oesophageal Speech*. Groningen: Hoitsema.

DAMSTE, P.H. (1962). Congenital short palate without cleft. In L. Croatto and C. Croatto-Martolini (Eds) *Proceedings of the 12th International Speech and Voice Therapy Conference*, Padua.

DAMSTE, P.H. (1964). Virilisation of the voice due to anabolic steroids. *Folia Phoniatr.* **16**, 10.

DAMSTE, P.H. (1967). A voice change in adult women caused by virilizing agents. *J. Speech Dis.* **32**, 126.

DAMSTE, P.H. (1983). Diagnostic behaviour patterns with communicative abilities. In D.M. Bless and J.H. Abbs (Eds) *Vocal Fold Physiology: Contemporary research and clinical issues.* San Diego: College-Hill Press.

DAMSTE, P.H. and LERMAN, J.W. (1975). *An Introduction to Voice Pathology. Functional and Organic.* Springfield, IL: Thomas.

DARLEY, F.L., ARONSON, A.E. and BROWN, J.R. (1969). Differential diagnostic patterns of dysarthria. *J. Speech Hear. Res.* **12**, 246.

DARLEY, F.L., ARONSON, A.E. and BROWN, J.R. (1975). *Motor Speech Disorders*. Philadelphia: W.B. Saunders.

DAWSON, J. (1919). *The Voice of the Boy*. New York: Kellog.

DE SOUZA, F.M. (1980). Thyroidectomy. In G.M. English (Ed.) *Otolarynology*, Vol. 5 (1988). New York: Harper & Row.

DEAL, J. and DARLEY, F. (1972). The influence of linguistic and situational variables on phonemic accuracy in apraxia of speech. *J. Speech Hear. Res.* **15**, 639.

DEDO, H.H. (1976). Recurrent laryngeal nerve section for spastic dysphonia. *Ann. Otol.* **85**, 451.

DEDO, H.H. and IZDEBSKI, K. (1983a). Problems with surgical (RLN section) treatment of spastic dysphonia. *Laryngoscope* **93**, 268.

DEDO, H.H. and IZDEBSKI, K. (1983b). Intermediate results of 306 recurrent laryngeal nerve sections for spastic dysphonia. *Laryngoscope* **93**, 9.

DEDO, H.H. and SHIPP, T. (1980). *Spastic Dysphonia – A Surgical and Voice Therapy Treatment Program*. Houston, Texas: College-Hill Press.

DEDO, H.H., URREA, R.O. and LAWSON, L. (1973). Intracordal injection of Teflon in the treatment of 135 patients with dysphonia. *Ann. Otolaryngol.* **82**, 1.

DEKELBOUM, A.M. (1965). Papillomas of the larynx. *Arch. Otolaryngol.* **81**, 390.

DELAHUNTY, J.E. (1972). Acid laryngitis. *J. Laryngol. Otol.* **86**, 335.

DELAHUNTY, J.E. and ARDRAN, G.M. (1970). Globus hystericus – a manifestation of reflux oesophagitis. *J. Laryngol.* **84**, 1049.

Di CARLO, L.M., AMSTER, W.W. and HERER, G.R. (1955). *Speech After Laryngectomy*. Syracuse: Syracuse University Press.

DIEDRICH, W.M. and YOUNGSTROM, K.A. (1966, 1977). *Alaryngeal Speech*. Springfield, IL: Charles C. Thomas.

DONALD, P.J. (1982). Voice change surgery in the transsexual. *Head Neck Surg.* **4**, 433.

DORNHURST, A.C. and NEGUS, V.E. (1954). Speech after removal of the oesophagus and the larynx and part of the pharynx. *Br. Med. J.* **2**, 16.

DOWNIE, A.W., LOW, J.M. and LINDSAY, D.D. (1981). Speech disorders in Parkinsonism – usefulness of delayed auditory feedback in selected cases. *Br. J. Dis. Commun.* **16**, 135.

DUFF, J. (1968). Laryngeal trauma. *J. Laryngol.* **82**, 825.

EDELS, Y. (Ed.) (1983). *Laryngectomy: Diagnosis to rehabilitation*. London: Croom Helm.

EDELS, Y. (1983). Pseudo-voice: its theory and practice. In Y. Edels (Ed.) *Laryngectomy: Diagnosis to rehabilitation*. London: Croom Helm.

EDWARDS, J.R. (1982). Language attitudes and their implications among English speakers. In R.L. Street and J. Cappella (Eds) *Sequence and Pattern in Communicative Behaviour*. London: Edward Arnold.

EDWARDS, M. (1980). Assessment and remediation of speech. In M. Edwards and A. Watson (Eds) *Cleft Palate: Advances in management.* London: Churchill Livingstone.

EDWARDS, M. (1984). *Disorders of Articulation: Aspects of dysarthria and verbal Dyspraxia*. Vienna: Springer-Verlag.

EDWARDS, N. (1976). The artificial larynx. *Br. J. Hosp. Med.* **16**, 145.

EDWARDS, N. (1983). The surgical approach to speech rehabilitation. In Y. Edels (Ed.) *Laryngectomy: Diagnosis to rehabilitation*. London: Croom Helm.

ELLIS, M. (1952a). Chronic specific laryngitis. In W.G. Scott-Brown (Ed.) *Diseases of the Ear, Nose and Throat*. London: Butterworths.

ELLIS, M. (1952b). Acute diseases of the larynx. In W.G. Scott-Brown (Ed.) *Diseases of the Ear, Nose and Throat*. London: Butterworths.

ELLIS, P.D.M. and BENNETT, J. (1977). Laryngeal trauma and prolonged endo-tracheal intubation. *J. Laryngol.* **91**, 69.

ELLIS, P.D.M. and PALLISTER, W.K. (1975). Recurrent laryngeal nerve palsy and endotracheal intubation. *J. Laryngol.* **89**, 823.

ELLIS, R. (1979). The Exeter nasal anemometry system. In R. Ellis and F.C. Flack (Eds) *Diagnosis and Treatment of Palato-glossal Malfunction*. London: College of Speech Therapists.

ELLIS, R.E., FLACK, F.C. CURLE, H.J. and SELLEY, W.G. (1978). A system for the assessment of nasal airflow during speech. *Br. J. Dis. Commun.* **13**, 31.

ENDERBY, P. (1983). *Frenchay Dysarthria Assessment*. San Diego: College-Hill Press.

ENDERBY, P. (1984). Assisting the patient who has difficulty with swallowing. *College of Speech Therapists Bulletin* no. 388.

ENDERBY, P. (Ed.) (1987). *Assistive Communication Aids for the Speech Impaired.* Edinburgh: Churchill Livingstone.

ENDERBY, P., HATHORN, I.S. and SERVANT, S. (1984). The use of intra-oral appliances in the management of acquired velopharyngeal disorders. *Br. Dent. J.* **157**, 157.

EYSENCK, H.J. (1960). *Behaviour Therapy and the Neuroses*. Oxford: Pergamon.

FAABORG-ANDERSON, K. and NYKOBING, F. (1965). Electromyography of laryngeal muscles: techniques and results. *Aktuelle Probleme in Phoniatrics and Logopedics*, Vol. 3. Basel: Karger.

FAHMY, M. (1950). The theory of habit control and negative practice as a curative method in the treatment of stammering. *Speech* **14**, 24.

FAIRBANKS, G. (1942). An acoustical study in the pitch of infant wails. *Child Develop.* **13**, 227.

FAIRBANKS, G. (1960). *Voice and Articulation Drill Book,* 2nd edn. New York: Harper.

FAIRBANKS, G., HERBERT, E.L. and HAMMOND, J.M. (1949). An acoustical study of vocal pitch in seven- and eight-year-old girls. *Child Develop.* **20**, 71.

FAIRBANKS, G., WILEY, J.H. and LASSMAN, F.M. (1949). An acoustical study of vocal pitch in seven- and eight-year-old boys. *Child Develop.* **20**, 63.

FALK, A. and BIRKEN, E.A. (1985). Hyperthyroidism: a surgeon's perspective. In G.M. English (Ed.) *Otolaryngology*, Vol. 4 (1988). New York: Harper & Row.

FAWCUS, M. (Ed.) (1986a). The causes and classification of voice disorders. In *Voice Disorders and Their Management*. London: Croom Helm.

FAWCUS, M. (Ed.) (1986b). Hyperfunctional voice: the misuse and abuse syndrome. In *Voice Disorders and Their Management*. London: Croom Helm.

FEE, W.E. (1984). Hypopharyngeal reconstruction. *Arch. Otolaryngol.* **110**, 384.

FERGUSON, D. (1988). Indoor air pollution - the concern of architects. *Building Owner and Manager*.

FIGI, F.A. (1953). Hemilaryngectomy with immediate skin graft for the removal of carcinoma of the larynx. *Ann. Otol.* **62**, 400.

FIGI, F.A. and NEW, G.B. (1929). Carcinoma of the larynx in the young. *Arch. Otolaryngol.* **51**, 386.

FISHER, A.J., CALDARELLI, D.D., CHACKO, D.C. and HOLINGER, L.D. (1986). Glottic cancer - surgical salvage for radiation failure. *Arch. Otolaryngol. Head Neck Surg.* **112**, 519.

FLACH, M. SCHWICKARDI, H. and SIMON, R. (1969). What influence do menstrua tion and pregnancy have on the trained singing voice? *Folia Phoniatr.* **21**, 199.

FLETCHER, S.G. (1970). Tonar. The oral nasal acoustic ratio. *Cleft Palate J.* **7**, 601.

FLETCHER, S.G. (1972). Contingencies for bio-electric modification of nasality. *J. Speech Hear. Dis.* **37**, 329.

FOGH-ANDERSEN, P. (1980). Incidence and aetiology. In M. Edwards and A.C.H. Watson (Eds) *Advances in the Management of Cleft Palate*. Edinburgh: Churchill Livingstone.

FONTAINE, A. and MITCHELL, J.C.E. (1960). Oesophageal voice: a factor of readiness. *J. Laryngol.* **74**, 870.

FORD, C.N. and BLESS, D.M. (1987). Collagen injection in the scarred vocal fold. *J. Voice* **1**, 116.

FORD, C.N., BLESS, D.M. and CAMPBELL, D.A. (1986). Studies of injectable soluble collagen for vocal fold augmentation. *Folia Phoniatr.* XXth IALP Congress, Tokyo, **2**, 283.

FORD, C.N., GILCHRIST, K.W. and BARTELLI, T.E. (1987). Persistence of injectable collagen in the human larynx: a histopathologic study. *Laryngoscope* **97**, 724.

FORDER, R.J. (1983). Laryngeal granuloma as a complication of the CO_2 laser. *Laryngoscope* **93**, 944.

FORMBY, D. (1967). Maternal recognition of infant's cry. *Develop. Med. Child Neurol.* **9**, 293.

FOSTER, T.D. (1980a). Growth and development. In M. Edwards and A.C.H. Watson (Eds) *Advances in the Management of Cleft Palate*. Edinburgh: Churchill Livingstone.

FOSTER, T.D. (1980b). The role of orthodontic treatment. In M. Edwards and A.C.H. Watson (Eds) *Advances in the Management of Cleft Palate*. Edinburgh: Churchill Livingstone.

FOURCIN, A.J. (1974). Laryngographic examination of vocal fold vibration. In B. Wyke (Ed.) *Ventilatory and Phonatory Control Mechanisms*. Oxford: Oxford University Press.

FOURCIN, A.J. and ABBERTON, E. (1971). First applications of a new laryngograph. *Med. Biol. Illus.* **21**, 172.

FOURCIN, A.J. and ABBERTON, E. (1977). The laryngograph and the Voiscope in speech therapy. *Proceedings of XVIth IALP Congress*, Copenhagen, p. 116.

FRASER, G. (1987). Cochlear implantation: more than just an operation. In J.G. Kyle (Ed.) *Adjustment to Acquired Hearing Loss: Analysis, change and learning*. Proceedings of Conference, Centre of Deaf Studies, University of Bristol.

FREEMAN, F.J., SCHAEFFER, S., CANNITO, M.P. and FINITZO, T. (1987). Episodic reactive dysphonia: a case study. *J. Commun. Dis.* **20**, 259.

FREUD, S. (1943). *A General Introduction to Psycho-Analysis*. New York: Garden City.

FRITZELL, B. (1969). The velopharyngeal muscles in speech. An electromyographic and cineradiographic study. *Acta Otolaryngol. Suppl.* 250.

FRITZELL, B., SUNDBERG, J. and STRANGE-EBBESEN, A. (1982). Pitch change after stripping oedematous vocal folds. *Folia Phoniatr.* **34**, 29.

FRITZELL, B., FEUER, E., HAGHUND, S., KNUTSSON, E. and SCHIRATZKI, H. (1982). Experience with recurrent laryngeal nerve section for spastic dysphonia. *Folia Phoniatr.* **34**, 160.

FROESCHELS, E. (1948). *Twentieth Century Correction*. New York: Philosophical Library.

FRY, D. (1977). How did we learn to do it? In *Homo Loquens*. Cambridge: Cambridge University Press.

FRY, D.B. (1979). *The Physics of Speech*. Cambridge: Cambridge University Press.

FUKADA, H., SAITO, S., KITAHARA, S., ISOGAI, Y., MAKINO, K., TSUZUKI, T., KOGAWA, N. and ONO, H. (1983). Vocal fold vibration in excised larynges viewed with an X-ray, stroboscope and an ultra-high-speed camera. In D.M. Bless and J.H. Abbs (Eds) *Vocal Fold Physiology*. San Diego: College-Hill.

GACEK, H.R. (1976). Hereditary abductor vocal cord paralysis. *Ann. Otol.* **85**, 90.

GARDENER, W.H. (1978). *Laryngectomee Speech and Rehabilitation*, 2nd edn. Springfield, IL: C.C. Thomas.

GARDENER, W.H., HILL, S.D. and CARANO, H.N. (1962). Oesophageal speech for a 12-year-old boy: a case report. *J. Speech Hear. Dis.* **27**, 227.

GARFIELD DAVIES, D. (1969). Fibrosarcoma and pseudosarcoma of the larynx. *J. Laryngol.* **83**, 423.

GARFIELD DAVIES, D. (1988). Spastic dysphonia. *Voice Research Society Newsletter*. **3**(1), 21.

GATELY, G. (1971). A technique for teaching the laryngectomised to trap air for the production of oesophageal speech. *J. Speech Dis.* **76**, 485.

GATES, G.A. and MONTALBO, P.J. (1987). The effect of Low-dose ß-Blockade on performance anxiety in singers. *J. Voice* **1**, 105.

GEDDA, J., FIORI-RATTI, I. and BRUNO, G. (1960). La voix chez les juneaux monozygotique. *Folia Phoniatr.* **12**, 81.

GELDER, M., GATH, D. and MAYOU, R. (1983). *Oxford Textbook of Psychiatry*. Oxford: Oxford University Press.

GILES, H. and POWESLAND, P.F. (1975). *Speech Style and Social Evaluation*. London: Academic Press.

GIMSON, A.C. (1962). *An Introduction to the Pronunciation of English*. London: Edward Arnold.

GODA, S. (1966). Speech therapy with selected patients with congenital velopharyngeal inadequacy. *Cleft Pal. J.* **3**, 268.

GOLDBERG, M., NOYEK, A.M. and PRITZKER, P.H. (1978). Laryngeal granuloma secondary to gastroesophageal reflux. *J. Otolaryngol.* 7, 196.

GOLDWYN, E. (1989). *The Poison that Waits*. London: Horizon No. 2, BBC Publications.

GOODE, R.L. (1975). Artificial laryngeal devices in post-laryngectomy rehabilitation.

Laryngoscope **83**, 677.

GORDON, M. (1977). Physical measurements in a clinically orientated voice pathology department. *Proceedings of XVIIth IALP Congress* **1**, 401.

GORDON, M. (1986). Assessment of the dysphonic patient. In M. Fawcus (Ed.) *Voice Disorders and Their Management*. London: Croom Helm.

GORDON, M.T., MORTON, F.M. and SIMPSON, J.C. (1978). Airflow measurements in diagnosis assessment and treatment of mechanical dysphonia. *Folia Phoniatr.* **30**, 161.

GOULD, W.J. (1981). The pulmonary–laryngeal system. In K.N. Stevens and M. Hirano (Eds) Vocal Fold Physiology. Tokyo: University of Tokyo Press.

GOULD, W.J. and OKAMURA, H. (1972). Status lung volumes in singers. *Ann. Otol.* **82**, 89.

GRAY, H. (1949). In T.B. Johnson and J. Whillis (Eds) *Gray's Anatomy: Descriptive and applied*, 30th edn. London: Longman, Green and Co.

GREENE, M.C.L. (1955). Puberphonia. *Proceedings of the College of Speech Therapists*, Oxford Conference. London: College of Speech Therapists.

GREENE, M.C.L. (1957). Speech of children before and after removal of tonsils and adenoids. *J. Speech Dis.* **22**, 361.

GREENE, M.C.L. (1960). Speech analysis of 263 cleft palate cases. *J. Speech Hear. Dis.* **25**, 144.

GREENE, M.C.L. (1961). Symposium on speech defects. Part III Speech therapy problems. *Radiography* **27**, 338.

GREENE, M.C.L. (1962). Possible areas of co-operation between speech therapists and teachers of the deaf. *Speech Pathol. Ther.* **5**, 57.

GREENE, M.C.L. (1967). Management of aphonia after surgical treatment of carcinoma of larynx, pharynx and oesophagus. *Br. J. Dis. Commun.* **2**, 30.

GREENE, M.C.L. (1968). Vocal disabilities of singers. *Proc. R. Soc. Med.* **61**, 1147.

GREENE, M.C.L. (1976). Basic structure in teaching reading and spelling to children with severe speech and language disorders in a special class. *Proceedings of XVIth IALP Congress*, Interlaken, 1974, pp. 135–141.

GREENE, M.C.L. (1980a). *The Voice and Its Disorders*, 4th edn. London: Pitman Medical.

GREENE, M.C.L. (1980b). Speech rehabilitation after laryngectomy. In *The Voice and Its Disorders*, 4th edn. London: Pitman Medical.

GREENE, M.C.L. (1982). Ageing of the voice: a review. In M. Edwards (Ed.) *Communicative Changes in Elderly People*. London: College of Speech Therapists.

GREENE, M.C.L. (1983a). Development of speech and language: normal and abnormal. In G.M. English (Ed.) *Otolaryngology*, Vol. 3 (1988). Philadelphia: Harper & Row.

GREENE, M.C.L. (1983b). The voice and voice disorders. In G.M. English (Ed.) *Otolaryngology*, Vol. 3 (1988). Philadelphia: Harper & Row.

GREENE, M.C.L. (1984). Functional dysphonia and the hyperventilation syndrome. *Br. J. Dis. Commun.* **19**, 263.

GREENE, M.C.L. (1986). Disorders of voice. In H. Halpern (Ed.) *Studies in Communication Disorders*. Austin, Texas: Pro-Ed.

GREENE, M.C.L. and CANNING, A. (1959). The incidence of nasal and lateral defects in cleft palate. *Folia Phonaitr.* **11**, 208.

GREENE, M.C.L. and CONWAY, J. (1963). Learning to talk: a study in sound of infant speech development. Folkways Records (NY) Fx 6271.

GREENE, M.C.L. and WATSON, B.W. (1968). The value of speech amplification in Parkinson's Disease patients. *Folia Phoniatr.* **20**, 250.

GREENE, M.C.L., ATKINSON, P. and WATSON, B.W. (1974). A substitute voice after surgical removal of the larynx. *J. Laryngol.* **88**, 1103.

GREENE, M.C.L., TIMMONS, B.H. and GLOVER, J.H.M. (1983). Anxiety state and chronic hyperventilation syndrome: relevance in speech and voice disorders. *Proceedings of XIXth IALP Congress* **2**, 704.

GREENE, M.C.L., TIMMONS, B.H. and GLOVER, J.H.M. (1984). The significance of anxiety and breathing disorders in functional dysphonia. Third International workshop on respiratory psychophysiology, Bordeaux. *Bull. Eur. Physiopathol. Respir.* **20**, 94.

GREWEL, F. (1957a). Classification of dysarthria. *Acta Psych. Neurol. Scand.* **32**, 325.

GREWEL, F. (1957b). Dysarthria in post-encephalitic Parkinsonism. *Acta Psych. Neurol. Scand.* **32**, 440.

GREWEL, F. (1960). Speech, language and hearing disorders in encephalopathy. *Folia Phoniatr.* **12**, 282.

GRUNWELL, P. (1982). *Clinical Phonology*. London: Croom Helm.

GUDYKUNST, W.B. (1986). Intergroup communication. In H. Giles (Ed.) *Social Psychology of Language and Communicative Studies*. London: Edward Arnold.

GUSSAK, G.S., JUROVICH, G.J. and LATERMAN, A. (1986). Laryngeal trauma: a protocol approach to a rare injury. *Laryngoscope* **96**, 660.

GUTHRIE, D. (1966). Forty-two years survival after laryngectomy. *J. Laryngol.* **80**, 851.

HABIB, M.A. (1977). Intra-articular steroid injection in acute rheumatoid arthritis of the larynx. *J. Laryngol. Otol.* **91**, 909.

HAGHUND, H., LUNDQUIST, P.G. and CANTRELL, K. (1981). Interferon therapy in juvenile laryngeal papillomatosis. *Arch. Otolaryngol.* **107**, 327.

HAHN, F.W., MARTIN, J.I. and LILLIE, J.C. (1970). Vocal cord paralysis with endotracheal intubation. *Arch. Otolaryngol.* **92**, 226.

HALPERN, H. (1981). Therapy for agnosis, apraxia and dysarthria. In R. Chapey (Ed.) *Language Intervention Strategies in Adult Aphasia*. Baltimore: Williams & Wilkins.

HAMAKER, R.C., SINGER, M.I., BLOM, E.D. and DANIELS, H.A. (1985). Primary voice restoration at laryngectomy. *Arch. Otolaryngol.* **3**, 182.

HAMMARBERG, B. (1986). Perceptual and acoustic analysis of dysphonia. *Studies in Logopedics and Phoniatrics*, No. 1. Huddinge University Hospital, Sweden.

HARDY, J.C., NETSELL, R., SCHWEIGER, J.W. and MORRIS, H.L. (1969). Management of velopharyngeal dysfunction in cerebral palsy. *J. Speech Dis.* **34**, 123.

HARRIS, H.H. and AINSWORTH, J.Z. (1965). Immediate management of laryngeal and tracheal injuries. *Laryngoscope* **75**, 1103.

HARRIS, L.L., VOGTSBERGER, K.N. and MATTOX, D.E. (1985). Group psychotherapy for head and neck cancer patients. *Laryngoscope* **95**, 585.

HARRIS, T. (1987). The place of stroboscopy in the examination of the larynx. *Voice Research Society Newsletter* **1**(2), 15.

HARRISON, D.F.N. (1964). Pharyngo-oesophageal replacement in post-cricoid and oesophageal carcinoma. *Ann. Otol.* **73**, 1026.

HARTMAN, D.E. and ARONSON, A.E. (1983). Psychogenic aphonia masking mutational falsetto. *Arch. Otolaryngol.* **109**, 415.

HARTMAN, D.E. and VISHWANAT, B. (1984). Spastic dysphonia and essential (voice) tremor treated with Primidone. *Arch. Otolaryngol.* **110**, 394.

HARTMAN, E. and VON CRAMON, D. (1984a). Acoustic measurement of voice quality in dysphonia after severe closed head trauma: a follow-up study. *Br. J. Dis. Commun.* **19**, 253.

HARTMAN, E. and VON CRAMON, D. (1984b). Acoustic measurement of voice quality in central dysphonia. *J. Commun. Dis.* **17**, 425.

HEATH, A. (1987). The deafened: a special group. In J.G. Kyle (Ed.) *Adjustment to Acquired Hearing Loss: Analysis, change and learning*. Proceedings of Conference, Centre of Deaf Studies, University of Bristol.

HEAVER, L. (1958). Psychiatric observations on the personality structure of patients with habitual dysphonia. *Logos* **1**, 21.

HEAVER, L. and ARNOLD, G.E. (1962). Rehabilitation of alaryngeal aphonia. *Post. Grad. Med.* **32**, 11.

HEINEMANN, M. (1969). Myxoedem und Stimme. *Folia Phoniatr.* **21**, 55.

HENDERSON, R. (1954). *Kathleen Ferrier*. London: Hamilton.

HENLEY, J. and SOULIERE, C. (1986). Tracheoesophageal speech failure in the laryngectomee: the role of the constrictor myotomy. *Laryngoscope* **96**, 1016.

HILDERNESSES, L.W. 1956). Voice diagnosis. *Acta Physiol. Pharmacol. Neer.* **5**, 73.

HILDICK-SMITH, M. (1980). *Management of Parkinson's Disease*. Postgraduate Medical Centres Publications.

HIRANO, M. (1974). Morphological structure of the vocal cord as a vibrator and its variations. *Folia Phoniatr.* **26**, 89.

HIRANO, M. (1981). *Clinical Examination of Voice*. Vienna: Springer-Verlag.

HIRANO, M., KOIKE, Y. and VON LEDEN, H. (1968). Maximum phonation time and air usage during phonation. *Folia Phoniatr.* **20**, 185.

HIRANO, M., KURITA, S. and NAKASHIMA, T. (1983). Growth, development and aging of human vocal folds. In D.M. Bless and J.H. Abbs (Eds) *Vocal Fold Physiology*. San Diego: College-Hill Press.

HIRANO, M., SHIGEJIRO, K. and TERASAWA, R. (1985). Difficulty in high-pitched phonation by laryngeal trauma. *Arch. Otolaryngol.* **107**, 59.

HIRANO, M., SHIN, T. and NOZOE, I. (1977). Prognostic aspect of recurrent laryngeal nerve paralysis. *Proceedings of IALP Congress*, Copenhagen. *Phonia-Arthria* **1**, 95.

HIROSE, H. (1985) Laryngeal electromyography. In G.M. English (Ed.) *Otolaryngology*, Vol. 3 (1988). Philadelphia: Harper & Row.

HIROSE, H. and SAWASHIMA, M. (1981). Functions of the laryngeal muscles in speech. In K.N. Stevens and M. Hirano (Eds) *Vocal Fold Physiology*. Tokyo: University of Tokyo Press.

HIROSE, H., SAWASHIMA, M. and YOSHIOKA, H. (1983). Simultaneous EMG and fiberscopic study of laryngeal adjustment for initiation of utterances. In D.M. Bless and J.H. Abbs (Eds) *Vocal Fold Physiology*. San Diego: College-Hill Press.

HIROTO, I. (1981). Introductory remarks. In K.N. Stevens and M. Hirano (Eds) *Vocal Fold Physiology*. Tokyo: University of Tokyo Press.

HIROTO, I., HIRANO, M. and TOMITA, H. (1968). Electromyographic investigation of human vocal cord paralysis. *Ann. Otol.* **77**, 296.

HIRSCHBERG, J. (1986). Velopharyngeal insufficiency (VPI). *Folia Phoniatr.* **38**, 221.

HIXON, T.J. (1987). *Respiratory Function in Speech and Song*. London: Taylor & Francis.

HIXON, T.J., GOLDMAN, M.D. and MEAD, J. (1973). Kinematics of the chest wall during speech production: volume displacements of the rib cage, abdomen and lung. *J. Speech Hear. Res.* **16**, 78.

HIXON, T., HAWLEY, J. and WILSON, K. (1982). An around the house device for the clinical determination of respiratory driving pressure. *J. Speech Hear. Dis.* **47**, 413.

HIXON, T.J., MEAD, J. and GOLDMAN, M.D. (1976). Dynamics of the chest wall during speech production: function of the thorax, rib cage and abdomen. *J. Speech Hear. Res.* **19**, 297.

HODGE, K.M. and GANZEL, T.M. (1987). Diagnostic and therapeutic efficiency in croup and epiglottitis. *Laryngoscope* **97**, 621.

HODSON, C.J. and OSWALD, M.V.O. (1958). *Speech Recovery after Total Laryngectomy*. Edinburgh: Livingstone.

HOLBROOK, A., ROLNICK, M.I. and BAILEY, C.W. (1974). Treatment of vocal abuse disorders using a vocal intensity controller. *J. Speech Hear. Dis.* **39**, 298.

HOLINGER, L.D. (1979). Congenital anomalies of the larynx. In G.M. English (Ed.) *Otolarynology*, Vol. 3. Philadelphia: Harper & Row.

HOLINGER, L.D. and WOLTER, R.K. (1979). Neurologic disorders of the larynx. In G.M. English (Ed.) *Otolaryngology*, Vol. 3 (1988). Philadelphia: Harper & Row.

HOLINGER, L.D., HOLINGER, P.C. and HOLINGER, P.H. (1976). Etiology of bilateral abductor vocal cord paralysis: a review of 389 cases. *Ann. Otol.* **85**, 428.

HOLINGER, P.H. (1959). In G.T. Pack and I.M. Ariel (Eds) *Treatment of Cancer and Allied Diseases*, Vol. 3, Chap. 34. London: Pitman.

HOLINGER, P.H. (1975). A century of progress of laryngectomies in the northern hemisphere. *Laryngoscope* **85**, 322.

HOLINGER, P.H., SCHILD, J.A. and MAURIZ, D.G. (1968). Laryngeal papilloma. Review of etiology and therapy. *Laryngoscope* **78**, 1462.

HOLLIEN, H. (1980). Developmental aspects of neonatal vocalization. In T. Murry and J. Murry (Eds) *Infant Communication*. San Diego: College-Hill Press.

HOLLIEN, H. (1983a). In search of vocal frequency control mechanisms. In D.M. Bless and J.H. Abbs (Eds) *Vocal Fold Physiology*. San Diego: College-Hill Press.

HOLLIEN, H. (1983b). Control of vocal frequency. In D.M. Bless and J.H. Abbs (Eds) *Vocal Fold Physiology*. San Diego: College-Hill Press.

HOLLIEN, H. and SHIPP, T. (1972). Speaking fundamental frequency and chronological age in males. *J. Speech Hear. Res.* **15**, 155.

HONJO, I. and ISSHIKI, N. (1980). Laryngoscopic and voice characteristics of aged persons. *Arch. Otolaryngol.* **106**, 149.

HONJO, I., OKAZAKI, N. and KUMAZAWA, I. (1979). Experimental study of the eustachian tube function with regard to its related muscles. *Acta Otolaryngol.* **87**, 84.

HUNT, R.B. (1964). Rehabilitation of the laryngectomee. *Laryngoscope* **74**, 382.

HUTZINGA, E. (1966). Historical vignette: Sir Felix Seman. *Arch. Otolaryngol.* **84**, 473.

HYMAN, M. (1979). Factors influencing intelligibility of alaryngeal speech. In R.L. Keith and F.L. Darley (Eds) *Laryngectomy Rehabilitation*. San Diego: College-Hill Press.

INGRAM, T.T.S. and BARN, J. (1961). A description and classification of common speech disorders associated with cerebral palsy. *Cerebr. Palsy Bull.* **3**, 57.

INNOCENTI, D.M. (1983). Chronic hyperventilation syndrome. In P.A. Downie (Ed.) *Cash's Textbook of Chest, Heart and Vascular Disorders for Physiotherapists*, 3rd edn. London: Faber & Faber.

ILLINGWORTH, R.S. (1980). The development of communication in the first year and factors which affect it. In T.M. Murry and J. Murry (Eds) *Infant Communication Cry and Early Speech*. San Diego: College-Hill Press.

INGRAM, T.T. (1960). Paediatric aspects of developmental dysphasia, dyslexia and dysgraphia. *Cerebr. Palsy Bull.* **2**, 254.

ISSHIKI, N. (1964). Regulatory mechanism of voice intensity variation. *J. Speech Hear. Res.* **17**, 17.

ISSHIKI, N. (1965). Vocal intensity and air flow rate. *Folia Phoniatr.* **17**, 19.

ISSHIKI, N. (1968). Airflow in esophageal speech. In J.C. Snidecor (Ed.) *Speech*

Rehabilitation of the Laryngectomised, 2nd edn. Illinois: Thomas.

ISSHIKI, N. (1980). Recent advances in phonosurgery. *Folia Phoniatr.* **32**, 119.

ISSHIKI, N., HONJO, I. and MORIMOTO, M. (1967). Cineradiographic analysis of movement of the lateral pharyngeal wall. *Plas. Reconstr. Surg.* **44**, 357.

ISSHIKI, N. OKAMURA, H. and ISHIKAWA, T. (1975). Thyroplasty Type 1. Lateral compression for dysphonia due to vocal cord paralysis and atrophy. *Acta Otolaryngol.* **80**, 465.

ISSHIKI, N., OKAMURA, H. and MORIMOTO, M. (1967). Maximum phonation time and airflow rate during phonation. Simple clinical tests for vocal functon. *Ann. Otol.* **76**, 998.

ISSHIKI, N., TANABE, M. and SAWADA, M. (1978). Arytenoid adduction for unilateral vocal cord paralysis. *Arch. Otolaryngol.* **104**, 555.

IZDEBSKI, K., DEDO, H.H. and SHIPP, T. (1981). Dysphonia patients treated by recurrent laryngeal nerve section. *Otolaryngol. Head Neck Surg.* **89**, 96.

IZDEBSKI, K., ROSS, J.C and LEE, S. (1987). Fungal colonisation of tracheoesophageal voice prosthesis. *Laryngoscope* **97**, 594.

JACKSON, C. and JACKSON, C.L. (1935). Contact ulcer of the larynx. *Arch. Otolaryngol.* **22**, 1.

JACKSON, C. (1940). Myasthenia laryngis: Observations on the larynx as an air column instrument. *Arch. Otolaryngol.* **22**, 1.

JACKSON, M.C.A. (1987). The high male voice. *Folia Phoniatr.* **39**, 18.

JACOBS, A.H. and ABRAMSON, A.L. (1980). Speech therapy after total laryngectomy and oesophageal replacement in a preschool patient: a case study. *Int. J. Ped. Otorhinolaryngol.* **2**, 21.

JACOBSON, E. (1929). *Progressive Relaxation*. Chicago: University of Chicago Press.

JANET, P. (1920). *The Major Symptoms of Hysteria*. New York: Macmillan.

JAYSON, M.I.V. (1987). *Back Pain: The facts,* 2nd edn. Oxford: Oxford University Press.

JIU, J.B., SOBOL, S.M. and GROZEA, P.N. (1985). Vocal cord paralysis and recovery with thyroid lymphoma. *Laryngoscope* **95**, 57.

JOHNS, D.F. (Ed.) (1985). *Clinical Management of Neurogenic Communicative Disorders*. Boston: Little, Brown.

JOHNS, D.F. and SALYER, K.E. (1978). Surgical and prosthetic management of neurogenic speech disorders. In D.F. Johns (Ed.) *Clinical Management of Neurogenic Communicative Disorders*. Boston: Little, Brown.

JOHNSON, H. (1987). *Hugh Johnson's Wine Companion*. London: Michael Beazley.

JONES, D. (1948). *An Outline of English Phonetics*. Cambridge: Heffer.

JULIAN, W., MacCURTAIN, F. and NOSCOE, N. (1981). Anatomical factors influencing voice quality. *J. Physiol.* **315**, 10.

JURIK, A.G., PEDERSEN, U. and NØRGÅRD, Å. (1985). Rheumatoid arthritis of the cricorytenoid joints: a case of laryngeal obstruction due to acute and chronic joint changes. *Laryngoscope* **95**, 846.

KABAT, H. and KNOTT, M. (1953). Proprioceptive facilitation techniques for treatment of paralysis. *Phys. Ther. Rev.* **2**, 33.

KAHANE, J.C. (1983). A survey of age-related changes in the connective tissues of the human larynx. In D.M. Bless and J.H. Abbs (Eds) *Vocal Fold Physiology*. San Diego: College-Hill Press.

KAHANE, J.C. (1986). Anatomy and physiology of the speech mechanism. In H. Halpern (Ed.) *Studies in Communication Disorders*. Austin, Texas: Pro-Ed.

KAHANE, J.C. and KAHN, A.R. (1984). Weight measurements of infant and adult intrinsic laryngeal muscles. *Folia Phoniatr.* **36**, 129.

KALIN, R. (1982). The social significance of speech in medical, legal and occupational settings. In E.B. Ryan and H. Giles (Eds) *Attitudes towards Language Variation*. London: Edward Arnold.

KALLEN, L.A. (1934). Vicarious vocal mechanisms. *Arch. Otolaryngol.* **20**, 460.

KARELITZ, S. and FISICHELLI, V.R. (1962). The cry thresholds of normal infants and those with brain damage. *J. Pediatr.* **61**, 679.

KEITH, R.L. and DARLEY, F.L. (1979). *Laryngectomee Rehabilitation*. San Diego: College-Hill Press.

KELMAN, A.W., GORDON, M.T., SIMPSON, I.C. and MORTON, F.M. (1975). Assessment of vocal function by airflow measurements. *Folia Phoniatr.* **27**, 250.

KELMAN, A.W., GORDON, M.T., MORTON, F.M. and SIMPSON, I.C. (1981). Comparison methods of assessing vocal function. *Folia Phoniatr.* **33**, 51.

KENNEDY, J.T. and KRAUSE, C.J. (1974). Survival rates in conservative surgery of the larynx. *Arch. Otolaryngol.* **99**, 274.

KENT, R.D. and ROSENBEK, J.C. (1983). Acoustic patterns of apraxia of speech. *J. Speech Hear. Res.* **26**, 231.

KERTESZ, A. (1983). Subcortical lesions and verbal apraxia. In J.S. Rosenbek, M.R. McNeil, A.E. Aronson (Eds) *Apraxia of Speech: Physiology, Acoustics, Linguistics, Management*. San Diego: College-Hill Press.

KING, E.B. (1953). Bilateral abductor paralysis. *Ann. Otol.* **62**, 196.

KINSEY, A.C., POMEROY, W.B. and MARTIN, C. (1948). *Sexual Behaviour in the Human Male.* Philadelphia: Sanderson.

KIRCHNER, J.A. (1966). Atrophy of laryngeal muscles in vagal paralysis. *Laryngoscope* **77**, 1753.

KIRCHNER, J.A. (1983). Factors influencing glottal aperture. In D.M. Bless and J.H. Abbs (Eds) *Vocal Fold Physiology*. San Diego: College-Hill Press.

KIRIKAE, I. (1981). Discussion following W.J. Gould's paper on 'The pulmonary-laryngeal system'. In K.N. Stevens and M. Hirano (Eds) *Vocal Fold Physiology*. Toyko: University of Tokyo Press.

KIRK, S.A. and KIRK, W. (1971). *Psycholinguistic Learning Disabilities: Diagnosis and remediation*. Chicago: University of Illinois Press.

KITZING, P. (1985). Stroboscopy - a pertinent laryngological examination. *J. Otolaryngol.* **14**, 151.

KLEINSASSER, O. (1968). *Microlaryngoscopy and Endolaryngeal Microsurgery*, translated by P.W. Hoffman. Philadelphia: W.B. Saunders.

KNOTT, M. and VOSS, D. (1963). *Proprioceptive Muscular Facilitation*. Philadelphia: Harper & Row.

KOIKE, Y., HIRANO, M. and VON LEDEN, H. (1967). Vocal initiation: acoustic and aerodynamic investigations in normal subjects. *Folia Phoniatr.* **19**, 173.

KOUFMAN, J.A. (1986). Laryngoplasty for vocal cord medialization: an alternative to Teflon. *Laryngoscope* **96**, 726.

KRAMARAC, C. (1982). Gender: how she speaks. In E.B. Ryan and H. Giles (Eds) *Attitudes towards Language Variation*. London: Edward Arnold.

KUNZEL, H.J. (1982). First applications of a biofeedback device for the therapy of velopharyngeal incompetence. *Folia Phoniatr.* **34**, 92.

LABARRAQUE, M.L. (1952). Les Phonophobies. *Ann. d'Otolaryngol. (Paris)* **69**, 200.

LADEFOGED, P. (1974). Respiration, laryngeal activity and linguistics. In B. Wyke (Ed.) *Ventilatory and Phonatory Control Systems*. Oxford: Oxford University Press.

LAGUAITE, J.K. and WALDROP, W.F. (1963). Acoustic analysis of fundamental frequency of voices before and after therapy. *N.Z. Speech Ther. J.* **18**, 23.

LALL, M. and EVISON, G. (1966). Voice production following laryngo-pharyngooesophagectomy. *J. Laryngol.* **80**, 1208.

LANCER, J.M. (1986). Photography and the flexible fibreoptic rhinolaryngoscope. *J. Laryngol Otol.* **100**, 41.

LANDES, B.A. (1977). Management of hyperfunctional dysphonia and vocal tension. In M. Cooper and M.H. Cooper (Eds) *Approaches to Vocal Rehabilitation*. Illinois: Thomas.

LANGLEY, J. (1988). *Working with Swallowing Disorders*. Winslow, Bucks: Winslow Press.

LANGLOIS, A., BAKEN, R.J. and WILDER, C.N. (1980). Pre-speech respiratory behaviour during the first year of life. In T. Murry and J. Murry (Eds) *Infant Communication: Cry and speech*. Houston, Texas: College-Hill Press.

LANGLOIS, A., WILDER, C.N. and BAKEN, R.J. (1975). Pre-speech respiratory patterns in the infant. *Am. Ass. Speech Hear.* **17**, 668.

LANGNICKEL, R. (1976). An endolaryngeal method of vertico lateral transposition of the vocal cord for bilateral abductor paralysis. *Laryngoscope* **86**, 1021.

LAST, R.J. (1984). *Anatomy, Regional and Applied*, 7th edn. Edinburgh: Churchill Livingstone.

LAUDER, E. (1965). The role of the laryngectomee in post-laryngectomy voice instruction. *J. Speech Dis.* **30**, 145.

LAUDER, E. (1968). The laryngectomee and the artificial larynx. *J. Speech Dis.* **33**, 147.

LAVER, J.D. (1980). *The Phonetic Description of Voice Quality*. Cambridge: Cambridge University Press.

LE QUESNE, L.P. (1964). Pharyngeal repair by immediate pharyngogastric anastomosis. *Proc. R. Soc. Med.* **57**, 1103.

LEDER, S.B. and LERMAN, J.W. (1985). Some acoustic evidence for vocal abuse in adult speakers with repaired cleft palate. *Laryngoscope* **95**, 837.

LEDERER, F.L. (1948). Present concepts of laryngeal disease. *J. Speech Dis.* **13**, 11.

LEHMANN, Q.H. (1965). Reverse phonation. A new manoeuvre for examining the larynx. *Radiology* **84**, 215.

LELL, W.A. (1941). Diagnosis and direct laryngoscopy: treatment of functional dysphonia. *Arch. Otolaryngol.* **34**, 141.

LENCIONE, R.M. (1980). Associated conditions. In M. Edwards and A.C.H. Watson (Eds) *Advances in the Management of Cleft Palate*. Edinburgh: Churchill Livingstone.

LENNEBERG, E.H. (1967). *Biological Foundaton of Language*. New York: John Wiley & Sons.

LENNEBERG, E.H., REBELSKY, F. and NICHOLS, I. (1965). The vocalisation of infants born to deaf and hearing parents. *Human Dev.* **8**, 23.

LEONARD, J.R., HOLT, G.P. and MARAN, A.G. (1972). Treatment of vocal cord carcinoma by vertical laryngectomy. *Ann. Otol.* **81**, 469.

LEOPOLD, D.A. (1983). Laryngeal trauma: a historical comparison of treatment methods. *Arch. Otolaryngol.* **109**, 106.

LEVIN, N.M. (Ed.) (1962a). Surgery of the larynx, trachea and neck. In *Voice and Speech Disorders: Medical aspects*. Illinois: Thomas.

LEVIN, N.M. (Ed.) (1962b). Esophageal speech. In *Voice and Speech Disorders: Medical aspects.* Illinois: Thomas.

LEVITT, S. (1962). *Physiotherapy in Cerebral Palsy.* Illinois: Thomas.

LEWIS, B.I. (1959). Hyperventilation syndrome. A clinical and physiological evaluation. *Calif. Med.* **91**, 121.

LEWIS, M.M. (1936). *Early Response to Speech and Babbling in Infant Speech.* London: Keegan Paul.

LEWIS, R.S. (1965). Pharyngeal reconstruction after pharyngolaryngectomy. *J. Laryngol.* 79, 771.

LI, S.L. (1985). Functional tracheoesophageal shunt for vocal rehabilitation after laryngectomy. *Laryngoscope* **95**, 1267.

LIBERMAN, A.M. (1957). Some results of research on speech perception. *J. Acoust. Soc. Am.* **29**, 117.

LIEBERMAN, P. (1967). Intonation in infant speech: physiologic, acoustic and perceptual criteria. In *Intonation, Perception and Language*. Research monograph No. 18. Cambridge, Massachusetts: MIT Press.

LINFORD REES, W.L. (1982). *A Short Textbook of Psychiatry*, 3rd edn. London: Hodder & Stoughton.

LIPPOLD, O. (1971). Physiological tremor. *Sci. Am.* **224**, 65.

LOGEMANN, J. (1983a). *Evaluation and Treatment of Swallowing Disorders*. San Diego: College-Hill Press.

LOGEMANN, J. (1983b). Vocal rehabilitation after extensive surgery for post-cricoid carcinoma. In Y. Edels (Ed.) *Laryngectomy: Diagnosis to rehabilitation*. London: Croom Helm.

LUCHSINGER, R. (1962). Voice disorders on an endocrine basis. In N.M. Levin (Ed.) *Voice and Speech Disorders: Medical aspects.* Illinois: Thomas.

LUCHSINGER, R. (1965a). Vocal disorders from laryngeal paralysis. Paralytic dysphonia. In R. Luchsinger and E. Arnold (Eds) *Voice, Speech and Language*. London: Constable.

LUCHSINGER, R. (1965b). Vocal disorders of emotional origin: psychogenic dysphonia. In R. Luchsinger and E. Arnold (Eds.) *Voice, Speech and Language*. London: Constable.

LUCHSINGER, R. (1965c). Physiology and pathology of respiration and phonation. The qualities of the voice. In R. Luchsinger and E. Arnold (Eds) *Voice, Speech and Language*. London: Constable.

LUCHSINGER, R. and ARNOLD, E. (Eds) (1965). *Voice, Speech and Language*. London: Constable.

LUDLOW, C.L. and BASSICH, C.J. (1965). Relationship between perceptual ratings and acoustic measurements of hypokinetic speech. In M.R. McNeil, J.C. Rosenbeck and A.E. Aronson (Eds) *The Dysarthrias: Physiology, acoustics, perception, management*. San Diego: College-Hill Press.

LUDLOW, C.L. and CONNOR, N.P. (187). Spasmodic dysphonia. *J. Speech Hear. Res.* **30**, 197.

LUM, C. (1976). The syndrome of habitual chronic hyperventilation. In O. Hill (Ed.) *Modern Trends in Psychosomatic Medicine*, Vol. III. London: Butterworths.

LUM, C. (1981). Hyperventilation and anxiety state (Editorial). *J. R. Soc. Med.* **74**, 1.

LURIA, A.R. (1961). *The Role of Speech in the Regulation of Normal and Abnormal Behaviour*. Oxford: Pergamon.

LURIA, A.R. (1966). *Higher Cortical Functions* London: Tavistock.

McCROSKEY, R.L. and MULLIGAN, M. (1963). The relative intelligibility of oesophageal speech and artificial larynx. *J. Speech Dis.* **16**, 9.

MacCURTAIN, F. and FOURCIN, A.J. (1982). Applications of the electrolaryngograph wave form display. In L. Van Lawrence (Ed.) *Transcripts of the Tenth Symposium on Care of the Professional Voice*, Part 2, p. 51. New York: The Voice Foundation.

McDONALD, E.T. and BAKER, H.K. (1951). Cleft palate speech: an integration of research and clinical observation. *J. Speech Dis.* **16**, 9.

McGLONE, R. and HOLLIEN, H. (1963). Vocal pitch characteristics of aged women. *J. Speech Dis. Res.* **6**, 164.

MACKENZIE, C. (1987). Communication disorders in Legionnaire's Disease. *Br. J. Dis. Commun.* **22**, 253.

McNEIL, M.R., ROSENBEK, J.C. and ARONSON, A.E. (eds). (1984). *The Dysarthrias: Physiology, acoustics, perception, management.* San Diego: College-Hill Press.

McWILLIAMS, B.J. (1954). Some factors in intelligibility of cleft palate speech. *J. Speech Dis.* **19**, 524.

McWILLIAMS, B.J. (1960). Cleft palate management in England. *Speech Pathol. Ther.* **3**, 3.

McWILLIAMS, B.J., BLUESTONE, C.D. and MUSGROVE, R.H. (1969). Diagnostic implications of vocal cord nodules in children with cleft palate. *Laryngoscope* **79**, 2072.

McWILLIAMS, B.J., LAVORATO, A.S. and BLUESTONE, C.D. (1973). Vocal cord abnormalities in children with velopharyngeal valving problems. *Laryngoscope* **83** 1745.

McWILLIAMS, B.J., MORRIS, H.L. and SHELTON, R.L. (1984). *Cleft Palate Speech.* Philadelphia: B.C. Decker.

MAGARIAN, G.J. (1983). Hyperventilation syndrome: infrequently recognised common expressions of anxiety and stress. *Medicine* **61**, 219.

MALCOLMSON, K.G. (1968). Globus hystericus vel pharyngis. *J. Laryngol.* **82**, 219.

MANIGLIA, A.J. (1985). New Technique of tracheoesophageal fistula for vocal rehabilitation after total laryngectomy. *Laryngoscope* **95**, 1064.

MARAN, A.G., HAAST, N.H. and LEONARD, J.R. (1968). Reconstruction surgery for improved glottic closure. *Laryngoscope.* **78**, 1916.

MARLAND, P.M. (1952). *The Treatment of Dysphonia due to Recurrent Laryngeal Nerve Palsies.* College of Speech Therapists Oxford Conference Report.

MARLAND, P.M. (1953). Speech therapy for cerebral palsy based on reflex inhibition. *Speech* **17**, 65.

MARTIN, A.D. (1974). Some objections to the term apraxia of speech. *J. Speech Hear. Dis.* **39**, 53.

MASSENGIL, R. (1972). *Hypernasality*. Illinois: Thomas.

MEAD, J., HIXON, T. and GOLDMAN, N. (1974). Configuration of the chest wall during speech. In B. Wyke (Ed.) *Ventilatory and Phonatory Control Systems*. London: Oxford University Press.

MECHAM, M.J. (1987). Cerebral palsy. In H. Halpern (Ed.) *Studies in Communication Disorders*. Austin, Texas: Pro-Ed.

MENDELSOHN, M.S. and McCONNEL, F.M.S. (1987). Function in the pharyngoesophageal segment. *Laryngoscope* **97**, 483.

MERWIN, G.E., GOLDSTEIN, L.P. and ROTHMAN, H.B. (1985). A comparison of speech using artificial larynx and tracheoesophageal puncture with valve in the same speaker. *Laryngoscope* **95**, 730.

MICHEL, J., HOLLIEN, H. and MOORE, P. (1966). Speaking fundamental characteristics of 15-, 16- and 17-year-old girls. *Language and Speech* **9**, 46.

MICHELSSON, K. and SIRVIO, P. (1976). Cry analysis in congenital hypothyroidism. *Folia Phoniatr.* **28**, 40.

MICHELSSON, K. and WASZ-HOCKERT, O. (1980). The value of cry analysis in neonatology and early infancy. In T. Murry and J. Murry (Eds) *Infant Communication: Cry and early speech*. Houston, Texas: College-Hill Press.

MICHELSSON, K., RAES, J. and RINNIE, A. (1984). Cry score: an aid in infant diagnosis. *Folia. Phoniatr.* **36**, 219.

MIHASHI, S., OKADA, M., KURITA, S., NAGATA, K., ODA, M., HIRANO, M. and NAKASHIMA, T. (1981). Vascular network of the vocal fold. In K.N. Stevens and M. Hirano (Eds) *Vocal Fold Physiology*. Tokyo: University of Tokyo Press.

MILLER, A.H. (1967). First experience with the Asai Technique for vocal rehabilitation after total laryngectomy. *Ann. Otol.* **76**, 829.

MILLER, A.H. (1968). First experience with the Asai Technique for vocal rehabilitation after total laryngectomy. In J.C. Snidecor (Ed.) *Speech Rehabilitation of the*

Laryngectomised 2nd edn. Illinois: Thomas.

MILLER, C.J. (1972). The speech therapist and the group treatment of young cerebral palsied children. *Br. J. Dis Commun.* 7, 176.

MITCHELL, S.W. (1908). Treatment by rest, seclusion etc. in relation to psychotherapy. *J. Am. Med. Ass.* **50**, 2033.

MOHR, R.M., QUENELLE, D.J. and SHUMRICK, D.A. (1983). Vertico-frontolateral laryngectomy (hemilaryngectomy) – indications, technique and results. *Arch. Otolaryngol.* **109**, 384.

MOLOY, P.J. and CHARTER, R. (1982). The globus symptom. *Arch. Otolaryngol.* **108**, 740.

MONOSON, P. and ZEMLIN, W.R. (1984). Quantitative study of whisper. *Folia Phoniatr.* **36**, 53.

MONRAD-KROHN, G.H. (1947a). Dysprosody or altered 'melody of language'. *Brain* **70**, 405.

MONRAD-KROHN, G.H. (1947b). The prosodic quality of speech and its disorders. *Acta Psychiatr. Neurol.* **22**, 255.

MONTGOMERY, W.W. (1963). Cricoarytenoid arthritis. *Laryngoscope* **73**, 801.

MOOLENAAR-BIJL, A.J. (1956). Voice correction under pathological conditions. *Acta Physiol. Neer.* **5**, 85.

MOORE, D.M., BERKE, G.S., HANSON, D.G. and WARD, P.H. (1987). Videostroboscopy of the canine larynx: the effects of asymmetric laryngeal tension. *Laryngoscope* **97**, 543.

MOORE, W.E. (1939). Voice quality and anxiety. *J. Speech Dis.* **4**, 33.

MORLEY, M.E. (1957). Developmental articulatory apraxia. In *The Development and Disorders of Speech in Childhood* London: Livingstone.

MORLEY, M.E. (1970). *Cleft Palate and Speech*, 7th edn. Edinburgh: Churchill Livingstone.

MORLEY, M.E. (1980). Cleft palate – an historical perspective. In M. Edwards and A.C.H. Watson (Eds) *Advances in Management of Cleft Palate*. Edinburgh: Churchill Livingstone.

MORRIS, G.H. (1985). The remedial episode as a negotiation of rules. In R.D. Street, J.R. Cappella and J.N. Cappella (Eds) *Sequence and Pattern in Communicative Behaviour.* London: Edward Arnold.

MORRISON, M.D., NICHOL, H. and RAMMAGE, L.A. (1986). Diagnostic criteria in functional dysphonia. *Laryngoscope* **94**, 1.

MOSES, P.J. (1954). *The Voice of Neurosis*. New York: Grune & Stratton.

MOSES, P.J. (1958). Rehabilitation of the post-laryngectomised patient. *Ann. Otol.* **67**, 538.

MOSES, P.J. (1959). The vocal expression of emotional disturbances. *Kaiser Foundation Med. Bull.* 7, 107.

MOSES, P.J. (1960). The psychology of the castrato voice. *Folia Phoniatr.* **12**, 204.

MUELLER, P.B. (1971). Parkinson's Disease: motor speech behaviour in a selected group of patients. *Folia Phoniatr.* **73**, 333.

MUELLER, P.B. (1973). Paralytic dysphonia: a case presentation. *Folia Phoniatr.* **25**, 104.

MUELLER, P.B. (1978). *Communicative Disorders in a Geriatric Population*. Report. ASHA Convention, San Francisco.

MUELLER, P.B., SWEENEY, R.J. and BARIBEAU, L.J. (1985). Senescence of the voice: morphology of excised male larynges. *Folia Phoniatr.* **37**, 134.

MURAKAMI, Y., SAITO, S., IKARI, T., HARAGUCHI, S., OKADA, K. and MARUYAMA, T. (1982). Esophageal reconstruction with a skin-grafted pectoralis major muscle flap. *Arch. Otolaryngol.* **108**, 719.

MURPHY, G.E., BOSNA, A.L. and OGURA, J.H. (1964). Determinants of rehabilitation following laryngectomy. *Laryngoscope* **74**, 1535.

MURRY, T. (1980). Acoustic and perceptual characteristics of infant cries. In T. Murry and J. Murry (Eds) *Infant Communication: Cry and early speech*. Houston, Texas: College-Hill Press.

MURRY, T. and MURRY, J. (Eds) (1980). *Infant Communication: Cry and early speech*. Houston, Texas: College-Hill Press.

MURRY, T., HOIT DALGAAD, J. and GRACCO, V.L. (1983). Infant vocalisation: a longitudinal study of acoustic and temporal parameters. *Folia Phoniatr.* **35**, 245.

MUSGROVE, J. (1952). Nervous diseases of the larynx. In W.G. Scott-Brown (Ed.) *Diseases of the Ear, Nose and Throat*. London: Butterworths.

MYEARS, D.W., MARTIN, R.J., ECKERT, R.C. and SWEENEY, M.K. (1985). Functional versus organic vocal cord paralysis: rapid diagnosis and decannulation. *Laryngoscope* **95**, 1235.

MYERSON, M.C. (1952). Smoker's larynx. *Ann. Otol.* **59**, 541.

MYSAK, E.D. (1959a). Pitch and duration characteristics of older males. *J. Speech Res.* **2**, 46.

MYSAK, E.D. (1959b). Significance of neuro-physiological orientation to cerebral palsy habilitation. *J. Speech Dis.* **24**, 221.

MYSAK, E.D. (1968). Dysarthria and oropharyngeal reflexology. *J. Speech Hear Dis.* **28**, 252.

MYSAK, E.D. and HANLEY, T. (1959). Aging processes in speech: Pitch and duration characteristics. *J. Gerontol.* **13**, 309.

NAHUM, M.C. (1967). Vocal rehabilitation for contact ulcer of the larynx. *Arch. Otolaryngol.* **85**, 41.

NASSAR, W.Y. (1977). Polytef (Teflon) injection of the vocal cords: experience with 34 cases. *J. Laryngol.* **91**, 341.

NEGUS, V.E. (1931). Observations on Semon's Law derived from evidence of comparative anatomy and physiology. *J. Laryngol.* **46**, 1.

NEGUS, V.E. (1949). *The Comparative Anatomy and Physiology of the Larynx*. London: Heineman Medical.

NEGUS, V.E. (1957a). The function of the paranasal sinuses. *Arch. Otolaryngol.* **66**, 430.

NEGUS, V.E. (1957b). The mechanism of the laryx. *Laryngoscope* **67**, 1961.

NEW, G.B. and DEVINE, K.D. (1949). Contact ulcer granuloma. *Ann. Otol.* **58**, 548.

NEWMAN, J., NGUYEN, A. and ANDERSON, R. (1987). Lipo-suction of the head and neck. In G.M. English (Ed.) *Otolaryngology*, Vol. 4 (1988). Philadelphia: Harper & Row.

NEWSON-DAVIS, J. (1970). Diseases of the nervous system: apraxia. In E.J.M. Campbell, E. Agostini and J.N. Davis (Eds) *The Respiratory Muscles: Mechanics and neural control*, 2nd edn. London: Lloyd-Luke.

NISHIJIMA, W., TAKODA, S. and HASEGAWA, M. (1984). Occult gastrointestinal tract lesions associated with the globus symptom. *Arch. Otolaryngol.* **110**, 246.

NORGATE, S. (1984). *Laryngectomy is Not a Tragedy*. Edinburgh: Churchill Livingstone.

OATES, J.M. and DACAKIS, G. (1983). Speech pathology consideration in the management of transsexualism - a review. *Br. J. Dis. Commun.* **18**, 3.

OSGOOD, C.E. (1953). *Method and Theory in Experimental Psychology*. Oxford: Oxford Press.

OSTWALD, P.F. (1963). *Soundmaking: The acoustic communication of emotion*. Illinois: Thomas.

OSTWALD, P.F., FREEDMAN, D.G. and KURTZ, J.H. (1962). Vocalization of infant twins. *Folia Phoniatr.* **14**, 1.

OYER, H.J. and DEAL, L.V. (1985). Temporal aspects of speech and the aging process. *Folia Phoniatr.* **37**, 109.

PAGET, R. (1930). *Human Speech* London: Kegan Paul.

PANJÉ, W.R. (1981). Prosthetic vocal rehabilitation following laryngectomy: the voice button. *Ann. Otolaryngol.* **90**, 116.

PANTOJA, E. (1968). The laryngeal cartilages. *Arch. Otolaryngol.* **87**, 416.

PARKER, A. (1974). Voice and intonation training for deaf children using laryngographic display. *Proceedings of the 8th International Congress on Acoustics*. London: Chapman & Hall.

PARKES, C.M. (1975). The emotional impact of cancer on patients and their families. *J. Laryngol.* **89**, 1271.

PARNES, S.M. and SATYA-MURTI, S. (1985). Predictive value of laryngeal electromyography in patients with vocal cord paralysis of neurogenic origin. *Laryngoscope* **95**, 1323.

PARSONS, T. (1987). *Voice and Speech Processing*. New York: McGraw Hill.

PAPSIDERO, M.J. and PASHLEY, N.R.J. (1980). Acquired stenosis of the upper airway in neonates: an increasing problem. *Ann. Otol.* **89**, 512.

PEACHER, W.G. and HOLINGER, P. (1947). Contact ulcer of the larynx: the role of vocal re-education. *Arch. Otolaryngol.* **46**, 617.

PEACHER, W.G. (1949). Neurological factors in the etiology of delayed speech. *J. Speech Dis.* **14**, 147.

PEACHER, W.G. (1961). Vocal therapy for contact ulcer: a follow-up of 70 patients. *Laryngoscope* **71**, 137.

PERKINS, W.H. and KENT, R.D. (1986). *Textbook of Functional Anatomy of Speech, Language and Hearing*. San Diego: College-Hill Press.

PERRY, A. (1983). The speech therapist's role in surgical and prosthetic approaches to speech rehabilitation, with particular reference to the Blom–Singer and Panjé techniques. In Y. Edels (Ed.) *Laryngectomy: Diagnosis to rehabilitation*. London: Croom Helm.

PERRY, A. (1987). Technical assistance for patients with voice disorders. In P. Enderby (Ed.) *Assistive Communication Aids for the Speech Impaired*. Edinburgh: Churchill Livingstone.

PERRY, A. and EDELS, Y. (1985). Recent advances in the assessment of 'failed' oesophageal speakers. *Br. J. Dis. Commun.* **20**, 229.

PETERSON, H.A. (1973). A case report of speech and language training for a two-year-old laryngectomised child. *J. Speech Hear. Dis.* **38**, 275.

PIAGET, J. (1952). *Play, Dreams and Imitation in Childhood*, translators C. Gattegno and M.E. Hodgson. London: Heineman.

PIGOTT, R.W. (1974). The results of nasopharyngoscopic assessment of pharyngoplasty. *Scand. J. Plas. Reconstr. Surg.* **8**, 148.

PIGOTT, R.W. (1977). The development of endoscopy of the palatopharyngeal isthmus. *Proc. R. Soc.* **195**, 269.

PIGOTT, R.W. (1980). Assessment of velopharyngeal function. In M. Edwards and A.C.H. Watson (Eds) *Advances in Management of Cleft Palate*. Edinburgh: Churchill Livingstone.

PIGOTT, R.W. and MAKEPEACE, A.P.W. (1975). The technique of recording nasal pharyngoscopy. *Br. J. Plas. Surg.* **28**, 26.

PIGOTT, R.W., BENSEN, J.F. and WHITE, F.D. (1969). Nasendoscopy in the diagnosis of velopharyngeal incompetence. *Plas. Reconstr. Surg.* **43**, 141.

POLLACK, D. (1952). Post arytenoidectomy voice therapy. *Speech* **16**, 4.

POWERS, G.R. (1986). Cleft palate: physical management. In H. Halpern (Ed.) *Studies in Communicative Disorders Series*. Austin, Texas: Pro-Ed.

PRATER, R.J. and SWIFT, R.W. (1984). *Manual of Voice Therapy*. Boston: Little, Brown.

PRESSMAN, J.J. and BAILEY, B.J. (1968). The surgery of cancer of the larynx with special reference to subtotal laryngectomy. In J.C. Snidecor (Ed.) *Speech Rehabilitation of the Laryngectomized*. Illinois: Thomas.

PROCTOR, D.F. (1974). Glottic aerodynamics and phonation. In B. Wyke (Ed.) *Ventilatory and Phonatory Control Systems* London: Oxford University Press.

PROCTOR, D.F. (1980). *Breathing, Speech and Song*. Vienna: Springer-Verlag.

PRONOVOST, W.L. (1967). Voice therapy for the hearing impaired. In M. Cooper and M. Cooper (Eds) *Approaches to Vocal Rehabilitation* Springfield, IL: Thomas.

PROSEK, R.A., MONTGOMERY, A.A., WALDEN, B.E. and SCHWARTZ, D.M. (1978). E.M.G. biofeedback in the treatment of hyperfunctional voice disorders. *J. Speech Dis.* **43**, 282.

PTACEK, P., SANDER, E.K., MALONE, W.H. and JACKSON, C.C.R. (1966). Phonatory and related changes with advanced age. *J. Speech Hear. Dis.* **9**, 353.

PUNT, N. (1968). Applied laryngology: singers and actors. *Proc. R. Soc. Med.* **61**, 1152.

PUNT. N.A (1983). Laryngology applied to singers and actors. *J. Laryngol. Otol.* Suppl. 6.

RABBETT, W.F. (1965). Juvenile laryngeal papillomatosis. The relation of irradiation and malignant degeneration. *Ann. Otol.* **74**, 1149.

RAMIG, L.A. and RINGEL, R.L. (1983). Effects of physiological aging on selected acoustic characteristics of voice. *J. Speech Hear. Res.* **26**, 22.

RAMIG, L.A., SCHERER R.C., TITZE, R. and RINGEL, S.P. (1988). Acoustic analysis of voices of patients with neurologic disease: rationale and preliminary data. *Ann. Otol. Rhinol. Laryngol.* **97**, 164.

RANDALL, P. (1980). Secondary surgery. In M. Edwards and A.C.H. Watson (Eds) *Advances in Management of Cleft Palate*. Edinburgh: Churchill Livingstone.

RANGER, D. (1964). Problems of repair after pharyngolaryngectomy. *Proc. R. Soc. Med.* **57**, 1099.

RANGER, D. (1983). Extensive surgery for post-cricoid carcinoma. In Y. Edels (Ed.) *Laryngectomy: Diagnosis to rehabilitation.* London: Croom Helm.

REICH, A.R. and McHENRY, M.A. (1987). Respiratory volumes in cheerleaders with a history of dysphonic episodes. *Folia Phoniatr.* **39** 71.

RENFREW, C.E., MITCHELL, J.C.E. and WALLACE, A.R. (1957). Listening. *Speech* **21**, 34.

RETHI, A. (1963). L'innervation du larynx. *Acta O.R.L.* Ibero-Amer. **2**, 43.

RHEINGOLD, H.L., GEWIRTZ, J.L. and ROSS, H.W. (1959). Social conditioning of vocalization in the infant. *J. Compar. Physiol. Psychol.* **52**, 68.

RINGEL, R.L. and CHODZHO-ZAJKO, W. (1987). Vocal indices of biological age. *J. Voice* **1**, 31.

RINGEL, R. and CHODZHO-ZAJKO, W. (1988). Some implications of current gerontological theory for the study of voice. *Communication Sciences and Disorders and Aging.* Washington DC: American Speech–Language–Hearing Association.

RINGEL, R. and KLUPPEL, D. (1964). Neonatal crying: A normative study. *Folia Phoniatr.* **16** 1.

RITTER, F.N. (1967). The effects of hyperthyroidism upon the ear, nose and throat. *Laryngoscope* **77**, 1427.

RIPPON, T.S. and FLETCHER, P. (1940). *Reassurance and Relaxation*. London: Routledge.

ROBB, M.P. and SAXMAN, J.H. (1985). Developmental trends in vocal fundamental frequency of young children. *J. Speech Hear. Dis.* **28**, 421.

ROBBINS, J., FISHER, H.B., BLOM, E.D. and SINGER, M.I. (1984). Selected acoustic features of tracheoesophageal, esophageal and laryngeal speech. *Arch. Otolaryngol.* **110**, 670.

ROBBINS, K.T. and HOWARD, D. (1983). Multiple laryngeal papillomatosis requiring laryngectomy. *Arch. Otolaryngol.* **109**, 765.

ROBE, E., MOORE, P. and BRUMLIK, J. (1960). A study of spastic dysphonia. *Laryngoscope* **70**, 219.

ROBE, E.Y., MOORE, P., ANDREWS, A.H. and HOLINGER, P.H. (1956). A study of the role of certain factors in the development of speech after laryngectomy. 1. Type of operation. 2. Site of pseudoglottis. 3. Co-ordination of speech with respiration. *Laryngoscope* **66**: 173, 382, 481.

ROBERTSON, M.S. and ROBINSON, J.M. (1984). Immediate pharyngoesophageal reconstruction. *Arch. Otolaryngol.* **110**, 386.

ROBERTSON, S.J. (1986). *Dysarthria Profile*. Winslow, Bucks: Winslow Press.

ROBERTSON, S.J. and THOMSON, F. (1984). Speech therapy in Parkinson's Disease: a study of the efficacy and long term effects of intensive treatment. *Br. J. Dis. Commun.* **19**, 213.

ROBERTSON, S.J. and THOMSON, F. (1986). *Working with Dysarthrics – A Practical Guide to Therapy for Dysarthria*. Winslow, Bucks: Winslow Press.

ROSENBEK, J.C. and LaPOINTE, L. (1985). The dysarthrias. In D.F. Johns (Ed.) *Clinical Management of Neurogenic Communicative Disorders* Boston: Little, Brown and Co.

RYAN, E.B., GILES, H. and SEBASTIAN, R.J. (1982). An integrative perspective for the study of attitudes toward language variation. In E.B. Ryan and H. Giles (Eds) *The Psychology of Language*, Vol. 1, *Attitudes towards Language Variation*. London: Edward Arnold.

RYAN, W.J. (1972). Acoustic aspects of aging voice. *J. Gerontol.* **27**, 265.

SALMON, S.J. (1978). Patients talk back. In S.J. Salmon and L.P. Goldstein (Eds) *The Artificial Larynx Handbook*. New York: Grune & Stratton.

SAMUEL, S. and ADAMS, F.G. (1976). The role of oesophageal and diaphragmatic movements in alaryngeal speech. *J. Laryngol* **90**, 1105.

SAPIR, S. and ARONSON, A.E. (1985a). Aphonia after closed head injury: aetiologic considerations. *Br. J. Dis. Commun.* **20**, 289.

SAPIR, S. and ARONSON, A.E. (1985b). Clinician reliability in rating voice improvement after laryngeal nerve section for spastic dysphonia. *Laryngoscope* **95**, 200.

SAPIR, S. and ARONSON, A.E. (1987). Coexisting psychogenic and neurogenic dysphonia: a source of diagnostic confusion. *Br. J. Dis. Commun.* **22**, 73.

SATALOFF, R.T., REINHARDT, J.H. and O'CONNOR, M.J. (1984). Rehabilitation of a quadriplegic professional singer: Use of a device to provide abdominal muscle support. *Arch. Otolaryngol.* **110**, 682.

SCHAEFFER, S.D, (1983). Neuropathology of spasmodic dysphonia. *Laryngoscope* **93**, 1183.

SCHAEFFER, S.D. and JOHNS, D.F. (1982). Attaining functional oesophageal speech. *Arch. Otolaryngol.* **108**, 647.

SCHAEFFER, S.D., FINITZO-HIEBER, T., GERLING, I.J. and FREEMAN, F.J. (1983a). Brainstem conduction abnormalities in spasmodic dysphonia. In D.M. Bless and J.H. Abbs (Eds) *Vocal Fold Physiology*. San Diego: College-Hill Press.

SHAEFFER, S.D., FINITZO-HIEBER, T., GERLING, I.J. and FREEMAN, F.J. (1983b). Brainstem conduction abnormalities in spasmodic dysphonia. *Ann. Otol. Rhinol. Laryngol.* **92**, 59.

SCHERER, K.R. (1978). Personality inference from voice quality: the loud voice of extroversion. *Eur. J. Soc. Psychol.* **8**, 467.

SCHERER, K.R. and GILES, H. (1979). *Social Markers in Speech*. Cambridge: Cambridge University Press.

SCHOW, R.L. and NERBONNE, M.A. (1981). Hearing levels among elderly nursing home residents. *J. Speech Hear. Dis.* **45**, 124.

SCOTT, S. and CAIRD, F.I. (1981). Speech therapy for patients with Parkinson's Disease. *Br. Med. J.* **283**, 1080.

SCOTT, S. and CAIRD, F.I. (1983). Speech therapy in Parkinson's Disease. *J. Neurol. Psychol.* **46**, 140.

SCOTT, S., CAIRD, F.I. and WILLIAMS, B.O. (1984). Evidence for an apparent sensory speech disorder in Parkinson's Disease. *J. Neurol. Neurosurg. Psych.* **47**, 840.

SCOTT, S., CAIRD, F.I. and WILLIAMS, B.O. (1985). *Communication in Parkinson's Disease*. London: Croom Helm.

SCOTTON, C.M. (1985). What the heck, sir: style shifting and lexical colouring as features of powerful language. In R.L. Street Jr and J.N. Cappella (Eds) *Sequence and Pattern in Communicative Behaviour*. London: Edward Arnold.

SEDLACKOVA, E. (1960). Les dysphonies hypercinetiques des enfants causees par surmenage vocal. *Folia Phoniatr.* **12**, 48.

SEEMAN, M. (1922). Speech and voice without larynx. An experimental and clinical study of the development of speech without larynx. *Cas. Lek. Ces.* **41**, 369.

SEEMAN, M. (1959). *Sprachstorungen bei Kindern*. Marhold Saale.

SELLEY, N.G. (1979). Dental and technical aids for treatment of patients suffering from velopharyngeal disorders. In R.E. Ellis and F.C. Flack (Eds) *Diagnosis and Treatment of Palatoglossal Malfunction*. London: College of Speech Therapists.

SELLEY, N.G. (1985). Swallowing difficulties in stroke patients: a new treatment. *Age Ageing* **14**, 361.

SENTURIA, B.H. and WILSON, F.B. (1968). Otorhinolaryngologic findings in children with voice deviations. *Ann. Otol. Rhinol. Laryngol.* **72**, 1027.

SETH, G. and GUTHRIE, D. (1953). *Speech in Childhood*. London: Oxford University Press.

SESSIONS, D.G., MANESS, G.M. and McSWAIN, B. (1965). Laryngofissure in the treatment of carcinoma of the vocal cord: a report of 40 cases and review of the literature. *Laryngoscope* **75**, 490.

SHANKS, S.J. (1979). A programmed approach to voice therapy. In F.B. Wilson and M. Rice (Eds) *Evaluation of Appraisal Techniques in Speech and Language Pathology*. Reading, Mass: Addison Wesley.

SHAW, H.J. (1966). Partial laryngectomy. *J. Laryngol.* **80**, 839.

SHAW, H.J. and FRIEDMAN, I. (1964). Diffuse keratosis of the larynx with multicentric malignant change and metastatic neuropathy. *J. Laryngol.* **80**, 403.

SHEPPARD, W.C. and LANE, H.I. (1968). Development of prosodic features of infant vocalizing. *J. Speech Hear. Res.* **11**, 94.

SHEPPERD, H.W.H. (1966). Androgenic hoarseness. *J. Laryngol.* **80**, 403.

SHERRINGTON, C. (1947). *The Integrative Action of the Nervous System*. Cambridge: Cambridge University Press.

SHIPP, T. (1975). Vertical laryngeal position during continuous and discrete vocal frequency change. *J. Speech Hear. Res.* **18**, 707.

SHIPP, T. and HOLLIEN, H. (1969). Perception of the aging male voice. *J. Speech Hear. Res.* **12**, 703.

SHIPP, T. and IZDEBSKI, K. (1975). Vocal frequency and vertical larynx positioning by singers and non-singers. *J. Acoust. Soc. Am.* **58**, 1104.

SHIPP, T. and McGLONE, R.E. (1971). Laryngeal dynamics associated with voice frequency change. *J. Speech Hear. Res.* **14**, 761.

SHRIMTZEN, R.J. (1979). Velopharyngeal insufficiency in the absence of overt or submucous cleft. In R.E. Ellis and F.C. Flack (Eds) *Diagnosis and Treatment of Palatoglossal Malfunction*. London: College of Speech Therapists.

SIEGAL, G.M. (1969). Vocal conditioning in infants. *J. Speech Dis.* **34**, 3.

SIEGMAN, A.W. (1987). The tell-tale voice: non-verbal messages of verbal communication. In A.W. Siegman and S. Feldstein (Eds) *Non-verbal Behaviour and Communication*. New York: Lawrence Erlbaum.

SILVER, F.M., GLUCKMAN, J.L. and DONEGAN, J.O. (1985). Operative complications of tracheoesophageal puncture. *Laryngoscope* **95**, 1360.

SILVERMAN, E. and ZIMMER, C.H. (1975). Incidence of chronic hoarseness among school age children. *J. Speech Dis.* **40**, 211.

SIM, M. (1981). Psychopathia sexualis. In *Guide to Psychiatry*. Edinburgh: Churchill Livingstone.

SIMPSON, J.C. (1971). Dysphonia: the organisation and working of a dysphonia clinic. *Br. J. Dis. Commun.* **6**, 70.

SIMPSON, J.C., SMITH, J.C.S. and GORDON, M.T. (1972). Laryngectomy: the influence of muscle reconstruction on the mechanism of oesophageal voice production. *J. Otolaryngol.* **86**, 961.

SINGER, M.I. and BLOM, E.D. (1980). An endoscopic technique for restoration of voice after laryngectomy. *Ann. Otol.* **89**, 529.

SINGER, M.I., BLOM, E.D. and HAMAKER, R.C. (1983). Voice rehabilitation after total laryngectomy. *J. Otolaryngol* **12**, 329.

SINGER, M.I., BLOM, E.D. and HAMAKER, R.C. (1986). Pharyngeal plexus neurectomy for alaryngeal speech rehabilitation. *Laryngoscope* **96**, 50.

SINGER, M.I., HAMAKER, R.C. and MILLER, S.M. (1985). Restoration of the airway following bilateral recurrent laryngeal nerve paralysis. *Laryngoscope* **95**, 1204.

SKINNER, B.F. (1953). *Science and Human Behaviour*. New York: Macmillian.

SKINNER, B.F. and VAUGHAN, B.F. (1983). *Enjoy Old Age: A programme of self management*. New York: W.W. Norton.

SKOLNICK, M.L. (1970). Videofluoroscopic examination of the velopharyngeal portal during phonation in lateral and basal projections. *Cleft Palate J.* **7**, 803.

SKOLNICK, M.L. and McCALL, G.N. (1973). A radiographic technique for demonstrating the causes of persistent nasality in patients with pharyngeal flaps. *Br. J. Plas. Surg.* **26**, 12.

SKYNNER, A.C.R. (1976). *One Flesh, Separate Persons: Principles of family and marital psychotherapy*. London: Constable.

SKYNNER, R. and CLEESE, J. (1983). *Families and How to Survive Them*. London: Methuen.

SLONIM, N.B. and HAMILTON, L.H. (1976). *Respiratory Physiology*. St Louis: C.V. Mosby.

SMITH, P.M. (1979). Sex markers in speech. In K.R. Scherer and H. Giles (Eds) *Social Markers in Speech*. Cambridge: Cambridge University Press.

SMITH, S. and THYME, K. (1976). Statistic research on changes in speech due to pedagogic treatment (the Accent Method). *Folia Phoniatr.* **28**, 98.

SMURTHWAITE, H. (1919). War neurosis of the larynx and speech mechanism. *J. Laryngol.* **34**, 13.

SNIDECOR, J.C. (1968). *Speech Rehabilitation of the Laryngectomised*, 2nd edn. Illinois: Thomas.

SNIDECOR, J.C. and CURRY, E.T. (1959). Temporal pitch aspects of superior esophageal speech. *Ann. Otol.* **68**, 623.

SNIDECOR, J.C. and CURRY, E.T. (1960). How effectively may the laryngectomee speak? In L. Stein (Ed.) *Proceedings of the 11th International Speech and Voice Conference*. New York: Karger.

SNIDECOR, J.C. and ISSHIKI, N. (1965). Air volume and air flow relationships of 6 male oesophageal speakers. *J. Speech Dis.* **30**, 205.

SOKOLOWSKY, R.R. and JUNKERMANN, E.B. (1944). War aphonia. *J. Speech Dis.* **9**, 193.

SONNINEN, A. (1960). Laryngeal signs and symptoms of goitre. *Folia Phoniatr.* **12**, 41.

SORENSEN, H. (1982). Laser surgery in benign laryngeal disease. *Acta Otolaryngol.* **94**, 537.

SPARKS, R.W. (1981). Melodic intonation therapy. In R. Chapey (Ed.) *Language Intervention Strategies in Adult Aphasia*. Baltimore: Williams & Wilkins.

SPARKS, R.W. and HOLLAND, A. (1976). Method: melodic intonation therapy. *J. Speech Hear. Dis.* **41**, 287.

SPENCER, P.S., NUNN, P.B., HUGON, J., LUDOLPH, A.C., ROSS, S.M., ROY, D.N. and ROBERTSON, R.C. (1987). Guam amyotrophic lateral sclerosis Parkinsonian-dementia linked to a plant excitant neurotoxin. *Science* **237**, 517.

SPIEGEL, J.R., SATALOFF, R.T. and GOULD, W.J. (1987). Treatment of vocal fold paralysis with injectable collagen: clinical concerns. *J. Voice* **1**, 119.

STARK, R.E. (1978). Features of infant sounds: the emergence of cooing. *J. Child. Lang.* **5**, 379.

STARK, R.E. (1979). Pre-speech segmental feature development. In P. Fletcher and M. Garman (Eds) *Language Acquisition*. Cambridge: Cambridge University Press.

STARK, R.E. and NATHANSON, S. (1975). Unusual features of cry in an infant dying suddenly and unexpectedly. In J. Bosma and J. Showacre (Eds) *Development of Upper Respiratory Anatomy and Function: Implications for SID.* Washington: US Dept. Health and Education.

STARK, R.E., ROSE, S.N. and McLAGAN, M. (1975). Features of infant sounds: the first eight weeks of life. *J. Child. Lang.* **2**, 205.

STEER, M.D. and HANLEY, T.D. (1959). Instruments of diagnosis, therapy and research. In L.E. Travis (Ed.) *Handbook of Speech Pathology*. London: Peter Owen.

STEINSCHNEIDER, A. (1972). Prolonged apnea and the sudden infant death syndrome: clinical and laboratory observations. *Pediatrics* **50**, 646.

STEINSCHNEIDER, A. and RABUZZI, D. (1976). Apnea and airway obstruction during feeding and sleep. *Laryngoscope* **86**, 1359.

STEMPLE, J.C. (1984). *Clinical Voice Pathology: Theory and management*. Columbus, OH: Merrill.

STETSON, R.H. (1937). Esophageal speech for any laryngectomised patient. *Arch. Otolaryngol.* **26**, 132.

STOICHEFF, M.L. (1981). Speaking fundamental frequency characteristics of non-smoking female adults. *J. Speech Hear. Res.* **24**, 437.

STONES, J. and DRAKE, T.M. (1984). *An intensive course of therapy for patients with Parkinson's Disease*. Bulletin 387, College of Speech Therapists.

STREET, R.L. and HOPPER, R., (1982). A model of speech style evaluation. In E.B. Ryan and H. Giles (Eds) *Attitudes towards Language Variation*. London: Edward Arnold.

STUART, D.W. (1966). Surgery in cancer of the cervical oesophagus: plastic tube replacement. *J. Laryngol.* **80**, 382.

SUMMERS, I.R. and MARTIN, M.C. (1980). A tactile sound level monitor for the profoundly deaf. *Br. J. Audiol.* **14**, 30.

SUNDBERG, J. (1974). Articulatory interpretation of the singing formant. *J. Acoust. Soc. Am.* **55**, 838.

SUNDBERG, J. (1977). The acoustics of the singing voice. *Sci. Am.* **236**, 82.

SWIFT, A.C. and ROGERS, J. (1987). Vocal cord paralysis in children. *J. Laryngol.* **101**, 169.

TAKANO-STONE, J. (1987). Intervention for psychosocial problems associated with sensory disabilities in old age. In B. Heller, L. Flohr and L.S. Zeagans (Eds) *Psychosocial Interventions with Sensorially Disabled Persons.* New York: Grune & Stratton.

TANABE, M., HAJI, T., HONJO, I. and ISSHIKI, N. (1985). Surgical treatment for androphonia: an experimental study. *Folia Phoniatr.* **37**, 15.

TANABE, M., HONJO, I. and ISSHIKI, N. (1985). Neoglottic reconstruction following total laryngectomy. *Arch. Otolaryngol.* **3**, 39.

TARDY-MITZELL, S., ANDREWS, M.L. and BOWMAN, S.A. (1985). Acceptability and intelligibility of tracheoesophageal speech. *Arch. Otalaryngol.* **3**, 213.

TARNEAUD, J. (1961). *Traité Pratique de Phonologie et de Phoniatrie*. Libraire Maloine, Paris.

TASHJIAN, L.S and PEACOCK, J.E. (1984). Laryngeal candidiasis. *Arch. Otolaryngol.* **110.**, 806.

TAUB, S. (1966). The Taub oral panendoscope. A new technique. *Cleft Palate J.* **3**, 328.

TAUB, S. (1975). Air bypass prosthesis for vocal rehabilitation of laryngectomees. *Ann. Otolaryngol.* **84**, 45.

TERRACOL, J., GUERRIER, Y. and CAMPS, F. (1956). Le sphincter glottique; etude anatomoclinique. *Ann. Otolaryngol. (Paris)* **73**, 451.

THOMSON, St S.C., NEGUS, V.E. and BATEMAN, G.H. (1955). *Diseases of the Nose and Throat* 6th edn. London: Cassell.

THOMSON, W.J.R. (1976). Lungs. *Black's Medical Dictionary*, 31st edn. London: A and C Black.

THYME, K. (1980). Trials of the Accent Method. *Proceedings XVIII IALP Congress*, Washington. Vol. 1, p. 633.

TITZE, I. (1981). The role of computational simulation in evaluation of physical properties of the vocal folds. In K.N. Stevens and M. Hirano (Eds) *Vocal Fold Physiology*. Tokyo: University of Tokyo Press.

TITZE, I.R. (1984). Parameterization of the glottal area, glottal flow and vocal fold area. *J. Acout. Soc. Am.* **75**, 570.

TOSI, O. (1979). *Voice Identification: Theory and legal applications*. Baltimore: University Park Press.

TRAVIS, L.W., HYBELS, R.L. and NEWMAN, M.H. (1976). Tuberculosis of the larynx. *Laryngoscope* **86**, 549.

TRUDEAU, M.D., HIRSCH, S.M. and SCHULLER, D.E. (1986). Vocal restorative surgery: why wait? *Laryngoscope* **96**, 975.

TUCKER, H.M. (1976). Human laryngeal re-innervation. *Laryngoscope* **85**, 769.

TUCKER, H.M. (1978). Human laryngeal reinnervation: longterm experience with the nerve-muscle pedicle technique. *Laryngoscope* **85**, 598.

TUCKER, H.M. (1980). Laryngeal paralysis: etiology and management. In G.M. English (Ed.) *Otolaryngology*, Vol. 3 (1988). Philadelphia: Harper & Row.

TUDOR, C. and SELLEY, W.G. (1974). A platal training appliance and a visual aid for use in treatment of hypernasal speech. *Br. J. Dis. Commun.* **9**, 117.

TURNER, L. (1952). Chronic infective conditions of the larynx and tuberculosis of the larynx. In D. Guthrie (Ed.) *Logan Turner's Diseases of the Nose, Throat and Ear*, 5th edn. Bristol: John Wright.

VALANNE, E., VUORENKOSKIV, V., PARTANEN, T.J., LIND, J. and WASZ-HÖCKERT, O. (1967). The ability of human mothers to identify the hunger cry signal of their own new born infants during the lying-in period. *Experimentia* **23**, 768.

VAN DEN BERG, J.W. (1962). Modern research in experimental phonetics. *Folia Phoniatr.* **14**, 81.

VAN GELDER, L. (1974). Psychosomatic aspects of endocrine disorders of the voice. *J. Commun. Dis.* 7, 257.

VAN RIPER, C. (1947). *Speech Correction*. New York: Prentice Hall.

VAN RIPER, C. and IRWIN, J.V. (1958). *Voice and Articulation Drill Book*. New York: Prentice Hall.

VAN THAL, J.H. (1934). *Cleft Palate Speech*. London: Allen & Unwin.

VAN THAL, J.H. (1961). Dysphonia. *Speech Pathol. Ther.* 4, 11.

VAN THAL, J.H. (1962). Four generations of aphonia. *Proceedings of the XIIth IALP Congress*, Padua.

VAUGHAN, C.W. and STRONG, M.S. (1981). The morphology of the phonatory organs and their neural control. In K.N. Stevens and M. Hirano (Eds) *Vocal Fold Physiology*. Tokyo: University of Tokyo Press.

VAN THAL, J.H. (1934) *Cleft Palate Speech*. London: Allen & Unwin.

VAN THAL, J.H. (1961). *Dysphonia. Speech Pathol. Ther.* 4, 11.

VAN THAL, J.H. (1962). Four generations of aphonia. *Proceedings of the XIIth IALP Congress*, Padua.

VAUGHAN, C.W. and STRONG, M.S. (1981). The morphology of the phonatory organs and their neural control. In K.N. Stevens and M. Hirano (Eds) *Vocal Fold Physiology*. Tokyo: University of Tokyo Press.

VENNARD, W. and VON LEDEN, H. (1967). The importance of intensity modulation in the perception of a trill. *Folia Phoniatr.* **19**, 19.

VERDOLINI, K., SKINNER, M.W., PATTON T. and WALKER, P.A. (1985). Effect of amplification on the intelligibility of speech produced with an electrolarynx. *Laryngoscope* **95**, 720.

VERMEULING, V.R. (1966). Laryngeal carcinoma in the young. *Laryngoscope,* **77**, 1724.

VON LEDEN, H. (1961). The mechanism of phonation. *Arch. Otolaryngol.* **74**, 660.

VON LEDEN, H. and MOORE, P. (1960). *Contact Ulcer of the Larynx*. Motion Picture Voice Research Lab., Northwestern Medical School, Chicago.

VON LEDEN, H. and MOORE, P. (1961). The mechanics of the cricoarytenoid joint. *Arch. Otolaryngol.* **73**, 541.

VOSS, D.E., IONTA, M.K. and MYERS, B.J. (1985). *Proprioceptive Neuromuscular Facilitation Patterns and techniques*. New York: Harper & Row.

VRABEC, D.P. and DAVISON, F.W. (1980). Inflammatory diseases of the larynx. In G.M. English (Ed.) *Otolaryngology*, Vol. 3 (1988). Philadelphia: Harper & Row.

VRTICKA, K. and SVOBODA, M. (1961). A clinical X-ray study of 100 laryngectomised speakers. *Folia Phoniatr.* **13**, 174.

VRTICKA, K. and SVOBODA, M. (1963). Time changes in the X-ray picture of the hypopharynx, pseudoglottis and esophagus in the course of vocal rehabilitation in 70 laryngectomised speakers. *Folia Phoniatr.* **15**, 1.

WALSHE, F.M.R. (1952). Anatomical or localising factors in diagnosis. In *Diseases of the Nervous System*, 7th edn. Edinburgh: Livingstone.

WANG, N-M., YEUNG, K.W. and CHEN, T-A. (1986). Voice disorders in children with velopharyngeal valving problems. *Proceedings of the XXth IALP Congress*, Tokyo.

WARD, P.H., HANSON, D.G. and ABEMAYER, E. (1985). Transcutaneous Teflon injection of the paralysed vocal cord: a new technique. *Laryngoscope* **95**, 644.

WASZ-HÖCKERT, O., LIND, J., VUORENSKI, V., PARTENEN, T.J. and VALANNE, E. (1968). *The Infant Cry: A spectrographic and auditory analysis. Clinics in Developmental Medicine* No. 29. Spastics International Medical Publication in association with Heineman Medical.

WATKIN, K. and EWANOWSKI, S. (1985). Effects of aerosol corticosteroids on the voice: triamcinolone acetonide and beclomethasone dipropionate. *J. Speech Hear. Res.* **28**, 301.

WATSON, A.C.H. (1980). Primary surgery. In M. Edwards and A.C.H. Watson (Eds) *Advances in the Management of Cleft Palate*. Edinburgh: Churchill Livingstone.

WEDIN, S. (1972). Rehabilitation of speech in cases of palato-pharyngeal paresis with the aid of an obturator prosthesis. *Br. J. Dis. Commun.* 7, 117.

WEINBERG, B. (1980). *Readings in Speech Following Total Laryngectomy*. Baltimore: University Park Press.

WEINBERG, B., SHEDD, D.P. and HORII, Y. (1978). Reed-fistula speech following pharyngolaryngectomy. *J. Speech Hear. Dis.* **43**, 401.

WEISBERG, P. (1963). Social and non social conditioning of infant vocalizations. *Child Devel.* **34**, 377.

WEISMER, G. (1984). Articulatory characteristics of Parkinsonian dysarthria: segmental and phrase-level timing, spirantization and glottal-supraglottal coordination. In M.R. McNeill, J. Rosenbek and A.E. Aronson (Eds) *The Dysarthrias: Physiology, acoustics, perception, management*. San Diego: College Press.

WEISS, D.A. (1950). The pubertal change of the human voice (mutation). *Folia Phoniatr.* **2**, 126.

WEISS, D.A (1955). The psychological relations to one's own voice. *Folia Phoniatr.* **7**, 209.

WEISS, D.A. (1964). *Cluttering*. New York: Prentice Hall.

WEISS, D.A. and BEEBE, H. (1951). *The Chewing Approach to Speech and Voice Therapy*. New York: S. Karger.

WENDLER, J. and ANDERS, L.C. (1986). Hoarse voices: on the reliability of acoustic and auditory classifications. *Proceedings of the XXth IALP Congress*, Tokyo.

WEPMAN, J.M., McGAHAN, J.A., RICKARD, J.C. and SHELTON, N.W. (1953). The objective measurement of progressive eosophaeal speech development. *J. Speech Hear. Dis.* **18**, 247.

WEST, J.B. (1979). *Respiratory Physiology*, 2nd edn. Baltimore: Williams & Wilkins.

WEST, R., ANSBERRY, M. and CARR, A. (1957). *The Rehabilitation of Speech*, 3rd edn. New York: Harper.

WETMORE, S.J., KRUEGER, K., WESSON, K. and BLESSING, M.L. (1985). Long term results of the Blom–Singer speech rehabilitation procedure. *Arch. Otolaryngol.* **3**, 106.

WHITED, R.E. (1985). A study of post-intubation laryngeal dysfunction. *Laryngoscope* **95**, 727.

WIEMANN, J.M. (1985). Interpersonal control and regulation in conversation. In R.L. Street and J.N. Cappella (Eds.) *Sequence and Pattern Communicative Behaviour*. London: Edward Arnold.

WILDER, C. (1983). Chest wall preparation for phonation in female speakers. In D.M. Bless and J.H. Abbs (Eds) *Vocal Fold Physiology*. San Diego: College-Hill Press.

WILLIAMS, G.T., FARQUHARSON, I.M. and ANTHONY, J. (1975). Fibreoptic laryngoscopy in the assessment of laryngeal disorder. *J. Laryngol.* **89**, 299.

WILLIAMS, S.E. and WATSON, J.B. (1985). Differences in speaking proficiencies in three laryngectomee groups. *Arch. Otolaryngol.* **3**, 216.

WILLIAMS, S.E. and WATSON, J.B. (1987). Speaking proficiency variations according to method of alaryngeal voicing. *Laryngoscope* **97**, 737.

WILLIAMSON, J. (1984). Drug induced Parkinson's Disease. *Br. Med. J.* **288**, 1457.

WILLIS, C.R. and STUTZE, M.L. (1972). The clinical use of the Taube oral panendoscope in the observation of velopharyngeal function. *J. Speech Dis.* **37**, 495.

WILSON, C.P. (1952). Trauma, stenosis and benign tumours of the larynx. In W.G. Scott-Brown (Ed.) *Diseases of the Ear, Nose and Throat*, Vol. 1. London Butterworths.

WILSON, D.K. (1987). *Voice Problems of Children*, 3rd edn. Baltimore: Williams & Wilkins.

WILSON, F., OLDING, D.J. and MUELLER, K. (1980). Recurrent laryngeal nerve dissection. A case report involving return of spastic dysphonia after initial surgery. *J. Speech Hear. Dis.* **45**, 112.

WINITZ, H. (1969). *Articulatory Acquisition and Behaviour*. New York: Prentice Hall.

WIRZ, S. (1986). The voice of the deaf. In M. Fawcus (Ed.) *Voice Disorders and Their Management*. London: Croom Helm.

WIRZ, S., SUBTELNY, J. and WHITEHEAD, R. (1979). A perceptual and spectrographic study of the tense voice in normal and deaf speakers. *Folia Phoniatr.* **33**, 23.

WITTKOWER, E.D. and MANDELBROTE, B.M. (1955). Thyrotoxicosis. In D. O'Neill (Ed.) *Psychosomatic Medicine*. London: Butterworths.

WOLFE, S.G. (1952). Causes and mechanisms in rhinitis. *Laryngoscope* **62**, 601.

WOLFE, V. and BACON, M. (1976). Spectrographic comparison of 2 types of spastic dysphonia. *J. Speech Hear. Dis.* **41**, 326.

WOLFE, V.I., GARVIN, J.S., BACON, M. and WALDROP, W. (1975). Speech changes in Parkinson's Disease during treatment with L-Dopa. *J. Commun. Dis.* **8**, 271.

WOLMAN, L., DORKE, C.S. and YOUNG, A. (1965). The larynx in rheumatoid arthritis. *J. Laryngol.* **79**, 403.

WOLPE, J. (1958). *Psychotherapy by Reciprocal Inhibition*. California: Stanford University Press.

WOODMAN, D. (1946). A modification of the extralaryngeal approach to arytenoidectomy for bilateral abductor paralysis. *Arch. Otolaryngol.* **43**, 63.

WOODMAN, D. (1953). Bilateral abductor paralysis: a survey of 521 cases of arytenoidectomy via the open approach as reported by ninety surgeons. *Arch. Otolaryngol.* **58**, 150.

WOODMAN, D. and PENNINGTON, C.L. (1976). Bilateral abductor paralysis: 30 years experience with adenoidectomy. *Ann. Otol. Rhinol. Laryngol.* **85**, 437.

WOODMAN, De G. and POLLACK, D. (1950) Bilateral abductor paralysis. The post operative care and speech therapy following arytenoidectomy. *Laryngoscope* **60**, 832.

WYKE, B. (1967). Recent advances in the neurology of phonation and reflex mechanisms in the larynx. *Br. J. Dis. Commun.* **21**, 1.

WYKE, B. (1969). Deus ex machina vocis: an analysis of laryngeal reflexes in speech. *Br. J. Dis. Commun.* **4**, 3.

WYKE, B. (Ed.) (1972). *Ventilatory and Phonatory Control Systems*. London: Oxford University Press.

WYKE, B. (1983). Neuromuscular control systems in voice production. In D.M. Bless and J.H. Abbs (Eds) *Vocal Fold Physiology*. San Diego: College-Hill Press.

WYNTER, H. and MARTIN, S. (1981). The classification of deviant voice quality through auditory memory. *Br. J. Dis. Commun.* **16**, 204.

YANAGIHARA, N. (1967a). Hoarseness: investigation of the physiological mechanism. *Ann. Otol.* **76**, 472.

YANAGIHARA, N. (1976b). Significance of harmonic changes and noise components in hoarseness. *J. Speech Hear. Res.* **10**, 531.

YANAGIHARA, N. and KOIKE, Y. (1967). The regulation of sustained phonation. *Folia Phoniatr.* **19**, 1.

YANAGIHARA, N., KOIKE, Y. and VON LEDEN, H. (1966). Phonation and respiration - Function study in normal subjects. *Folia Phoniatr.* **18**, 323.

YOUNG, E. and HAWK, S.S. (1955). *Children with Delayed or Defective Speech: Motokinaesthetic factors in their training*. California: Stanford University Press.

YUMOTO, E. (1983). The quantitative evaluation of hoarseness - a new harmonics to noise ratio method. *Arch. Otolaryngol.* **109**, 48.

YUMOTO, E., SASAKI, Y. and OKAMURA, H. (1984). Harmonics-to-noise ratio and psychophysical measurement of the degree of hoarseness. *J. Speech Hear. Dis.* **27**, 2.

ZAGZEBSKI, J.A., BLESS, D.M. and EWANOWSKI, S.J. (1983). Pulse echo imaging of the larynx using rapid ultrasonic scanners. In D.M. Bless and J.H. Abbs (Eds) *Vocal Fold Physiology*. San Diego: College-Hill Press.

ZALIOUK, A. (1960). Falsetto voice in deaf children. In *Aktuelle Probleme der Phoniatrie und Logopedie*, Vol. 1. Zurich: Karger.

ZALIOUK, A. (1963). The tactile approach to voice placement. *Folia Phoniatr.* **15**, 147.

ZEMLIN, W.R., DAVIS, P. and GAZA, C. (1984). Fine morphology of the posterior cricoarytenoid muscle. *Folia Phoniatr.* **36**, 233.

ZENKER, W. (1964). Vocal muscle fibres and their motor end-plates. In D. Brewer (Ed.) *Potentials in Voice Physiology*. New York: State University Press.

ZILSTORFF, K. (1968). Vocal disabilities of singers. *Proc. R. Soc. Med.* **61**, 1147.

ZWITMAN, D.H. (1979). Bilateral cord dysfunctions: abductor type spastic dysphonia. *J. Speech Hear. Dis.* **44**, 373.

ZWITMAN, D.H., SONDERMAN, J.C. and WARD, P.H. (1974). Variations in velopharyngeal closure assessed by endoscopy. *J. Speech Dis.* **39**, 366.

ZYSKI, B.J., BULL, G.L., McDONALD, W.E. and JOHNS, M.E. (1984). Perturbation analysis of normal and pathologic larynges. *Folia Phoniatr.* **36**, 190.

Index (Author)

Index (Subject)